Culture and Health

A Critical Perspective Towards Global Health

SECOND EDITION

Malcolm MacLachlan

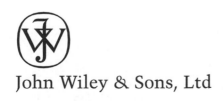

John Wiley & Sons, Ltd

Other Wiley Editorial Offices

John Wiley & Sons Inc., 111 River Street, Hoboken, NJ 07030, USA

Jossey-Bass, 989 Market Street, San Francisco, CA 94103–1741, USA

Wiley-VCH Verlag GmbH, Boschstr. 12, D-69469 Weinheim, Germany

John Wiley & Sons Australia Ltd, 42 McDougall Street, Milton, Queensland 4064, Australia

John Wiley & Sons (Asia) Pte Ltd, 2 Clementi Loop #02–01, Jin Xing Distripark, Singapore
129809

John Wiley & Sons Canada Ltd, 22 Worcester Road, Etobicoke, Ontario, Canada M9W 1L1

Wiley also publishes its books in a variety of electronic formats. Some content that appears in
print may not be available in electronic books.

Library of Congress Cataloging-in-Publication Data

MacLachlan, Malcolm.
    Culture and health : a critical perspective towards global health / Malcolm MacLachlan. –
2nd ed.
        p. cm.
    Includes bibliographical references and index.
    ISBN-13: 978-0-470-84736-7 (cloth : alk. paper)
    ISBN-10: 0-470-84736-0 (cloth : alk. paper)
    ISBN-13: 978-0-470-84737-4 (pbk : alk. paper)
    ISBN-10: 0-470-84737-9 (pbk : alk. paper)
    1. Transcultural medical care.   2. Ethnic groups – Health and hygiene.   3. Minorities –
Health and hygiene. I. Title.

RA418.5.T73M33 2006
362.1089 – dc22

                                                                        2005030937

British Library Cataloguing in Publication Data

A catalogue record for this book is available from the British Library

ISBN-10 0–470–84736–0 (hbk) 0–470–86737–9 (pbk)
ISBN-13 978-0-470-84736-7 (hbk) 978-0-470-84737-4

Typeset in 10/12 pt Palatino by SNP Best-set Typesetter, Ltd., Hong Kong
Printed and bound in Great Britain by Antony Rowe Ltd, Chippenham, Wiltshire
This book is printed on acid-free paper responsibly manufactured from sustainable forestry
in which at least two trees are planted for each one used for paper production.

Culture and Health

SECOND EDITION

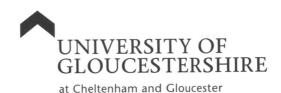

UNIVERSITY OF
GLOUCESTERSHIRE

at Cheltenham and Gloucester

Dedication

To my parents;
for the fun
of life

Contents

About the Author

Professor Malcolm MacLachlan is with the Centre for Global Health and School of Psychology, Trinity College Dublin. He originally trained and worked as a clinical psychologist, and then as a management consultant, in the UK, before taking up a lectureship at Chancellor College, University of Malawi. There he worked on a range of health promotion projects concerning HIV/AIDS and various tropical diseases, as well as with Mozambican refugees, and held a visiting position at Zomba Mental Hospital. Since moving to Trinity, he has held visiting positions at the Universities of Limpopo, Cape Town and Stellenbosch, all in South Africa, and at the College of Medicine, University of Malawi. Over the last 10 years he has also researched health-related aspects of rapid social change and increased multiculturalism in Europe, particularly Ireland. His major research interests concern cultural aspects of health, the psychosocial rehabilitation of people with physical disability and the human dynamics of international aid.

Professor MacLachlan is a Fellow of Trinity College Dublin and the Psychological Society of Ireland, and was elected to membership of the Royal Irish Academy in 2005. He has worked with a broad range of international and development organisations including UNICEF, OECD, WHO and UNESCO, the Academy for Educational Development, Finnish Refugee Council, American Refugee Committee, Banja La Mtsogolo, Concern and Development Co-operation Ireland. He was also a member of an EU-funded specialist group on Psychotrauma and Human Rights. He is Co-Director of the Masters Degree in Global Health at Trinity. He has the entirely unintentional distinction of a peculiar type of multicultural education – being a graduate from universities in Scotland, England, Ireland and Wales.

Critical acclaim for the First Edition

Psychology

... ideal for undergraduate students in psychology and the health sciences, while still having a great deal to offer to professionals.

Christina Lee, *Australian Psychologist*, July 1998, p. 158

This book is a welcome addition to the literature, written by an author who is evidently an expert in this field.

Rachel Tribe, *Behaviour Research & Therapy* **36**, 1998

... *Culture and Health*, is a welcome addition. It attempts to glean the relevant and most pertinent literature related to cultural influences on both mental and physical health into a single resource for the health practitioner. As one of the first, and perhaps to date only, book resource to do so, it attempts to fill an important gap in our knowledge, and provide an important service to those who work with cultural issues in their everyday professional practices, as well as to those who teach in these areas.

David Matsumoto, *Journal of Health Psychology* **4**(1): 109–10

... health workers have a great deal to learn from this volume ... of great value and interest are the many illustrations of health related cultural phenomena ... which includes both illnesses and 'case studies'. The author uses these imaginatively to encourage the reader to challenge his or her assumptions of others and best practice ... the concluding 'guidelines for professional practice' ... are excellent tools for thinking critically about health care in a multicultural society ...

James Nazroo, *British Journal of Health Psychology* **4**(1), 1999

Psychiatry

I particularly liked MacLachlan's 'Problem Portrait Technique' as a helpful way of gaining an understanding of the individual patient's cultural background from the patient himself/herself. . . . Perhaps it should be a requirement of every mental health professional that we demonstrate that we have mastered this technique . . .

George Ikkos, *Psychological Medicine*, 1998, pp. 1248–9

. . . an enlightening view of different facets of culture and human inter-action . . . [which will] fill an important gap in the field of cross-cultural psychiatry. MacLachlan provides a theoretical overview with guidelines for professionals . . .

Dinesh Bhugra, *International Review of Psychiatry* **11**, 1999

This work is important for two reasons. In the first place, the author emphasises correctly an aspect that is often forgotten: that an individual is mainly ill, both somatic and mental, *in his culture*. . . . Secondly, the author warns that Western based diagnostic systems should not be uni-versalised. . . I would like to recommend this book.

H. Van Hoorde (translated) *Tijdschrift voor Psychiatrie*, 1998

Medicine

MacLachlan provides an excellent overview of the relationship that culture plays in the health and wellness of both individuals and the com-munities in which they live. . . . I found this book to be well balanced and well documented and I would be comfortable recommending it for both undergraduates and graduate students alike. . . . *Culture and Health* should be considered a 'must read' for any health professional, especially those who will practice in a multi-cultural environment.

Richard Mroz, *Social Science and Medicine* **48**: 857, 1999

MacLachlan is at his most interesting when recounting tales of cultural diversity

Kamran Abbasi, *British Medical Journal* **316**, 1998

Health services management

This publication addresses a particularly important issue, especially given the multicultural society within Europe, and deserves to be read by a managerial audience.

Press Release: European Healthcare Management Association, 1998
(Culture and Health was the runner-up for
the Association's Baxter Award)

Social work

... what I found particularly interesting was that it was not overly biased towards an academic discourse and had a clear(er) focus towards practitioners' needs. It does offer the practitioners ways to examine, compare and contrast their practice in relation to each subject area. Each chapter concludes with guidelines for professional practice that social workers in health settings and associated professionals will find useful.

Alison Cornwall-Dwyer, *British Journal of Social Work* **28**, 1998

International development

Although this text is relevant and timely as a useful academic text for students, it also incorporates a number of design and layout features which make it an invaluable field reference guide for clinicians working in a multicultural environment. As such, this book is highly recommended for students and practitioners in the health and social sciences.

Paul Watters, *Development Bulletin* **46**: 71, 1998

General book review publications

MacLachlan introduces various approaches used with immigrant and refugee populations for assessing problems and helping patients achieve treatment objectives. [The book is] ... broad in scope, addressing communication patterns and health care issues among a wide variety of racial, ethnic and religious groups

Multicultural Review, 1998

Covers the assessment and treatment of illness as well as the promotion of health, introducing new techniques such as the problem portrait technique for assessment, and critical incident analysis as a form of treatment

New York Review, 1998

Preface to the First Edition

This book offers a path through a forest. The many and varied relationships between culture and health are what populate this metaphorical forest. At different times of day the light will play tricks on you with shadows pointing you to travel in one direction or another. These can be likened to the truly multidisciplinary perspectives that are relevant to an understanding of culture and health. While I have tried to be aware of these, the path travelled in this book doubtless reflects my own training in clinical psychology and my subsequent experiences of working in different cultures. As with any path it cannot take in all that it passes by and so my description of culture and health is one which makes personal sense.

The terrain covered in this book is not comprehensive; it is highly selective. I do not want you, the reader, to travel this path and believe that you have seen through the forest, but to retrace some of my steps and follow different shadows and kinks of light.

This book is written at a time of explosive activity in research and writing about both culture and health, and an increasing realisation of the importance of their tantalising interplays. I have omitted to tackle some topics which are undoubtedly important – emotion, interpersonal relationships, attitudes toward ageing and psychometric assessment, to mention but a few. Some of these issues are dealt with by other books in this series, while others would not squeeze into the confines of space allotted me. Some of the ideas included are, however, 'new' and doubtless somewhat raw. These include the Problem Portrait Technique, the Faith Grid, the use of Critical Incidents as a form of therapy and the suggestion of health change progressing through Incremental Improvement. They are served up to be chewed over and, if need be, spat out! They are things which I picked up and put into my pocket as I picked out a pathway.

It has been difficult to know how to refer to cultural groupings. One of these is the idea of 'Western' cultures. Of course there is no such thing as 'the West'. What is west of you all depends on where you're standing. It can be the height of ethnocentricity to talk of the Middle East or indeed the Far East. If I say I live in the 'Far East', you may well ask where it is that I am far from and east of! Yet such misnomers can be widely understood summaries of an abstract concept. In this book I have opted to use the term 'West' to refer to a range of cultures which have some important characteristics in common. These countries include the United States of America, much of Europe, Australia, New Zealand and to a lesser extent some countries which have been strongly influenced by the values held by people from these 'Western' cultures. To remind us that there is no such place as 'the West' I have used the term with inverted commas.

During the writing of this book I have had the great good fortune to travel five continents, work in three different universities and live in four 'homes'. The influences on me have literally been too numerous to mention. The thoughts of many people have beat out my path and pulled back the undergrowth, so infusing me with the excitement and bewilderment which is born of true exploration. However, to move forward you must have some way of knowing where you have been. My editor, Daphne Keats, and publishers Comfort Jegede and Michael Combs at Wiley, have awoken me from slumber when I have dosed off in some cosy corner of a Malawian mountain or Irish hay field. Without the support and thoughtful commentaries of my wife, Eilish McAuliffe, and mother, Pat MacLachlan, the writing of this book would have been a very solitary pursuit. I am also very grateful to Lisa Cullen for her skill and patience in producing the tables and figures in this book. Finally, a thank you to all those colleagues and friends from different cultures, who over the years have tolerated many strange questions. Some of your answers are in this book.

Malcolm MacLachlan

Preface to the Second Edition

Since the first edition of *Culture and Health*, globalisation has increased apace. The ethos of diversity, whether in terms of multiculturalism, sexuality, gender roles or access for the disabled, is now much more pervasive then before. Confronted with the choice between a cultural mosaic and a cultural 'melting pot', the mosaic seems more resilient and more preferable. However, the term 'multiculturalism' stresses the need for an increasing array of distinct identities rather than being subsumed under a singular idea of 'diversity'. As is illustrated in this volume, cultural identity serves not just a group's need for cohesiveness, but also an individual's need for a coherent, and particular, world view.

In this second edition there are significant new additions and ideas. At a conceptual level, I have tried to think through the interrelationships of medical anthropology, medical sociology and health psychology, and acknowledge something that was implicit in the first edition – that, whatever the cultural or contextual parameters, *people have the right to their own health psychology* – to make what sense they can of the relationship between what they think, how they act and their well-being. I have also, however, tried to acknowledge my sympathy with a *critical* perspective, one that is concerned with broader social issues, less individualistic and less oriented towards biological and reductionist understandings of people's personal experiences. As such, I believe in a social constructionist perspective that is *critical for* rather than simply being *critical of* other perspectives on health.

In this second edition I also seek to emphasise the need for a *global health* perspective and that such a perspective must inherently recognise that this broad panoramic view is made up of different 'takes' from varying cultural positions. Although the idea of *health as a human right* is compelling, identifying just exactly what that means in different cultures is crucial if it is not to become yet another United Nations' 'feel-good' abstraction with few specifics to guide practitioners.

In the first edition of this book I paid insufficient attention to gender and poverty as 'cross-cutting' issues and I have sought to address this in the second edition. I have also tried to indicate how culture can often present ethical issues for which there may be no clear 'right answer'. All of the chapters have been updated and added to, and I have also added a completely new chapter on global health, because this movement is highly relevant and sympathetic to cultural perspectives on health. While in the first edition I used inverted commas and a capital first letter to describe the idea of, for example, the 'West', I have dropped these and now simply refer to the west, as is now the trend. Perhaps it is an alternative way of acknowledging that while such an *idea* exists, the *place* does not. My publishers have been extraordinarily patient in their waiting for this second edition and I am most grateful for the time that they have allowed me. Finally, my children, Anna, Tess and Lara (all new additions since the first edition), and my wife, Eilish, have been my travel companions across each continent and furnished me with perspectives that I was quite foreign to. And this is the essence and value of understanding how cultures influence our lives, our health and our experience of illness.

Malcolm MacLachlan

CHAPTER 1

Culture and health

Multiculturalism is the only way in which the whole of humanity can be greater than the sum of its parts. If we are to avoid being churned in a mono-cultural 'melting pot' this requires us all to acknowledge, tolerate and work with different interpretations of some of the things that we hold most precious. One of these things is health. The interplay between culture and health is truly complex and invites consideration of a kaleidoscope of causes, experiences, expressions and treatments for a plethora of human ailments. However, while cultural variations are intuitively intriguing and inviting to focus in on, especially in relation to health, they can also veil equally fundamental economic, political and social differences between peoples.

This book explores the complexity of human experiences of health and illness across cultures. The complexity includes the broader social context in which minority and majority groups operate. We must resist empirically stereotyping people as though they were 'cultural dopes' whose behaviour will conform to an abstracted 'cultural type'. Individuals must not be relegated to simple conduits of culture, but recognised as active sifters of the ideas presented to them through their family, community and social context, as well as their broader culture. Already we have taken as implicit some assumptions and definitions such as the meaning of the terms 'culture' and 'health'. However, before proceeding to define these I want to make clear the perspective taken in this book, and how it differs from other books by seeking to integrate the contributions of the various social health sciences to understanding the interplay of culture and health.

The social health sciences and culture

Within the social health sciences of sociology, anthropology and psychology the importance of cultural differences is treated in quite different ways. Although my background is in psychology, much of my thinking in this area is influenced by ideas from related disciplines. However, differences in how these disciplines make sense of and incorporate 'culture' into their understanding of health can be confusing and somewhat disorienting. Although I argue for the synthesis of these differences it is nevertheless also important to understand their distinctions. We shall therefore consider each of these 'treatments' of culture in turn. Table 1.1 gives several definitions of each of these

Table 1.1 Some definitions of medical sociology, medical anthropology and health psychology.

Definitions of medical sociology
Explores '. . . how diseases could be differently understood, treated and experienced by demonstrating how disease is produced out of social organisation rather than, nature, biology or individual lifestyle choices'.
White (2002, p. 4)

'The study of health care as it is institutionalised in a society and of health, or illness and its relationship to social factors'.
Ruderman (1981, p. 927)

'. . . is concerned with the social causes and consequences of health and illness'.
Cockerham (2001, p. 1)

Definitions of medical anthropology
'. . . how people in different cultures and social groups explain the cause of ill-health, the type of treatments they believe in, and to whom they turn if they do become ill . . .'
Helman (2000, p. 1)

'. . . the cultural construction of illness, illness experience, the body, and medical knowledge . . .'
Lindenbaum and Lock (1993, p. xi)

'A biocultural discipline concerned with both the biological and sociocultural aspects of human behaviour, and particularly with the ways in which the two interact throughout human history to influence health and disease'
Foster and Anderson (1978, pp. 2–3)

Definitions of health psychology
'. . . devoted to understanding psychological influences on how people stay healthy, why they become ill, and how they respond when they do get ill'.
Taylor (2003, p. 3)

'Health psychology emphasizes the role of psychological factors in the cause, progression and consequences of health and illness. The aims of health psychology can be divided into (1) understanding, explaining, developing and testing theory and (2) putting this theory into practice.'
Ogden (2000, p. 6)

'. . . the aggregate of the specific educational, scientific, and professional contributions of the discipline of psychology to the promotion and maintenance of health, the prevention and treatment of illness, and the identification of the etiological and diagnostic correlates of health, illness and related dysfunctions'.
Matarazzo (1980, p. 815)

disciplines, and it is apparent that there are significant differences between them, but also that definitions within disciplines vary. Different people interpret their own disciplines in different ways.

Medical sociology

Lupton (2003) distinguishes between three approaches within medical sociology:

1. *Functionalism* sees illness as a potential state of social deviance, e.g. a person adopting the 'sick role' relies on others rather than being independent of them. According to this view, the medical profession, as an institution of social control, serves to distinguish between normality and deviance.
2. The *political economy* approach, on the other hand, emphasises how socioeconomic context shapes health, disease and treatment. Here health is seen not only as a state of well-being, but also as having access to the basic resources required to promote health.
3. The third approach, and the most influential in contemporary medical sociology, is *social constructionism*, which understands medical knowledge and medical practice to be socially constructed, as opposed to being an independent and scientific body of knowledge.

Medical sociology's interests are in the structural organisation of health services in society, and how they relate to other social structures and how these contribute to or detract from health (Goldie, 1995).

The tradition within medical sociology has, however, been to focus on social structures in western societies (primarily Europe and North America – Matcha, 2000). Although, in principle, the social structure of any cultural group may be of interest to medical sociologists, it is primarily its structural component, rather than its cultural component, that is of concern here. However, another way of construing what medical sociology is about is that it is interested in *the culture of healthcare* within a society.

Medical anthropology

McElroy (1996) has identified three perspectives within medical anthropology:

1. *Ethnomedicine* is concerned with cultural systems of healing and the cognitive parameters of illness. The variety of meaningful constructions across cultures can be seen to challenge the reductionist epidemiology of biomedicine (Kleinman, 1980).
2. The *medical ecology* perspective is concerned more explicitly with the interaction of biological conditions and cultural contexts. It thus considers the interrelationships of ecological systems, human evolution, health and illness, where health may be seen as a measure of environmental adaptation. Medical anthropologists' interest in nutrition and cultural rules about what can and cannot be eaten fit well within this framework.
3. *Applied medical anthropology* seeks directly to affect people's health by taking account of their cultural beliefs. An example given by Helman (2000) is increasing the acceptability of oral rehydration therapy for diarrhoeal diseases by first understanding cultural reasons for it being rejected. As such, applied medical anthropology is directly concerned with intervention, prevention and health policy.

Medical anthropology is a biocultural discipline, which puts greater emphasis on understanding the meaning of events than on objectively trying to measure them. With its use of qualitative methods, medical anthropology seeks to provide an 'insider perspective' (Skultans & Cox, 2000), to understand the relationships between health and illness through the cultural lens of the people whom it studies. It also seeks to look beyond the ethnocentric nature of modern western biomedicine.

Health psychology

Health psychology is concerned with how an individual's personal characteristics and beliefs contribute to their personal health and illness experiences. How the beliefs of different cultures contribute to these individual beliefs and characteristics is of special interest to cultural health psychologists, who explore how psychological determinants of health vary in different cultural contexts. Health psychology takes a biopsychosocial approach to health and has positioned itself at the intersection between biological and social factors in health and illness (Kazarian & Evans, 2001). However, most theories in health psychology have been derived from mainstream psychology and have therefore adopted psychology's assumptions, methods and problems somewhat uncritically (Marks, 1996). This approach can therefore have an individualistic bias and broadly reflects western values. Furthermore, although health psychology claims to reject the biomedical approach, in clinical practice it rarely departs from traditional medical agendas (Marks, 1996). There have, however, been attempts to overcome these limitations by, for example, integrating health psychology and cultural psychology (Kazarian & Evan, 2001). The advent of a *critical health psychology* has also recently challenged and sought to depart from the limitations of health psychology, and has been argued as central to an emerging *cultural health psychology* (MacLachlan, 2004). Cultural psychology is concerned with the cultural environment of individuals (Marsella, Thorp & Ciborowski, 1979) and how they interact with it as individuals. As we noted, cultural health psychology recognises that people are not simply empty vessels with 'thinking spaces' filled by the flows of their culture, but rather people reflect on and make their own interpretations of cultural understandings and these are influenced by individual differences in, among other things, emotion and cognition. Health psychology is particularly concerned to measure these variables in as valid and reliable a way as possible.

Integrating social health sciences

To some extent the three social sciences outlined above have each responded to limitations inherent in the biomedical model, including neglecting the socioenvironmental context of health and illness, treating patients as passive objects, denying them their own interpretations of their experiences, and being intolerant of competing or pluralistic explanations and of alternative

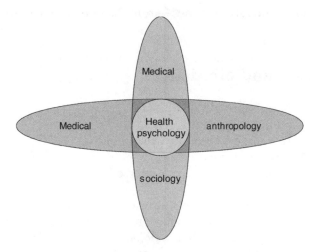

Figure 1.1 A schematic representation of the relationship between health psychology, medical anthropology and medical sociology.

forms of healing (Nettleton, 1995). Conrad (1997) talks of 'parallel play' in the way that the disciplines of anthropology and sociology continue side by side without interacting with each other, and the same can be said for psychology. Figure 1.1 schematically represents the interrelationship of these three health social sciences, which all have a legitimate claim to contribute to understanding health in a broader cultural context.

Health psychology focuses on the smallest unit in society, the individual, and how the individual's life experience and characteristics influence health. This experience is seen as *central* to, but not independent of, structural and cultural factors. Medical sociology provides a wider, societal frame of reference, one that addresses why certain groups are more vulnerable and less well treated than others in a given social system. As a result of medical sociology's interest in the structure and inequalities of a society's health system, I have represented this as a 'vertical' oval, which indicates that a particular health culture may be stratified at different levels. Medical anthropology's perspective allows for comparison of the cultural systems that construct differing social and health systems, and I have therefore represented this as a 'horizontal' oval, looking across societies. Although some might question the centrality that I, a psychologist, have given to psychology, I feel that it is justified on the grounds that, whatever one's structural or cultural context, individuals operate according to their own health psychology. In fact, to put it more emphatically – everybody is entitled to their own health psychology!

Culture forms the implicit backdrop to many of the variables studied in psychology, sociology and anthropology, and requires that our understanding of them be presented in a 'joined-up' fashion. In order for us to be able to provide any given individual from whatever cultural background with the optimal care, we have not only to appreciate this backdrop but also to embrace it in the most conducive manner – from the perspective of the person seeking healthcare.

Culture, race and ethnicity

> Paddy: 'Good morning Mick.'
> Mick: 'Good morning Paddy.'
> Paddy: 'Ah, but it's a great day for the race!'
> Mick: 'And what race would that be?'
> Paddy 'Why the human race, of course!'

Ahdieh and Hahn (1996) reviewed the way in which the terms 'race', 'ethnicity' and 'national origin' have been used over a 10-year period in articles published in the influential *American Journal of Public Health*. Their motivation for doing this was to determine the extent to which authors were complying with an objective set by the US public health service, for researchers explicitly to refer to racial or ethnic differences in health status. They found that researchers used such categories in their samples, either specifically (e.g. 'black', 'Chinese' or 'Hispanic') or more generically (e.g. 'race' or 'ethnicity'), only in half of the studies; in less than 1% of all the studies were 'race' and 'ethnicity' examined independently. Furthermore, less than 10% of those studies that did use terms relating to race, ethnicity or national origin explicitly defined what they meant by the term. Often the terms were used in combinations or interchangeably. It is also interesting to note that in those articles that did describe their samples using these terms, most did so only to control for their possible 'confounding' effects. Less than 10% of all the articles treated these categories as potential risk factors in themselves. Ahdieh and Hahn concluded that there was little consensus in the scientific community regarding the meaning or use of terms such as race, ethnicity or national origin.

The idea of different human 'races' is something that many people are uncomfortable with. This is probably because it is seen as suggesting that differences between human beings can be reduced to tiny biological variations in nucleic acid. Furthermore, these genetic differences are understood to determine human behaviour in a relatively immutable fashion. It is assumed that, if genetic differences exist, they must influence behaviour. These possible differences are at their most controversial when they are used to explain variations in antisocial behaviour, intelligence or health, between members of different cultural groups, i.e. when cultural differences are explained as resulting from different genetic constitutions. There seems to be an irresistible drive towards evaluating any possible differences in terms of them being 'good' or 'bad'.

The term 'ethnicity' is often used to remove the pejorative use of 'race' and in recognition that different 'races' may share a similar culture. Thus, members of an ethnic group are seen as sharing a common origin and important aspects of their way of living. The word 'ethnicity' is derived from the

Greek *ethnos*, meaning nation. Essentially, it refers to a psychological sense of belonging that will often be cemented by similar physical appearance or social similarities. This sense of belonging to a group can either stigmatise individual members or empower them through consciousness raising. Black consciousness in some countries can be seen as an attempt to empower members of a stigmatised minority group. Although it is tempting to gloss over the sensitive issue of race, its association with heredity makes it especially important to consider in relation to health.

Rushton (1995, p. 40) suggests that, in zoological terms, a race refers to a 'geographic variety or subdivision of a species characterised by a more or less distinct combination of traits . . . that are heritable'. He argues that differences in body shape, hair, facial features and genetics distinguish three major human races: Mongoloid, Caucasoid and Negroid. He further suggests that modern humans evolved in Africa some time after 200,000 years ago, with an African/non-African split occurring about 110,000 years ago and the Caucasoid split occurring about 41,000 years ago. Rushton suggests that the different evolutionary pressures produced by different geographical environments resulted in genetic differences across a number of traits. Through genetic drift, natural selection and mutation, particular characteristics were selected for in certain environments but not in others (e.g. white skin, large nostrils) and, as they gave individuals some advantage over those who did not have these characteristics, such characteristics later predominated in relatively geographically isolated gene pools. Thus, populations in diverse geographical areas came to differ in their physical appearance.

Variation in gene frequencies may affect health in very specific ways, e.g. bone marrow transplantations are used in the treatment of leukaemia and other haematological illnesses. National registers of potential bone marrow donors in Britain and North America consist primarily of, so-called, 'Caucasian' donors. Similar to blood, bone marrow comes in different types – human leukocyte antigen (HLA) types – that appear to be genetically determined. Only roughly a third of potential recipients of a bone marrow transplant find a good match among their relatives, the rest being dependent on unrelated donors who are identified through large-scale registries. Within the British and American registries the chances of finding a match for 'non-Caucasian' patients are considerably lower than they are for 'Caucasian' patients. Consequently, it has been argued that different ethnic groups should establish their own registries in order to improve the success rate for finding a matching donor (Asano, 1994; Liang et al., 1994).

There are of course numerous such links between genetic constitution and health. Another example is research suggesting that genetics may be relevant to the prevalence of seasonal affective disorder (SAD), which is usually taken to refer to the higher incidence of depression during winter months. It has been reported that descendants of Icelanders living in the Northern Territories of Canada have a lower incidence of SAD than descendants of either the indigenous population or other settlers. In seeking to explain this finding Magnusson and Axelsson (1993) have suggested that, in extreme northern latitudes, such as Iceland, the propensity not to get depressed during the dark winter months may have been positively selected for through reproduction. Therefore the indigenous Icelandic population would have evolved with a lower incidence of SAD in northern latitudes. Further south, in Canada, descendants of these Icelanders would therefore be less susceptible to SAD than the indigenous population or settlers whose ancestors originated from lower latitudes.

This is a particularly interesting argument for us because it concerns genetic variation within a particular 'racial' group – being 'Caucasians'. It also suggests that genetic variations are *not* synonymous with the traditional anthropological distinctions of Caucasoids, Negroids and Mongoloids. In other words, genetic variability is not a distinguishing feature of this classification. Furthermore, Haviland (1983) has also argued that genetic variation appears to be continuous rather than discontinuous. By this is meant that, although people from different parts of the world may differ in physical appearance, no one group differs to the extent that different gene frequencies are found. Instead there appears to be a continuum of phenotypic expression, with different 'racial' groups found at different points along a continuum. Thus bodily shape does not change abruptly as we move across the globe, but gradually with neighbouring peoples resembling each other.

The idea of a continuum must not, however, blind us to important health-related differences that do exist between people from different parts of the world. For example, why is it that diabetes is much more prevalent, and colorectal cancer much less prevalent, among Indian immigrants to Britain than it is among the British population as a whole (Bhopal, 2004)? Answers to such questions may provide vital insights into understanding such diseases. However, although the term 'race' offers an important perspective on health problems because it derives from genetics, it is increasingly important to recognise the existence of 'mixed race' and people's increasing inclination to describe themselves as 'other', under the 'race' category in many surveys. People may use a broad range of factors in defining whom they are and what they identify with, including ancestry, geographical origin, birthplace, language, religion, migration history, name, the way they look, etc. Bhopal (2004) suggests that a variety of forces will stimulate increasing interest in the issues of culture, ethnicity and race, including the new genetics, a focus on healthcare inequalities, globalisation, migration and increased movement of refugees and asylum seekers – all issues addressed in this book.

Interestingly, while concluding that there is no convincing biological or scientific basis for the actual existence of 'races' LaVeist (2002a, p. 120) states: 'even though race may be a biological fiction, it is nevertheless . . . a profoundly important determinant of health status and health care quality'. By this is meant people discriminate as if there were race-based differences between people and, in doing so, they create *actual* differences. Thus whether or not you are impressed by evidence for biological difference implying the existence of 'race', the *idea* of race is a reality that we need to take account of in healthcare.

Ultimately, the way in which people conceptualise the relationship between 'race' and health is important because it affects their ideas about health policy. If, for instance, they adopt a 'biological determinist' viewpoint they may believe that there are relatively few interventions that will reduce race-related health differentials. On the other hand, a strongly behavioural perspective might suggest that interventions focus only on modifying an individual's health-related behaviours. Alternatively, understanding at a purely societal level might suggest that appropriate interventions should all be beyond the engagement of individuals (LaVeist, 2002b).

Folk taxonomies

Physical differences can be observed in people from diverse geographical areas and these differences may have adaptive value. In the tropical regions of Africa and South America populations developed dark skins (densely pigmented with melanin which blocks sunlight), presumably as protection against the sun, whereas populations in the colder areas, such as northern Europe, which are dark for long periods of time and where people cover their skin for warmth, developed lighter skins (less densely pigmented with melanin), presumably because they did not require the same degree of protection from sunlight. Fish (1995) argues that in some 'folk taxonomies' (local ways in which people classify things) light versus dark skin is considered a racial difference. However, Fish also emphasises that other physical features that we associate with 'whiteness' or 'blackness' do not necessarily coincide with a black versus white distinction. He writes (1995, pp. 44–5):

> There are people, for example, with tight curly blond hair, light skin, blue eyes, broad noses, and thick lips – whose existence is problematic for our racial assumptions.

Ironically the white versus black distinction is not seen as reliable enough to distinguish between people of different 'race', because each 'race' has a huge (and overlapping) spectrum of skin colours.

'Inter-racial' marriage further increases the overlap between the skin colour of 'blacks' and 'whites' (or 'browns' and 'pinks'!) and so, to overcome this problem, in North America 'race' has been administratively defined according to the 'one-drop rule'. If you are an offspring of one black and one white parent then you are black; in fact, if you have 'one drop' of 'black blood' in you, you are black, even if your skin is white! This identification of 'race' with blood is not a universal assumption. Different societies construct different definitions of 'race'. For example, in Brazil racial categorisation draws equally on skin colour and hair form, but may also be influenced by an individual's wealth and profession. This means that a person can have a different racial identity, not only from his siblings, but also from either of his parents too.

'Black' versus 'white' is simply one way of describing the variation observed between people. 'Tall' versus 'short' could be another, with accompanying 'secondary' physical and psychological features. Indeed research has found that there are certain erroneous psychological traits associated with tallness (e.g. the impression of intelligence), just as there may be with skin colour. Thus people from different parts of the world differ in certain physical features and they also differ in how they explain this variation in human features. The *construction* of 'racial' differences in one culture can be quite different to its construction in another culture. Indeed in some countries people may now choose their 'race'.

Whether there is one human race or several does not seem to be a crucial issue for health. What is important is whether there are some groups of people whose genetic make-up disadvantages them in terms of health. Such disadvantage will always express itself alongside skin colour, eye colour, hair type, height, etc. What we should be interested in is whether there are links between disadvantageous genes and the location of any individuals or groups on the many continua of human genetic variation. Such links, through the provision of physical markers for disadvantageous genes, can be meaningful and useful if they lead to health-enhancing interventions. Sometimes such links may coincide with skin colour and at others they may coincide with other characteristics. However, this book is based on the premise that the great majority of variation in human health is not related to genetic variation as such, but to the different ways in which people exist in the world, i.e. to their culture.

Social variations

We have reviewed one aspect of our adaptation to different environments in the form of the different physical characteristics that humanity exhibits; another aspect of this variation is the plethora of social characteristics to be found among us. Social variations exist because hunter–gatherers in the Kalahari Desert and car production workers in Tokyo need to organise themselves in different ways in order to get the best out of their respective ecological niches. Given that human beings inhabit many different environments and that human characteristics vary along a multitude of continua, it is not surprising that our social features as well as our physical features should differ around the world. The way in which we organise ourselves socially also has a form of heredity – a means through which such organisation is passed on from one generation to the next.

Harris (1980, p. ix) suggests that cultural materialism is 'based on the simple premise that human social life is a response to the practical problems of earthly existence'. Harris draws on Marx's idea that the means of production found in a society will determine its functioning, or culture. Thus different geographical locations will require different social orders (cultures) for optimal functioning. Social orders are passed on from one generation to the next through a variety of mechanisms including traditions. Over the years people have organised themselves in certain ways in order to get the most out of their environment.

Historically society has presented successive generations with similar problems. Social structures, from one generation to the next, have often adopted similar solutions to the 'timeless' problems of survival, e.g. food, shelter and reproduction. It is easy to forget this in our modern ever-changing world, where many of us cannot keep up with the rush of innovative technologies that sweeps us along unknown paths. In the past a social culture could provide solutions to the problems of living, over many generations. Today the demands to adapt to a rapidly changing society can themselves constitute an acculturation experience (see later and see Chapter 4).

Culture as communication

So what about the term 'culture'? The term has been so widely used that its precise meaning will vary from one situation to another. In 1952 Kluckhohn and Kroeber reviewed 150 different definitions of 'culture' and the passage of time has not witnessed much consensus. Some academics have tried to put the plethora of definitions into conceptual categories. Allen (1992), for instance, distinguishes seven different ways in which the word 'culture' can be used:

1. Generic: referring to the whole range of learned as opposed to instinctive behaviour.
2. Expressive: essentially artistic expression.
3. Hierarchical: through which the superiority of one group over another is suggested in contrast to 'cultural relativism'.
4. Superorganic: analytically abstracting meaning concerning the context of everyday behaviour rather than the minutiae of the behaviour.
5. Holistic: recognising the interconnectedness of difference aspects of life such as economics, religion and gender.
6. Pluralistic: highlighting the coexistence of multiple cultures in the same setting.
7. Hegemonic: emphasising the relationship between cultural groups and power distribution.

Even this attempted simplification of 'culture' produces a rather complex matrix of overlapping concepts.

Here we emphasise a pragmatic role of culture, one that is especially pertinent to health. A culture presents us with a set of guidelines – a formula – for living in the world. Just as a biologist may need a particular 'culture' to allow the growth of a particular organism, social cultures nurture the growth of people with particular beliefs, values, habits, etc. But, above all, culture provides a means of communication with those around us. Different styles of communication reflect the customary habits of people from different cultures. In each case, however, the culture is the medium through which communication takes place. A culture that prohibits communication has no way of passing on its 'shared customs'.

At the most obvious level it may be the custom for a language to be spoken in one place but not in another. A gesture may mean one thing in Britain and quite another thing in Greece. An amusing example of this is the raised thumb used as a symbol of approval in Britain, but as an insult in Greece, where it is taken to mean 'sit on this!' Even in the same country gestures can be taken to have different meanings. In France, the ring sign created by bending and touching the tips of the thumb and index finger is interpreted to mean 'OK' in some regions and 'zero' in others (Collett, 1982). In a similar way a form of art may convey a particular message to one group of people and be apparently incomprehensible to others. Whether it is words, gestures, music, painting, work habits or whatever, a culture creates a certain way of communicating ideas between people. Culture then is the medium that people use for communication; it is the lubricant of social relationships.

Communication varies in many contexts. The form of communication may be quite different depending on whether you are at home or at work, with people of the same gender as yourself, whether they are elders or children, of the same class or caste, etc. We are each members of many cultures, or subcultures, as they are sometimes called. There are subcultures of region, religion, gender, generation, work, income and class, to name but a few of the obvious.

It is the amalgam of these 'memberships' that constitutes the (often differing) experiences of one's self. This allows us to know ourselves in different ways. Different cultures require us to 'show' different aspects of our selves. Different cultures, because they allow different forms of communication, allow us to relate to others in different ways and to be related to in different ways. Thus, experiencing a new culture can often allow one to experience a new aspect of oneself. Generally we have most in common with people who share the same culture(s) and we find communication easiest (but not necessarily 'best') with them, i.e. we share a customary way of relating to each other.

Sometimes the language used to relate to each other has great symbolic significance, as well as being the means of communication, e.g. the language of South Africa's Apartheid was Afrikaans, the language of the Boer oppressors. It was Afrikaans that sparked the 1976 Soweto riots which left 500 dead, when the then Nationalist Party government sought to make it the medium of black education throughout the townships. As Roup (2004) poignantly says 'the language of the oppressor in the mouth of the oppressed is the language of the slave' (p. 2). Of course many languages 'have blood on their vowels' (p. 1) and for most of them that blood has long since dried and stained their speaker's constructions of their own identity. No doubt this is also true in South Africa, where today they aspire to every child having the right to be educated in his or her 'mother' tongue, including – quite correctly – Afrikaans.

Not only is culture a 'voice' through which we can communicate, it is also the eyes and ears through which we receive communications. As such, customary forms of communication often 'frame' what we expect to see and hear, e.g. in one cultural context we expect to see a woman in a short white dress and people applauding (at the Wimbledon tennis championships), whereas in another cultural context we expect to see a woman in a long black dress and people crying and wailing (at a Greek funeral procession). As smell and touch are also forms of sensing the world, they too are part of the machinery of culture.

Our senses are the instruments through which we receive and exhibit our own and other people's cultures. What gets into us and what we give out (either knowingly or unknowingly) are the elements, or building blocks, of culture. When we 'just don't get it', no wonder things seem senseless – they are! Once the involvement of our biological sense organs is recognised as part of the process of culture, the psychological and physiological implications of culture become not only more apparent but also more credible.

Ways of thinking about culture

There are a great number of different ways of thinking about culture and thus far I have primarily emphasised its identity function, achieved through the means of communication. However, it is also useful to consider different ways in which 'culture' can affect people, in terms of both their apparent health and their broader sense of empowerment. In the following I discuss taxonomy that is intended to be neither comprehensive nor mutually exclusive, but that can nevertheless heighten awareness of the influence of culture on health (for a fuller description, see MacLachlan, 2004).

Cultural colonialism

In the nineteenth-century heyday of multiple European colonial powers (e.g. Britain, France, Belgium, Portugal, Holland, Italy), Europeans sought to 'farm' South America, Africa and Asia for the benefit of the European ruling classes. An important aspect of this venture was not only to understand 'the mind of the savage', but also to make sure that 'he' was healthy enough to be productive. Dubow (1995) suggests that, through the colonial research agenda, Africans became the 'objects' of three distinct 'scientific' projects: accumulating scientific knowledge of 'primitive minds'; Africa as a laboratory for the discovery of psychological universals; and the design of psychometric devices for the selection and training of African workers. These endeavours were exploitive and their primary relevance was to the academic, government and industrial communities of the time, and not to Africans (Nsamenang & Dawes, 1998). The *dramatic exotica* (Simons,

1985) of so-called 'culture bound syndromes', so often 'typical' of the colonies (see Chapter 3), although seemingly bizarre, do in fact usually have a meaningful *order* and perform a valuable *social function* within their cultural context. The idea of anthropology being the 'hand maiden' of colonialism is controversial (Asad, 1973), but persists and highlights the continuing sensitive issue of what function our understanding of cultural differences might serve.

Cultural sensitivity

This approach to healthcare is typical of the situation where ethnic minorities have particular requirements within a health system. These minority groups may be migrants or indigenous peoples whose culture has existed only on the periphery of mainstream society. The emphasis in this approach is to provide minorities with the same sort of health service as mainstream society, but to take into account the cultural 'peculiarities' of the minority groups. The best of intentions may, however, become problematic if, in an attempt to help identify service needs, for example, an ethnic minority group is surveyed for mental health problems and they are shown to have a high need for services, not because of inherent mental health problems but because of the cultural insensitivity of the instrument. An example of how this might come about is in the consideration of the criteria of the *Diagnostic and Statistical Manual*, 4th edition (DSM-IV) for personality disorder. There are behaviours that are characteristic of certain ethnic groups that increase the likelihood of such a diagnosis, *in the absence of mental health problems* (Alarcon & Foulks, 1995; see Chapter 4). Ultimately cultural sensitivity has to be more about an approach to human problems that is accepting of alternative causal models, than it is about modifying a mainstream theory or ethos to take account of cultural peculiarities.

Cultural migration

The focus here is on people who have left their own country either as temporary sojourners or permanent migrants, or sometimes as *forced* (involuntary) migrants or refugees. A major concern is how the stresses and strains of the adjustment to individual culture are dealt with and to what extent they create acculturative stress and associated problems: loss of familiar social networks and roles, communication difficulties, different attitudes regarding the relative status of older and younger people, vocational changes and changes in religious practices. Although it is important to consider the migration experience in terms of cultural change, it is also important to ground this in terms of a possibly more significant change in political, economic and social context (see Chapters 5).

Cultural alternativism

Kleinman (1980) identifies three overlapping sectors in healthcare: the popular, professional and folk sectors. If one adds the 'New Age' therapies to the 'traditional healers' of the folk sector, there is a plethora of approaches to healing that are attracting ever-increasing numbers of followers (Furnham & Vincent, 2001). Although many of these approaches may be beneficial in their own right, it may also be that they are attractive to people because they offer a different 'culture' of healthcare – perhaps one that stresses less the curing of disease and the control of symptoms, and more a caring concern with life domains beyond the physical domain, and viewing disease as symptomatic of underlying systemic problems (Gray, 1998). Furnham and Vincent (2001) suggest that a centrally attractive – and probably therapeutic in itself – feature of complementary medicine is the consultation process (see Chapter 6). In short, conventional medicine seems increasingly to focus on the clinician finding technical outcomes that will create better health, whereas alternative practitioners are more aware of the *process* of healing and use this to facilitate better health. While recognising that not all alternative therapies are complementary (e.g. St John's wort and some antidepressants are antagonistic), I use the term 'cultural alternativism' in the sense that those not choosing to stick solely with conventional healthcare are entering into an ethos of 'pick and mix', which offers many alternatives to orthodoxy, some of which may be complementary.

Cultural empowerment

In many historical and contemporary conflict situations 'the conquered' are often re-oriented to consider the world from the perspective of those who conquered them. This re-orientation effectively strips people of the value of their own culture. Even after the 'independence' of many former colonies, which had been culturally denuded of their traditional practices and customs, there remained a diminished sense of cultural worth. It was not, after all, so much that the colonials were giving up control, more that they were giving up residence, often maintaining strong economic and political influence. Recently indigenous psychologies have sought to give credence to more traditional and localised ways of understanding people, as an equally legitimate alternative to European and North American 'mainstream' psychology (Holdstock, 2000). Thus, reconnecting individuals with their cultural heritage may not only provide a medium for intervention, but also regenerate a collect sense of value and meaning in the world (see Chapter 6).

Cultural globalisation

Just when you thought we were finished with colonialism, it is back again! Giddens (1999, p. 4) describes how:

Globalisation is restructuring the way in which we live, and in a very profound manner. It is led from the West, bears the strong imprint of American political and economic power, and is highly uneven in its consequences.

Although there are many facets to globalisation (technological, cultural, political, economic), some of which can be quite positive, there are also many victims, especially of economic globalisation.

One of the most disturbing hallmarks of this globalisation is the huge inequities with which it is associated, e.g. the three wealthiest people in the world (Bill Gates, Warren Buffet and Sultan Hassanal Bolkiah, with a combined wealth of US$117 billion) are a few million ahead of the combined gross national product (GNP) of the world's 45 poorest *countries*, the population of which is close to 300 million (Hopkin, 2002). In 1997 the UN Development Report stated that, in Africa alone, the money spent on annual debt repayments could be used to save the lives of about 21 million children by the year 2000 – that did not happen. Indeed it has been argued by many that debt is now *the new colonialism* (see, for example, George, 1988; Somers, 1996). 'Third world' debt and globalisation are different branches of the same tree. Many 'third world' countries that have had to cut back spending on health and social welfare to liberalise their markets and invest in cash crop production – all in order to compete on the global market and to meet the requirements for structural adjustment loans (SALs) from the World Bank – the living conditions of the poorest deteriorate, and so does their health, unsurprisingly (see Chapter 9 and Marks, 2004).

Cultural evolution

Cultural evolution refers to the situation where values, attitudes and customs change within the same social system, over time. Thus different historical epochs, although being characteristic of the same 'national' culture (e.g. Victorian England compared with contemporary England), actually constitute very different social environments – cultures. Peltzer (1995, 2002), working in the African context, has described people who live primarily traditional lives, those who live primarily modern lives, and those who are caught between the two – transitional people. However, these 'transitional' people can be found throughout the world, including in its most 'advanced' industrial societies.

Inglehart and Baker (2000) examined three waves of the World Values Survey (1981–82, 1990–91 and 1995–98), encompassing 65 societies on 6 continents. Their results provide strong support for both massive cultural change and the persistence of distinctive traditional values with different world views. Rather than converging, many cultures are moving on 'parallel trajectories shaped by their cultural heritages. We doubt that the forces of modernisation will produce a homogenised world culture in the foreseeable future' (Inglehart & Baker, 2000, p. 49). Use of the term 'cultural evolution' does not necessarily imply attributes of biological evolution in the sense that the fittest for the changing environmental niche will prosper at the expense of those who are less adaptive. Yet adapting to culture change within one's own culture may be every bit as demanding as adapting to cultural change across geographical boundaries, even when the changes within a culture are broadly welcomed (see for instance, Gibson & Swartz, 2001, who give an account of the difficulties that some people in South Africa have faced in making sense of their past experience under Apartheid in the context of their current democratised experience) (see also Chapter 4).

The seven cultural themes described in Table 1.2 represent different forms that the interplay between culture and health can take. In a sense, just what culture 'is' is becoming increasingly contested, as the notion of 'culture' is being used to explain an increasingly diverse array of social phenomenon.

Table 1.2   A typology of themes relating culture, empowerment and health.

Cultural colonialism
Rooted in the nineteenth century when Europeans sought to compare a God-given superior 'us' with an inferior 'them' and to determine the most advantageous way of managing 'them' in order to further European elites.

Cultural sensitivity
Being aware of the minorities among 'us' and seeking to make the benefits enjoyed by mainstream society more accessible and modifiable for 'them'.

Cultural migration
Taking account of how the difficulties of adapting to a new culture influence the opportunities and well being of geographical migrants.

Cultural alternativism
Different approaches to healthcare offer people alternative ways of being understood and of understanding their own experiences.

Cultural empowerment
As many problems are associated with the marginalisation and oppression of minority groups, a process of cultural reawakening offers a form of increasing self and community respect.

Cultural globalisation
Increasing (primarily) North American political, economic and corporate power reduces local uniqueness, and reinforces and creates systems of exploitation and dependency among the poor, throughout the world.

Cultural evolution
As social values change within cultures, adaptation and identity can become problematic with familiar support systems diminishing and cherished goals being replaced by alternatives.

Adapted from MacLachlan (2004).

Even if one accepts this 'stretching' of 'culture' as an explanatory term, we still need to ask a fundamental question: what is culture for?

Culture as a defence

Marin (1999) has described how the U'wa (meaning intelligent people who know how to speak) of Columbia, a traditional indigenous society, responded to plans for oil exploration in their traditional territory: that should the plans go ahead they would collectively commit suicide:

> To be severed from their place, to be removed from the context of the stories which they have passed down from generation to generation, is to be killed as a people, and is, as they have made very clear, a fate worse than death.

> Marin (1999, p. 43)

In their own words the U'wa explain this stance:

> We must care for, not maltreat, because for us it is forbidden to kill with knives, machetes or bullets. Our weapons are thought, the word, our power is wisdom. We prefer death before seeing our sacred ancestors profaned.

> Cited in Marin (1999, p. 43)

But surely this is too extreme and, if people will die for their culture, is this not an indication that cultural identity can go too far?

Over the last 15 years a trio of experimental social psychologists have developed and demonstrated the value of terror management theory (TMT), based largely on the writings of Becker (1962, 1968, 1973) (for a review, see Solomon, Greenberg & Pyszczynski, 1991, 1998; Pyszczynski et al., 2004). A review of either Becker's work, or of the deft experimental evaluation of TMT, is beyond the scope of this book. The central premise of TMT is that our concerns about mortality – our death – play a pervasive and far-reaching role in our daily lives. One product of human intelligence is our capacity for self-reflection, along with an ability to anticipate the future, and the rather gloomy consequence of this is our unique capacity to contemplate the inevitability of our own death.

Along with Sigmund Freud and Otto Rank, Becker believed that humans would be rooted to inaction and abject terror if they were continually to contemplate their vulnerability and mortality. Thus cultural world views evolved and these were 'humanly created beliefs about the nature of reality shared by groups of people that served (at least in part) to manage the terror engendered by the uniquely human awareness of death' (Solomon et al., 1998, p. 12). The way in which reality is constructed through cultural world views helps to manage such 'terror' by answering universal cosmological questions: 'Who am I? . . . What should I do? What will happen to me when I die?'(Solomon et al., 1998, p. 13). In a sense, then, cultures give people a role to play: distracting them from the anxiety of worrying about what they fear most.

Cultures provide recipes for immortality, either symbolically (such as amassing great fortunes that out-survive their originator) or spiritually (such as going to heaven). While sticking to the 'rules' and interpretations of your culture can ensure immortality, it has an equally important 'here-and-now' function:

> The resulting perception that one is a *valuable* member of a *meaningful* universe constitutes *self-esteem*; and self-esteem is the primary psychological mechanism by which culture serves its death-denying function.
>
> Solomon et al. (1998, p. 13, italics in the original)

Whether self-esteem is seen as arising from the need to deny death or from needs for competence, autonomy and relatedness (Ryan & Deci, 2004), these different paths to self-esteem are clearly embedded within cultural norms and practices.

The U'wa may thus more fully appreciate the life-saving and death-denying function of culture than do many others. Too often and for too long psychologists have stripped hapless mortals of their shaky beliefs and sent them out to discover their 'true self' and their apparently obligatory, enormously creative inner potential (MacLachlan, 2004a). Sheldon Kopp's (1972) best-selling book, *If You See the Buddha on the Road, Kill Him*! is typical of a genre of psychologists 'individualising' and 'inverting' their clients and warning against pursuing happiness through 'following' anything outside their 'true' self. What such a perspective fails to recognise is that sometimes people can 'find' themselves and 'protect' themselves through a collective identity shared by others. As Isaiah Berlin states in *Two Concepts of Liberty*:

> When I am among my own people, they understand me, as I understand them; and this understanding creates within me a sense of being somebody in the world. (p. 43)

Singing other people's songs

Bandawe (2005) has discussed a common theme that pervades many of Africa's different cultures and also distinguishes them from many western cultures – the notion of *uMunthu* (although the actual term differs from place to place, for instance in South Africa it is *uBunthu*). In Chichewa (one of the Malawian languages), the philosophy is conveyed through the phrase '*Umuntu ngumuntu ngabantu*' (a person is a person through other persons). As Bandawe points out, this is very different from the strident individualism enshrined in Descartes' '*cogito ergo sum*' ('I think, therefore I am'), a perspective that pervades so much of western thinking about the self. The understanding of identity and the contents of what makes up that identity do of course overlap and are political, in the sense that they reflect the influence of power relationships on people's lives – in this case, their understanding of their own life.

A recent example of this is seen in a letter to the (South African) *Sunday Times* (20 March 2005) by Motsumi oa Mphirime, of Boksburg, who wrote in relation to accusations of racism in the Catholic Church:

> Anglicans and Catholics have for many years enjoyed the exclusivity of being the representatives of England and Rome in South Africa. Their 'organized' church sessions are deeply rooted in perceptions and ideologies that hold no interest for African people. Most white Priests look down on our traditional ways of worshiping through our ancestors, yet expect us to listen to their stories about the Jewish ancestors. . . . We need to realize that we have been singing other people's songs. (p. 20)

This idea of 'of singing other people's songs' is powerful because it recognises that language is one of the ways through which we construct our experience of the world. Through language cultural myths seem to be 'natural realities', when they are in fact 'cultured realities' (Althusser, 1999). So the natural interjection – 'ouch!' in English, is 'owa!' in German (Saussure, 1999). When you learn a language you are not just learning an instrumental form of communication, you are also passively assimilating a way of constructing reality, which, with practice, seems to constitute the 'natural order' of things.

Health, illness and wellness

Many people think of health as a lack of illness. This notion of health is encouraged by a purely disease (or medical) conception of health and illness. By this way of thinking, if you have an infection, a broken leg, an inheritable disease or a latent virus you are in an undesirable state and therefore ill. However, a moment's reflection on this rationale easily illustrates its shortcomings (Antonovsky, 1987). For instance, we may understand by the term 'benign' that somebody has a tumour but that it does not seem to be a problem at the moment. Is this being healthy or ill? Somebody may be HIV positive but not show any symptoms of AIDS. Is this being healthy or ill? A person who has experienced hallucinations and delusions, but who is presently free of them, may be diagnosed as 'schizophrenic in remission'. Is this being healthy or ill? Someone who has suffered brain damage at birth may have reduced mental capabilities but above-average physical capabilities. Is this being healthy or ill? The inadequacy of a healthy versus ill dichotomy is demonstrated dramatically by the brilliant Irish author Christie Nolan. He is constrained physically by a 'damaged' body but his intellectual insight and creative expression graphically demonstrate an unconstrained and 'undamaged' mind.

In 1948, when the World Health Organization (WHO) was founded, it gave us the following definition of health: 'a complete state of physical, mental and social well-being and not merely the absence of disease or infirmity'. Although this definition of health got away from the idea that health is an absence of illness, and that it is one (physical) dimensional, it has been criticised for the inclusion of the word 'complete'. As we have noted, health is a multidimensional state. It can be broken down not just into physical, mental and social domains, but also into further subdivisions within each of these. We can at once be relatively healthy in some aspects of life and relatively unhealthy in other aspects of it. There is no clear line that we cross to move from an unhealthy category into a healthy category. People, and their health, are more complicated than that.

In the Alma Ata declaration of 1978, the WHO put greater emphasis on the social dimensions of health by focusing on primary healthcare. This declaration stated that resources were too concentrated in centralised, professionally dominated, high-tech institutions – especially hospitals. Instead it emphasised the importance of community participation in healthcare and the importance of communities having some ownership over their health services. In focusing on the primacy of the community, this declaration allowed for the incorporation of community values. Different communities have different values. These differences often reflect different cultures or subcultures. Thus the movement towards community health also offered a mechanism for integrating cultural values into healthcare.

Perhaps the clearest integration of culture into a community-focused definition of health is the following, adopted by Health and Welfare Canada (cited in Kazarian & Evans, 2001, p. 7):

> ... a resource which gives people the opportunity to manage and even change their surroundings ... a basic and dynamic force in our lives, influenced by our circumstances, our beliefs, our culture and our social, economic and physical environment.

Community health and ecology

In his book *The Psychological Sense of Community* Sarson (1974) laments the downfall of the sense of community in contemporary North American society. A sense of community, or the experience of a feeling of belongingness, has real implications for health. A considerable amount of psychological research conducted over the past 30 years has illustrated how 'people need people', not just for the sake of their company, but also for the sake of their own health. A range of studies has illuminated how social support influences health, including physical health (Ornstein & Sobel, 1987; Uchino, Cacioppo & Kiecolt-Glaser, 1996), such that high levels of social support are associated with less stress, increased disease resistance, better adherence to treatment, easier labour and childbirth, less severe bereavement reactions and even reduced death rates.

As the importance of a sense of community, belongingness and social support has become increasingly recognised, health services have undergone a community re-orientation. The ethos of community care has shifted our focus to the preventive, therapeutic and rehabilitative value of those people around us. The community is also the natural ally of the primary healthcare philosophy. Around the world, in both the most and the least industrialised countries, for economic, clinical and theoretical reasons, healthcare has come home to the community.

Once again, if we turn to definitions, we find that it is not easy to say exactly what a 'community' is. The ideal community, according to Heller and Monahan (1977, p. 382), is 'one that maximizes citizen input by providing opportunities for individuals to participate and contribute to the welfare of that group'. This definition of the ideal community emphasises two important aspects. First, 'citizen input' and participation are key elements in what has been described as 'community involvement in health' (CIH – Oakley, 1989). Second, the recipients of good community health practices are the members of the community itself.

However, the community practitioner works in a context that incorporates much more than just community factors. This broader context can be described as the 'ecological' perspective (O'Conners & Lubin, 1984), suggesting that a person's behaviour is strongly influenced by their surroundings. Thus, while an individual's personality, attitudes, intelligence and other 'internal' attributes contribute to his or her behaviour, the context, or surroundings, also have an important influence. The ecological approach therefore focuses our attention less on the individual's psychology and more on factors such as the community and the culture with which the person identifies.

This aspect of taking into account the person's environment is perhaps one of the reasons why the ecological (or ecosystemic) approach is becoming increasingly popular and effective in the field of public health. The ecological perspective, in allowing us to move away from focusing on the individual, allows us to consider whether 'the community' is a healthy or unhealthy organisation in its own right. Winnett, King and Altman (1989, p. 130) state:

> The ability to foster communities that promote health is dependent upon stimulating opportunities for group membership and influence, meeting group needs, and promoting the sharing of social support.

Our conception of community health now involves not just how the health of an individual can be influenced by the community, but also whether or not the community itself is healthy. These two notions are of course closely related, not only in contemporary thinking, but also among the ancients.

The origins of the word 'community' are concerned with the idea of sharing a wall (T. Knight, 1994, personal communication). A wall, of course, is a barrier; it can serve to keep others out, but it also defines the common ground to those within it. According to the ancients this sharing of space referred not just to physical space but also to the psychological space created by a sense of enclosure. It was not only the physical space therefore that was shared by those behind the walls, but also the psychological responsibility of living within that space and of being with others. Once again, in ancient times, such communities, often protected by a circular wall, would congregate for meals and ceremonial occasions in the 'forum', which was built at the centre of the community. Such a community therefore literally shared the same forum or 'focus' (a word derived from forum). Another aspect of the meaning of 'focus' is the fire at the centre (around which people would crowd). Such a fire could literally keep the community alive and metaphorically keep alive the spirit of the community.

The ancients believed that places of great social value, such as a forum, were guarded by the gods. They would perform certain rituals in order to keep in good favour with the gods. In effect they would cultivate the favour of the gods. This was done by ensuring that only people who knew the correct etiquette were allowed to enter particular places such as the forum. Thus certain rituals would be performed on entering a forum, and their performance would signify the right of the individual to enter and take part in community activities. Such rituals and etiquette varied and distinguished one community from another. The word culture refers to the notion of cultivating – as in cultivating a crop – a relationship, not just with the gods, but also with other members of the community.

Evidently the ideas inherent in the words 'culture' and 'community' are intricately woven together in an ancient fabric of etymology. Of equal relatedness – and perhaps surprisingly to our 'modern' thinking – is the ancient understanding of health. Health was seen as an index of how useful or 'appropriate' a person was to their community. It was believed that if an individual's behaviour was out of 'balance' with the requirements of the community, then ill-health and suffering would result. Interestingly, according to this belief system, the individual who caused the imbalance was not necessarily the one who suffered. Instead another person, or group of people, could suffer because of the inappropriate behaviour of an individual. In ancient societies health was a very public concern. How individuals relate to each other can therefore be seen to be a common element in ancient notions of culture, community and health. An understanding of how the self relates to others will be shown to be of crucial importance for contemporary mental and physical health.

Gender

Culture is patterned by many features, perhaps the most prominent and important of these being how men and women are treated differently. Men and woman are distinguishable by both their biological sex and their social gender roles. In terms of biological sex women, particularly in poorer countries, face significant hazards as a consequence of child bearing and pregnancy. There are also significant differences in the incidence of some diseases, e.g. on average, men develop heart disease 10 years earlier than women, women are around 2.7 times more likely than men to develop an autoimmune disease, and male-to-female infection with HIV is more than twice as 'efficient' as female-to-male infection (Global Forum for Health Research (GFHR), 2004).

These differing roles, expectations and rights for men and women across all cultures are also related to health. There are no societies in which women are treated as the equals of men (UNDP, 1998). Herein lies one of the major challenges in working with different cultural groups and in different socioeconomic circumstances. The inequalities between men and women tend to be greatest in the world's poorest countries, and so women in these contexts are disadvantaged the most. This disadvantage extends from the preference for male children (and reported infanticide of baby girls) to the greater burden on mothers to care and provide for the family, and these responsibilities and pressures perhaps account for the much higher incidence of mental health problems among women than among men. Challenging such inequalities often means challenging the traditions that underpin the culture. Often it will not be possible to be sensitive to both conservation of culture and liberation of women from oppression and subjugation. Sometimes cultures will need to 'evolve' and the rights and positions of different genders be re-negotiated.

This evolution of gender roles need not be at the expense of men, however, because many traditional male gender roles emphasise the role of breadwinner, so putting men at increased risk of occupational accidents. Men are also more likely to take part in dangerous or violent activities, such as smoking, excessive drinking, driving too fast, engaging in unsafe sex, and taking their own lives through suicide (Smyth, MacLachlan & Clare, 2003; GFHR, 2004; see Chapter 4). The relationship between sex and gender roles itself deserves much more research and more thinking through by clinicians. Gender relationships are almost always unequal across cultures and they show distinctive patterns of exposure to and experience of many of the major physical and mental health problems that people experience. This is an issue to which I shall return throughout this book and is salient to the case study described in the next section.

An integrative model

There have been numerous attempts to synthesise a comprehensive understanding of all things that affect health. Generally these models integrate physiological, psychological and sociological influences on health. However, to attempt this is no easy task and sometimes the complexity of 'bringing it all together' can confuse the reader. A model should, after all, be easier to understand than reality. Otherwise what is the advantage of having a model? Hancock and Perkins (1985) have described 'the Mandala of health' as a way of understanding and remembering an array of factors that can influence health. The model sees human ecology as an interaction of culture and environment, incorporating a holistic view of health and recognising the biological sediment of organs, cells, molecules and atoms, which form the substrata

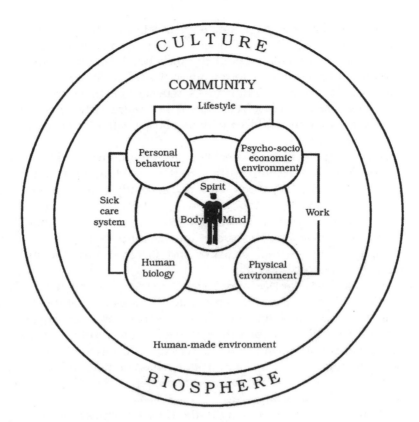

Figure 1.2   A model of the human ecosystem (reproduced from Hancock and Perkins (1985) with permission).

of us all. Figure 1.2 shows this model, which, by its symmetrical design, implicitly reminds us of the importance of balance between different systems and subsystems. The community interfaces between the culture and family, and allows for differences in lifestyle along with biological, spiritual and psychological experiences of life. These three 'divisions' are enclosed within a circle suggesting that they are often interdependent. Spiritual experiences may have biological and psychological aspects or consequences.

The Mandala provides an aide memoire but not an explanation. One of its merits is that it leaves you space to think. It cannot prescribe an action, but it can guide towards a more comprehensive understanding than might otherwise have been the case. The following case study provides a fairly tough test of the value of any model seeking to relate culture to health.

Case study: torture or tradition?

Lydia Oluloro asked for 'cultural asylum' in the USA from her native Nigeria and Yoruba tradition of female circumcision. Lydia had been married to a fellow Nigerian, Emmanuel, who held a US residency permit. After their divorce Emmanuel had failed to complete the necessary paperwork to allow Lydia and their two US-born children – Shade aged 6 and Lara aged 5 – to remain in the USA. One of the grounds for divorce was given as Emmanuel's repeated beatings of the children. Lydia, who had been given custody of the children, saw herself as caught between leaving the children with an abusive father or bringing them to an 'abusive culture'.

Female circumcision is described by some human rights activists as 'female genital mutilation'. Although the procedure itself, and the age at which it is done, vary across cultures, generally young girls have some part (sometimes all) of their external genitalia cut off. The clitoris and labia may be completely excised and the vulva stitched together. The girls are awake during the entire procedure, the purpose of which is to ensure virginity, reduce sexual pleasure and thereby make the girls better marriage prospects.

A.M. Rosenthal, a *New York Times* columnist, has called for UN intervention on the issue and for economic sanctions against those countries where the practice is common. She claims that many girls are left 'in lifelong pain and sexual deprivation' as well as 'more vulnerable to disease, infection and early death'. On the basis of Lydia Oluloro's argument that her two daughters would be at risk of genital mutilation if they returned to Nigeria, the family was allowed to remain in the USA. In short, they received 'cultural asylum'.

Many African women living in the USA are opposed to sanctions. Dr Asha Mohamud, a Somali-born paediatrician working in Washington, says that 'The practice is not being done to intentionally harm anyone. Mothers do it in good faith for their children.' Alice Walker, the author of the anti-genital mutilation book *Warrior Marks*, has been criticised by Dr Nahid Tobia, a Sudanese-born obstetrician who works in New York city: 'It suggests that, "I, Alice Walker, save the beautiful children who are being tortured by their own people". It's like saying Harlem women give their children AIDS because they don't love them. In reality it's more complex.' Indeed it is complex; some immigrants to the USA continue the practice of female circumcision, while others are disappointed that there is no formal provision made for it.

Although the above case was reported in *Time* Magazine in 1994, approximately 2 million cases of female circumcision/genital mutilation occur each year; it is practised in 28 African countries and almost universally in parts of North Africa (Rix, 2005). Interestingly, although it is not practised by most Muslims, it has acquired a religious dimension among those who do it, but Islamic leaders are divided on its practice (Rix, 2005).

Let us consider the utility of the Mandala for understanding culture, community and health in relation to each other in the context of this case study. The Mandala model of the human ecosystem depicts the interaction between culture – as the most abstract unit of social analysis – and the biosphere – as the most abstract unit of physical analysis. As we have already seen culture and the biosphere are linked in that certain behaviours and social structures are appropriate to certain environments, but not to others. The model thus emphasises that lifestyles and community customs need to be understood in a broader context. Clearly American and Nigerian values may differ because they are an expression of cultures that have adapted to different environments. Instead of taking the context of an individual's behaviour into account, we often attribute the cause of it solely and directly to the individual in question. This is one aspect of the 'fundamental attribution error'. If we lack an understanding of the cultural context in which a behaviour occurs, the behaviour may appear quite bizarre and unwarranted. The US court judged that the Oluloro children should not have to experience the circumcision custom of the Yoruba. The court judged the practice to be unwarranted. It could be argued that the court's decision can be understood only in the cultural context of the USA.

Apart from drawing our attention to the context provided by culture and biosphere, the Mandala model also suggests that the following sorts of questions (moving from the outside to the centre of the model) might be asked:

- Does the practice have other functions within the communities where it happens? (Does it act as a form of initiation right into womanhood? What are the consequences of not undergoing the ritual?)
- Does it have an economic value? (Is a dowry system part of the culture?)
- How does it affect how women see themselves?
- How does it affect future intercourse and/or ability to have children?
- Does it have any spiritual connotation?
- Are there health risks?

The Mandala model is an aid to the community practitioner to 'think through cultures' (see Shweder, 1991) and in doing so to be more able to evaluate and act in a culturally sensitive manner.

To argue that behaviour needs to be understood in its cultural context is not to argue for a liberal cultural relativism, where anything goes if it goes as part of 'the culture'. Although evaluating cultures is a rather treacherous endeavour, I would venture that the value of cultural practices should be judged in terms of whether or not they serve their people well. Beneficiaries may be at various levels, including the individual, family and community levels. If the practice fails to deliver some advantage at any of these levels, it is likely to be of dubious value. If it is of value at some levels and not at others, whether or not change should be negotiated should be judged not only from within the cultural system, but also on the basis of a broader understanding of human rights.

Culture and human rights

In the case study involving Shade and Lara Oluloro, a legitimate feminist argument is that 'leaving it up to the culture' is to deny these children their basic human rights. This is an appealing argument but it must also be recognised as a culturally based one, even though members of that culture may believe their values to be 'universal' human rights. Let us not side step the issue here. There is nothing wrong with attempting to change certain aspects of a culture – that is how different cultures have evolved over many generations. Cultures will survive by adaptation but not by stagnation.

One of the most promising developments regarding health in recent years has been its recognition – or more precisely the recognition of the resources that can produce and sustain health – as a human right (see Chapter 9), e.g. the Dublin Declaration, arising from an international conference on HIV/AIDS in 2004, has as its first of 33 principles the idea of protecting people from the threat of AIDS, as a *human right*. The Universal Declaration of Human Rights, adopted by the UN in 1948, asserts that 'all human beings are born free and equal in dignity and rights. They are endowed with reason and conscience and should act towards one another in a spirit of brotherhood [and sisterhood].'

Mary Robinson (2004), the former President of Ireland and UN High Commissioner for Human Rights, stresses that the declaration 'is not a Western human rights agenda, but a truly universal one', in that it puts equal emphasis on civil and political rights (such as fair trial, freedom from torture, freedom of the press) and on economic, cultural and social rights (such as the right to food, safe water, health, education and shelter). Robinson points out that to ignore progress on some rights, e.g. progress on education and health in China, and focus only on a lack of progress on other rights, e.g. civil rights in China, is to be disingenuous. Although the interpretation of how health as a human right might differ in different cultures, it is hoped that its status as a human right can be agreed across all cultures.

If, in some traditional societies, female circumcision is seen to confer 'eligibility' as a marriage partner because the woman has adhered to the cultural rites of passage, then, in some highly industrialised western societies, cosmetic interventions may be seen as conferring 'eligibility' in other ways. Kalp (1999) catalogues the 'improvements' of Holly Laganante, a 35-year-old woman from Chicago, who has had an eyelid lift, liposuction on her thighs, varicose vein removal and a forehead peel. She said 'It's been tough on me financially, but it's worth every penny . . . it's life-changing'. According to the American Society of Plastic and Reconstructive Surgeons, there was a 153% increase between 1992 and 1999 in such operations, with more than one million in the last year. California leads America in 'augs' (augmentations) where it is apparently not uncommon for 16-year-old high school girls to get breast enlargements – long before they may have finished physically maturing. McGrath and Mukerji (2000) reported that the eight operations most commonly done on teenagers of 18 or less were (in descending order):

- rhinoplasty ('nose jobs')
- ear surgery
- reduction mammoplasty (breast reduction)
- surgery for asymmetrical breasts
- excision of gynaecomastia (male breast reduction)
- augmentation mammoplasty (breast enlargement)

- chin augmentation
- suction-assisted lipoplasty (removal of fat under the skin).

Although these procedures may be necessary and appropriate in many cases, the difficulty is where to draw the line between cosmetic therapy and cosmetic recreation, and perhaps even a culturally sanctioned 'cosmetic mutilation'. McGrath and Mukerji (2000, p. 105, italics added) state: 'In the final analysis, *the purpose of plastic surgery is to change the patient's psyche* in a positive way.' It would seem that both genital mutilation and cosmetic surgery share the desire to change the way that people are seen psychologically, by physically altering them in some respect, causing them pain and changing physical aspects that work (in an anatomical sense) satisfactorily.

Airhihenbuwa (1995) has emphasised the importance of multiculturalism addressing all cultures, and not simply the majority culture using the concept of 'multiculturalism' to manage the health of other cultures. He has expressed justifiable concern that the agenda of health interventions is rooted in North American and European concerns to achieve what are seen within these cultures as positive outcomes, but which may not be seen as positive outcomes by other cultures. Whoever you are and wherever you are reading this book, a cultural analysis of health is every bit as applicable to your health and your culture as it may seem to be to the culture and health of far-off and exotic peoples. To understand ourselves we must stand outside ourselves and realise that our way is but one of many.

We have now reviewed the conceptions of culture and health to be used here. Culture is used broadly to refer to shared means of communication and social experience of living in the world, while also keeping in mind that culture influences health and people's sense of empowerment in a plethora of different ways. Health is seen as multidimensional, with each dimension represented on a continuum, rather than in an all-or-none (healthy or ill) dichotomy. I place health within the community context, because this recognises both ancient thought and contemporary practice, and I also see access to health services as a right and not a privilege. With these working definitions in mind there follows a preview of forthcoming chapters.

Preview

Cultural differences (Chapter 2)

Acculturation describes the process whereby individuals encounter more than one culture and respond to the interplay between them in various ways. The way in which acculturation takes place, and the stress experienced, can seriously affect health. The reaction to acculturation is, however, not easily predictable and family members may have vastly different acculturative experiences.

One feature of encountering a different culture may be having to under-stand a different perspective on the factors responsible for health and illness. Within most western societies the biomedical model predominates, which attributes health and illness to changes in our biochemical and physiological substrate, changes that often occur at such a microscopic level that belief in them is, for most people, an act of faith. On a worldwide scale, faith in other causal mechanisms, such as the intervention of displeased spirits or the use of witchcraft, is probably more widespread. It would seem vital therefore to understand not only the nature of a person's presenting complaint but also their explanation of it, because the two are almost certainly interwoven to some extent. Health professionals, often through ignorance and sometimes because of arrogance or insecurity, may try to impose their own model on their patients. Clinicians are often less tolerant of ambiguity and less accept-ing of more than one explanation for illness or suffering than are their patients. Within a multicultural society clinicians must recognise and show some tolerance towards a pluralistic approach to health.

In assessing any one individual there is always the difficulty of knowing to what extent they conform to cultural stereotypes. Stereotypes refer to con-ceptual and statistical averages, not to individuals. We must therefore find a way of mapping out how individuals' beliefs about their state of health relate to their own personal situation, the community in which they live, their culture, etc. The *problem portrait technique* is proposed as a tool for unravelling such interlocking influences. Through a collaborative interview methodology, the clinician may assess the relative strengths of many factors that simulta-neously influence a person's health-related behaviour. The problem portrait technique is a way of integrating individual (foreground) and culture (background).

Syndromes of culture (Chapter 3)

The idea of 'culture-bound syndromes' has been popular for many years. One interpretation of these exotic conditions has been that they embody social myths, perform certain social functions and/or reflect particular social pres-sures within the cultures where they are expressed. However, this sort of analysis may be made of any syndrome of illness. All illness or disorder occurs in a cultural context of some kind, and it is argued that, to some extent, cul-tural contexts influence the way in which suffering is caused, experienced and expressed, and the consequences of such suffering. In describing some syn-dromes as 'culture bound' it has been implied that some syndromes are not influenced by culture. Such an assumption is not warranted and in most cases is probably ethnocentric, in that it suggests that 'our' syndromes are not culture bound but universal, i.e. they really do exist!

If we accept the influence of social forces on our well-being, it follows that the problem with which a particular individual presents may reflect factors beyond the self. An individual may, for instance, become anxious because of unease within the community in which he or she lives. In such a case a person's suffering can be said to point beyond that person: he or she may be a social scapegoat. If an individual's suffering sometimes reflects community or cultural concerns, how should this concern be demonstrated? What form should suffering take? A society that is anxious about the way in which child-like girls enter adult-like womanhood may express this anxiety through an individual adolescent female's concern with her body shape, size or weight. In an extreme case an adolescent female may starve herself of food, perhaps unconsciously seeking to retain the body of a child-like girl. Here we may also talk of the body being used as a symbol, symbolising concerns within the culture. In this way cultural concerns may interfere with physical and mental functioning, either 'exploiting' existing ailments or shaping new ones into a form of cultural expression. The experiencing of a culture-bound syndrome by a person of a different culture may reflect their anxieties over self-identity and cultural identity. At times cultural-bound syndromes may also be seen as a means of cultural resistance to oppression or exploitation.

Mental aspects of health (Chapter 4)

The study of cross-cultural mental health takes place in different forms. Comparative mental health compares the nature of mental health and disorder in one culture with that in another, minority culture mental health considers what the consequences of being a member of a minority cultural group are for mental functioning, and transition mental health is concerned with how experiences of, say, refugeehood or migration affect mental health. Each of these perspectives is quite distinctive but in reality they also overlap. Thus immigrants are often members of minority cultural groups and may be reported as having a higher incidence of certain disorders than the majority cultural group. A multitude of factors influence consideration of mental health, and these factors should include social, economic and political forces that interact with cultural considerations as indicated in Table 1.2.

It is tempting for clinicians to try to classify the unknown through diagnostic systems that are familiar to them. A Chinese person presenting with stomachache after experiencing bereavement as a result of the death of a family member may be described as suffering from 'masked depression'. This insinuates that he is not suffering from the real thing but from something else that replaces it, for whatever reason. Contrariwise, in theory, a Chinese clinician may say that a French man who is depressed after experiencing a similar bereavement is suffering from 'masked stomachache'. Such an explanation would be unacceptable to most westerners because they assume the universal primacy of psychological processes. The only way out of such a riddle is to try to understand people's experience of suffering within the terms in which they experience it, i.e. within their cultural 'terms of reference'. Failure to do so is to strip suffering of its meaning and symbolism and in so doing affront the integrity of the sufferer. When cultural 'terms of reference' change within a society this may also dislodge individuals' sense of identity and threaten their mental health.

The communities in which people live should be seen as resources for community health. A sense of belonging and the opportunity to receive social support from similar people can have a positive effect on mental health. Also, living in areas where the number of people who constitute a minority cultural group is large appears to be much better for mental health than living in an area where your cultural group is in a small minority. Such considerations may help to buffer the stressful experience of transition that many immigrants experience on arriving in a new country or culture.

Physical aspects of health (Chapter 5)

Recent research has demonstrated that psychosocial stressors can influence physical well-being in a variety of ways. The fact that many of the salient psychosocial stressors are likely to vary across cultural groups also implicates cultural variations in physical disease processes. As already noted with mental health, a strong sense of community, or cultural identity, may benefit physical health. Research on 'cultural inwardness' has found that mortality from serious diseases is lower where traditional cultural values are cherished. It also seems clear that some cultural groups live a healthier life than others, e.g. Seventh Day Adventists appear to live longer and have fewer physical problems than most people. We must therefore be prepared to learn healthier ways of living from other cultures.

Reactions to illness will reflect the way in which cultures socially construct the meaning of illness behaviour. Consideration of the cultural aspects of pain, cancer, deafness and obesity illustrate the range of effects that culture has on quite diverse illness behaviour; how it affects sensation, help seeking, stigmatisation and indeed the creation of health problems.

Treatments (Chapter 6)

One reason why cultures vary in how their individual members present illness is that different cultures require different paths to be followed in order to become 'legitimately' ill. To be a good patient in Brazil you must understand the Brazilian way of being ill. If the patient and the clinician know the rules to be followed each can have faith in the other. The faith of a patient, or client, in a treatment is often referred to as the placebo effect. This effect applies not just to treatments but to clinicians as well. When a patient and a clinician come from different cultural groups, this may influence the degree of faith that a patient has in the treatment offered and in the clinician who is offering it. A *faith grid* can chart the interaction between clinician and patient.

Another aspect of the process of treatment concerns what sort of information is shared between clinician and client. A cultural difference in diagnostic disclosure (whether clinicians tell their clients the true diagnosis that they have made) is an example of this. Patients and clinicians are cast in different roles by different cultures and this affects clinical decision-making. Clinicians are a product of their culture and so too are their treatments. Sometimes inappropriate therapies can be oppressive. If a black person suffers from depression because of their experience of racism, a treatment that focuses only on his depression (e.g. antidepressants or cognitive therapy) problematises his legitimate distress. Such a treatment supports the view that the problem is with the individual rather than with the context in which that individual lives. The concept of transference can assist the clinician in understanding the personal history that individuals (both patients and clinicians) bring to clinical encounters of all kinds. Another technique that may be useful is the use of critical incidents as a therapeutic technique, whereby the clinician can help clients think through how the problems that they present reflect their own values in the context of their culture. Rather than focusing on the culture and then 'zooming in' on the individual, the critical incident technique offers the possibility of focusing on the individual and then 'panning out' to take in the cultural and social context.

A recent development in thinking about culture and treatment is the recognition of the possible role of culture as treatment. For minority groups who have been marginalised by majority society, and who may in the process have lost any strong sense of identity and experienced low self-esteem, rekindling of their culture as a medium to their own rehabilitation has been encouraged; an example of this is seen among the indigenous people of Canada and Australia. The current interest in the west in different ways of living life (e.g. Buddhism) suggests that cultures or subcultures that are used as 'treatment' do not have to be one's own culture to be effective. The therapeutic effect of culture may simply be that it gives a sense of belonging, an anchor in the sea of life. The rise of 'race-based' therapeutics does however question any construction of the relationship between culture and health that denies the existence of specific biological mechanisms associated with different skin colours. This in turn may raise ethical concerns regarding research and practice.

Health services (Chapter 7)

Health services of the twenty-first century must adopt a multicultural perspective. These services need to reach beyond just concerns with the way in which different cultures experience and express illness, and how clinicians and their clients communicate, to include a community's infrastructure of care (of all types) in planning for health. Multicultural care requires western-trained clinicians to ascertain where they 'fit in' to the overall system, and not to centre the healthcare system on themselves. The community must be the home of health. Even in a monocultural society clinicians of different professions will hold different (subcultural) beliefs about the mechanisms of, and remedies for, suffering. So too will the lay members of such a society, because their health beliefs are constituted from popular and folk beliefs, not just the beliefs of health professionals. As such the very notion of a monocultural society is a fallacy.

Greater tolerance of pluralistic approaches to suffering is now required. This tolerance must extend not only to making allowances for other explanations of and interventions for suffering, but also to acknowledging that different systems of cause and effect may be synthesised in ways that do not always make obvious sense to you or me (from whatever our cultural perspective may be). This is not to say that 'anything goes', but it does suggest that we should be open to empirically evaluating interventions that we may neither fully comprehend nor recommend. In this sense clinicians must be prepared to learn from their patients.

Promoting health (Chapter 8)

Intervention can occur not only as treatment but also as prevention. We can go beyond the idea of preventing things from going wrong to promoting things going right! For too long health services have reacted to illness and disorder rather than living up to what that phrase implies – servicing health. Unfortunately even the best of health promotion initiatives are inevitably developed within particular models and cultural contexts. Thus cultural minorities may be disadvantaged because such initiatives are less accessible to them. Culturally sensitive health promotion will require working through different media and in different ways in different cultures. Flexibility and adaptability will be central requirements for health promoters working with diverse cultures.

Specific risk factors have been identified for particular disorders. In the case of depression, for example, experiencing severe stressors, having low self-esteem and living in poverty have been identified (among others) as risk factors. The distribution of such stressors across different cultural groups may be uneven, particularly for minority immigrant groups. Once again we need to appreciate that cultural variation does not present itself in isolation from other factors that influence health. Cultural expectations may also constitute risk factors. It can be argued that the emphasis on individualism and achievement, which is found in many western cultures, predisposes westerners to individual failure and self-depreciation; this may constitute a loss of faith in the self, a key feature in the western experience of depression.

Cultures offer different solutions to living and therefore different pathways to healthy living. They need to be understood at a systems level and not simply by extracting a few cultural practices on which to focus. Health promotion efforts that do not acknowledge established cultural pathways risk derailing these important conduits of health. Clinicians once again need to see themselves as facilitators of health and not directors of it. Promoting public health must be seen as a long-term strategic goal, which will not be achieved in a biotechnological flash! Instead, such a goal is more likely to be achieved through slower *incremental improvements* in existing services where the pace of change reflects what communities are able to absorb while retaining their distinctive character and culture. Health promotion must also consider the opportunities and challenges presented by specific sub-cultural groups and what might be the most effective means of influencing behaviour in such groups, with research of the gay community in Sichaun province, China, being a particularly interesting example.

Global health (Chapter 9)

McAuliffe (2003) defines global health as an attempt to address health problems that transcend national boundaries, may be influenced by circumstances and experiences in other countries, and are best addressed by cooperative actions and solutions. The underlying assumption is that the world's health problems are shared problems and are therefore best tackled by shared solutions. An implicit aspiration within this perspective is to work towards removing inequalities and privileges in accessing health, i.e. to establish health as a human right. More recently the need for health as a prerequisite to economic development has been recognised, as has its importance in maintaining international security.

Many of the world's health problems are problems that thrive on poverty. This is not just a poverty of resources but also a poverty of research and, perhaps, interest too, e.g. 'the 10/90 gap' refers to the fact that only 10% of the world's health research funding is given over to addressing 90% of the world's disease burden, mostly found in the world's poorer countries. We consider the millennium development goals (MDGs) and the UN's targets for improved health by 2015 from a cultural perspective. Given such a diversity of goals and targets, the case of HIV/AIDS is considered as a result of its pervasiveness and devastation, and the richer world's continual ability to turn away from it.

The challenge of global health is to recognise that the factors that affect health in one country or context are much the same as those in another. Although the extent of health and social problems may differ, the background determinates are similar. In a world of increasing interconnectedness we need to develop shared solutions to these shared problems. We also need to keep the economic engine of globalisation from 'running away' with our world, and to ensure that its' proceeds are used to address, and not augment, existing inequities.

Conclusion

The indisputable process of internationalisation – the increasing contact between peoples of different countries – is often seen as making the world a smaller place, or reducing the differences between cultures. This is the 'melting-pot' perspective on our future. It asserts that the world's cultures will be thrown together with little to distinguish the behaviour of an Indian from that of a Spaniard, or an Irish from a Japanese person. An alternative is the 'kaleidoscopic' perspective, which is that we are not getting more similar, but instead more different. Internationalisation is producing more subcultures within our traditionally recognised cultures. The Indian, Spanish, Irish and Japanese ways of life – the cultures – will still remain fundamentally different, because these peoples operate in ecologically different contexts. For some people this 'selection box' of humanity presents threats and problems, yet for others it allows a world of variety, stimulation and opportunities.

Many modern industrialised cities are thronged with different cultures and communities. A community is not a geographical location; it is a state of mind, shared by a group of people. You and I may be next-door neighbours, but inhabit quite different communities. Whether you live in Berlin, Blantyre or Brisbane, your mere physical location does not give you a right of entrance into a 'local' community. Your membership of a community will depend on your methods of communication, practice of rituals, and adherence to certain 'rules'. 'Mainstream' health services, and the clinicians who work in them, often fail to cultivate meaningful relationships with people who are not part of a mainstream culture. This book aims to outline ways in which good health can be understood and cultivated both within and across cultures.

Guidelines for professional practice

1. The social health sciences of medical sociology, medical anthropology and health psychology each has a legitimate claim to a useful perspective on the relationship between culture and health. Each of these perspectives offers interesting insights at the structural, systems and individual level of analysis. Although individuals are entitled to their own health psychology, how they construct such beliefs will be influenced by the cultural systems in which they live and how they enact such beliefs will be influenced by the constraints of the society in which they live.

2. The terms 'culture', 'race' and 'ethnicity' are often used interchangeably, although they refer to quite different ideas. Race is, strictly speaking, a biological term and refers to heritable physical characteristics. Ethnicity is often used to refer to common physical features that are in turn associated with a psychological sense of similarity. Culture refers to shared customs of communication and common experiences of living in the world.

3. Variations in human physique are often taken as evidence for the existence of several distinct human races. However, it is also the case that human physique varies within the traditional anthropological categories of race. Furthermore, significant genetic differences may also occur *within* traditional race categories, and these differences appear to be related to health. Consequently, although physical and genetic differences certainly do occur between peoples of different geographical origin, the concept of race provides an inadequate framework for assessing these differences in relation to health.

4. Whatever concepts we use to describe human variation – 'race', 'ethnicity', 'culture' – they are themselves a product of how this variation is understood to occur. Different groups of people have different explanations for this variation. As such, these 'local' ways of understanding

human variation (folk taxonomies) are subjective interpretations. Different cultures understand human variation differently. What most of them do share, however, is the belief that their own interpretation is the correct one!

5. Human variation is also found in the ways in which groups of people organise themselves. Whatever form this organisation takes, its functioning is facilitated by communication. In this book culture is seen as the medium of communication shared by a group of people.

6. Our senses are the biological conduits of our cultural communications. There is no barrier between the psychosocial processes of relating to fellow human beings and the biological substrate of processing this information. Culture's influence on health is not restricted to mental functioning; it also affects physical functioning.

7. Traditional ideas about cultural differences associate them strongly with different geographical locales. This association no longer holds true and new types of culture–health relationships have emerged including 'alternative' healthcare, rapid social change, globalisation and empowerment.

8. Health is multidimensional and includes physical, psychological and social well-being. People can be healthy in some aspects of their life while being ill in others. On any one dimension, health and illness are not experienced in the absence of the other. Health is on a continuum; it is not a dichotomy. Thus patients are often healthy in many more ways than they are ill.

9. The community health philosophy invites consideration of how communities differ from each other. This is entirely consistent with examining cultural differences in health and recognising that cultures operate through local communities. However, when considering cultural differences, the clinician should also consider the social, economic and political contexts in which culturally different communities operate. Sometimes these latter differences can affect health more profoundly than can cultural differences themselves.

10. The belief that culture, community and health are related is not simply a reflection of modern practice; it was also a belief in ancient times. Our modern use of these terms often obscures their related etymologies. The way in which an individual relates to others is a common factor in culture, community and health.

11. The Mandala of health is a schematic for thinking through and attempting to integrate the many factors that can influence health. It is presented as a clinically useful aide memoir rather than a comprehensive academic model.

12. The status of health as a human right is becoming increasingly accepted both in international agreements and among practitioners. This perspective challenges the idea that health is a privilege that can be bought and recasts it as an obligation that must be met. Although this conception of health presents challenges across cultures, it also presents challenges within cultures and societies that take its 'purchase' for granted.

CHAPTER 2

Understanding cultural differences

In this chapter we consider cultural differences in terms of human interactions and health. Of fundamental importance for understanding the interplay between culture and health is the appreciation of the relationship between an individual and the society in which he or she lives – in essence, the relationship between the individual's personality and the society's personality, its culture. The social context of intergroup relationships can easily result in prejudice and racism. We consider how people from one culture may encounter those from another culture. Migration represents one of the most common vehicles of cross-cultural encounters. We review a model of acculturative experience, which outlines the different ways in which immigrants can exist within a host society. We also apply the model to adaptation to changes within the same society.

The variety of cultures that now constitutes many urban centres reflects a huge range of different beliefs about health and illness. We review a classic study of health beliefs across the world. Moving away from the diversity across cultures some psychologists have sought empirically to derive psychological dimensions that are common across many different cultures. Some of these dimensions appear to be relevant in areas as diverse as psychotherapy, teaching and physical illness. However, although large-scale empirical studies and the models derived from them appear to be useful at a broad level, they do not inform individual clinicians how they should respond to the person from a different culture to their own, who presents an ailment for healing. The problem portrait technique is described as a simple way of ascertaining the relationship between an individual and other social forces that may influence their health beliefs.

Personality and culture

'Culture is to society what memory is to the individual' (Kluckhohn & Kroeber, 1952). The need to understand population-level influences on individual's psychological functioning is addressed by the discipline of cross-cultural psychology (Berry et al., 2002). This perspective acknowledges the necessity of taking cultural context into account when trying to understand what individuals think and why they think it. Furthermore, it also recognises that collective culture and individual psychology are in a reciprocal relationship, i.e. they 'make each other up' (Shweder, 1991). There are two broad approaches to considering personality–culture relationships: one is how culture influences the development and expression of certain personality traits, and the other is how culture influences the way in which people understand themselves.

Much of the recent research on personality has focused on the 'big five' personality dimensions of extraversion, agreeableness, conscientiousness, neuroticism and openness to experience, and the claim that they are independent of culture (McCrea, 2000). However, the extent to which these five factors are universal is controversial and it is possible that there may be additional culture-specific factors, e.g. 'filial piety' (or respect for elders/authority) among the Chinese cultures (Berry et al., 2002). Although the 'big five' factors do emerge across cultures, most studies have not considered cultures very different from western samples, and few have included emic, or cultural-specific, traits in their overall analysis (Triandis & Suh, 2002). Regardless of the stability of the 'big five' (or any other) personality traits, what influence they may have, above and beyond situational determinants, e.g. in predicting health behaviour, remains open to question (Berry et al., 2002). Church (2000) has argued that, for example, in relatively more collectivist cultures (see later) situational determinates are relatively more influential, whereas in more individualist cultures (see later) cognitive consistency is relatively more influential in determining behaviour.

A related issue concerning the relationship between culture and personality is whether the idea of *what a person is* varies in different cultures. The idea of individuality, of people stopping at the skin, being bound by their biological limit, is key to a differentiated or independent self. Alternatively people may also be seen as *relational* (Kagitcibasi, 1996) or *interdependent* (Markus & Kitayama, 1991). I once heard an Indian psychologist describe people in the west as *individuals* and people in India as *dividuals*! Of course the extent to which a sense of self derives from individual or collective ideas (recall the concept of uMunthu in Chapter 1) is only one dimension along which culture may influence how 'the self' is seen, e.g. Nsamengang (1992) describes the influence of the world of spirits, and the ecological environment, as also being formative in many African conceptions of the self.

Managing cultural complexity

Moving from the complexities of understanding the self to understanding others, and in trying to deal with such complexity, we naturally try to simplify things. One way of achieving this is to lump together what appears to be similar, ignoring (apparently small) differences. Sometimes we can get so used to seeing the similarities that we expect to see, that we stop looking for – and fail to detect – important differences. In such cases the world can, in fact, become a more difficult place for us to manage, because we oversimplify it. The process of 'oversimplifying people' is referred to as stereotyping. Much of the psychological literature on stereotyping has concerned two related themes: 'in-groups' versus 'out-groups', and prejudice.

We tend to group people into different 'sorts'. People put into the same group as the self are members of our 'in-group', whereas those outside this selection are 'out-group' members (Tajfel, 1978). Furthermore, we tend to differentiate between the members of our in group, i.e. we see them as 'people in their own right'. In contrast, we often fail to differentiate between members of an out group – we see them as 'all the same'. In addition we generally see in-group members as better people than out-group members. Research has indicated a number of ways in which individuals can benefit psychologically from identifying with the members of a distinctive group (Baumeister, 1991). A frequent finding is that group membership bolsters the individual's impression of him- or herself. However, and somewhat obviously, such membership is beneficial only if the in group is seen to be a good group to be a member of. Groucho Marx's quip that 'I wouldn't be a member of any club that would have me!' reflects a crisis in self-esteem, not redeemable through group membership!

To feel good about our own group we elevate its status by focusing on the negative or undesirable qualities of other groups. This is referred to as 'out-group derogation' (Branscombe & Wann, 1992, for an example). Thus for your own good, and that of the other members of your in-group, it is as well to concentrate on the positive aspects of your own group and the negative aspects of other groups. Out-group members are therefore discriminated against, even when there are few obvious differences between them and 'in-group' members. It is not necessarily that people consciously sit down and decide that the group with which they identify is superior to other groups; rather in order to enhance and protect our own self-esteem we assume some 'natural superiority'. However, such a process of group identification is made easier if obvious differences do exist between the groups.

Recent neuropsychological research has supported the idea that cultural learning about particular 'racial' groups, as opposed to the novelty of out-group members, may also be an important factor. Lieberman et al. (2005), using fMRI (functional magnetic resonance imaging – brain imaging technology) found that both African–Americans and Caucasian–Americans reacted with greater activity in a particular brain region (the amygdala) when presented with African–American images than when presented with Caucasian images. How the brain mediates culturally related beliefs and attitudes towards others is of interest, as long as we remember that it only mediates these psychological states, rather than being their primary source. Such an assumption could be dangerous if people were to conclude that biologically – which some may take to mean 'naturally' – some groups of people are more 'frightening' than others!

It has been suggested that there is an intimate link between accepting others and being accepted by others. Berry (2005) discusses what he refers to as the 'multicultural assumption', a term he coined some 30 years ago, which states that 'only when people are secure in their own cultural identity will they be able to accept those who differ from them' (p. 14). This statement can be seen in positive terms: that a personal sense of security is a prerequisite for a tolerance of difference or diversity. It can also be seen in a more negative light: it is threats to, or anxiety about, one's own cultural identity that actually underpin prejudice towards others.

Cultural identity is often underpinned by physical appearance, dress norms, religious beliefs and customs, which are quite distinctive. When out-group members look or act differently from in-group members, the oversimplifications inherent in stereotyping can be heightened. 'Racism' and prejudice may be products of the stereotyping process. From time to time we are probably all guilty of misjudging others, on the assumption that they are either similar to us, or different from us, on the basis of their cultural background. Thus 'racism' – or the negative stereotyping of different cultural groups – should not be seen simply as, for instance, the product of aggression bred of social delinquency. Instead it should also be understood as a very common – if undesirable – 'by-product' of our attempts to manage a complex world.

Prejudice is as great a problem for the 'helping professions' as it is for anyone else. Furthermore, time pressure, the need to make quick clinical judgements, high cognitive load and task complexity, are each psychological factors that predispose individuals to the need to reduce complexity, simplify and stereotype (van Ryn & Burke, 2002), just to get through the day! Unfortunately, a genuine desire to help alleviate suffering affords no immunity from the psychological mechanisms, which may oversimplify the sufferer. If you were working in a multicultural setting, would you not just love to 'discover' a set of rules (generalisations) for working with one cultural group as opposed to another? Such 'rules' would probably take the form of caricatures: 'Italians exaggerate pain – especially Italian football players!'; 'Africans, being always happy, don't get depressed'; 'Chinese somatise their problems.' Indeed evidence could probably be found to back up claims that 'the average' person from a particular cultural background tends to behave in a certain way in a particular situation.

The problem with this is that its hard to know how 'average' is the person whom you are seeking to help. Thus the caricature 'solution' to working with people from different cultures is likely to build on our natural processes for simplifying and stereotyping. It makes individuals into what Garfinkel (1967) calls 'cultural dopes', who are expected to follow the rules of their culture. Unfortunately some cultural research falls into this category. What is needed instead is an approach to working with people from different cultures that will acknowledge the diversity, not only of peoples from different cultural groups or geographical regions, but also of the individuals within these groups.

Cultural encounters

People from different cultures encounter each other in various ways. Historically, we have travelled the world for adventure, commerce, and military and diplomatic reasons. In the twentieth and twenty-first centuries travel for leisure in the form of tourism has become more common. These days, students also frequently have periods of study abroad and professional workers take 'career breaks' or seek overseas work in order to experience something different. However, perhaps the greatest modes of intercultural contact are emigration and refugeehood. In some countries such as Australia, Canada and the USA immigrants far outnumber the indigenous people.

The encountering of another culture from the perspective of either the 'locals' or the 'foreigners' presents various difficulties. The discussion of the function of culture in Chapter 1 highlighted culture as a medium of communication. It was argued that such communication does not simply refer to language, or even non-verbal communication, important as these are in such encounters, but also refers to the way in which a person experiences the world in general, and the way in which other people experience and respond to that person. Bochner (1982) has outlined a taxonomy of the ways in which cross-cultural communication can occur. These cultural encounters can take place between members of the same society (e.g. black and white Australians) or between members of different societies (e.g. immigrants). Bochner also distinguishes between different aspects of the contact such as its time-span, purpose and frequency. Research has found that such factors can critically influence the behaviour of the parties involved (Smith & Bond, 1993).

We may have difficulty in communicating with people from another culture because they fail to meet our expectations:

> People are late for appointments, or early, or do not make appointments at all and simply arrive. People stand too close or too far away; talk too much, or too little, or too fast, or too slow, or about the wrong topics. They are too emotional, or too moderate, show too much or too little of a certain emotion, or show it at the wrong time, or fail to show it at the right time.
>
> Smith and Bond (1993, p. 177)

Smith and Bond suggest that such differences can lead to 'cross-cultural misattribution' where the explanations for an event given by a foreigner and a local may be quite different. Such difficulties in cultural encounters may have various effects on the individuals involved. For the foreigner a series of such encounters may give them some impression of how they are managing, or failing to manage, in a different culture.

Culture shock

Oberg (1960) was the first to use the term 'culture shock' in describing people's attempts to adapt to a new culture. However, his use of it implied a rather negative and passive reaction, and this interpretation has since been superseded by a much more positive interpretation where people are seen as attempting actively to deal with a succession of new challenges (Furnham & Bochner, 1986). The model outlined in Ward, Bochner and Furnham (2001) distinguishes an affective (how people feel), a behavioural (what people do) and a cognitive (what people think and how they perceive their situation) response to culture change. In this model the affective reaction is thought of as a response to trying to cope with a stressful situation, and individuals' personal coping characteristics are stressed as being important in their adjustment. The behavioural component relates to the notion of cultural learning, essentially that people need to have the opportunity of learning culturally relevant knowledge and social skills in order to be able to navigate their way through a socially quite different environment to that into which they were socialised. The behavioural and affective components of the 'culture shock' reaction are seen to be often mutually reinforcing, with positive affective reactions encouraging socially skilled behaviour and negative affective reactions increasing social anxiety. The third component of the 'culture shock' reaction, the cognitive component, is concerned with psychological processes involved in 'looking outward', e.g. stereotyping, prejudice and discrimination towards out groups (those not like me), and those involved in 'looking inward' such as identity formation and transition (see below). This overall affect–behaviour–cognitions, or ABC, model of 'culture shock' is illustrated in Figure 2.1.

Ward et al. (2001) use the concept of cultural distance to account for different reactions to encountering new cultures, and to different degrees of 'culture shock'. Cultural distance refers to the extent of the 'cultural gap' between par-

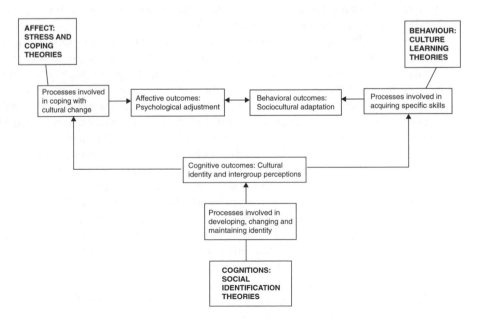

Figure 2.1   The ABC model of 'culture shock'. Reproduced from Ward et al., 2001.

ticipants. For example, there is less of a cultural gap between people from Australia and New Zealand/Aotearoa than between people from Malaysia and Mexico, because in the former there are more customs and beliefs in common, than in the latter. Interestingly one can actually have more 'cultural commonality' between people from elsewhere than between people from one's own country, e.g. those whose ancestors migrated to Australia or New Zealand/Aotearoa from Britain probably have much more in common with British 'natives' than with those who are 'native' to their own countries, the Aboriginal people of Australia or the Maori people of New Zealand/ Aotearoa. Thus 'culture shock' can apply as much to getting to know your 'neighbours' as it can to migrants getting to know a new country. However, as much of the research on cultural adaptation has concerned migrants, we now consider this case in more detail.

Acculturation

'Acculturation', a related term to culture shock, refers to the process of transition that is brought about by the meeting of peoples from two different cultures. Such transition may occur in either one, or both, of the cultures. Increasing internationalism and multiculturalism have produced a hive of activity in research and thinking on the effects of people from different cultures coming together. Berry and colleagues (see Berry, 1997a,b, 2003, for a review) have been researching a framework of acculturation that considers to what extent the newcomer modifies his or her cultural identity and characteristics when coming to a new country. The framework is shown in Figure 2.2. It fits the situation of an immigrant well.

Although this acculturation framework expresses the degree of cultural identity as a dichotomised choice, it should be thought of as, in fact, lying along a continuum. The framework (Berry & Kim, 1988; Berry, 1997, 2003) has been very influential and can provide some valuable insights into cross-cultural experiences. According to the framework a person decides whether or not to keep his or her original cultural identity and characteristics, and also whether or not to acquire the host culture's identity and characteristics (taking the case of an immigrant). Integration between the two cultures occurs when the decision is to identify with and exhibit the characteristics of both the original culture and the new host culture. Here the immigrant selects parts of both cultures and brings them together through their own behaviour and beliefs.

A second type of acculturation occurs when the immigrant retains his or her original cultural identity and does not want to adopt the host country's culture. It is important whether this happens on a voluntary or involuntary basis. If voluntarily chosen the individual is seeking separation from the new culture.

A third alternative is that the immigrant wishes to take on the identity and characteristics of the new culture and disown his or her original culture. This situation is described as assimilation.

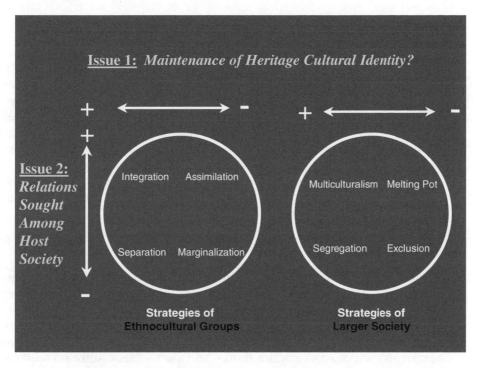

Figure 2.2 Acculturation strategies among immigrant groups and the receiving society. Adapted from Berry (1997).

The fourth option in the model is marginalisation. In this circumstance there is little interest in identifying with or displaying the characteristics of either the original culture or the new culture. In essence the person is living on the margins of both the old and new culture. Such a person may not be accepted or supported by either.

To illustrate the above four strategies Berry gives the example of an Italian family that has migrated to Canada:

> The father may lean toward integration in terms of job prospects, wanting to get involved in the economics and politics of his new society, and learning English and French, in order to obtain the benefits that motivated his migration in the first place. At the same time he may be a leader in the Italian–Canadian Community Association, spending much of his leisure and recreational time in social interaction with other Italian–Canadians. Hence he has a preference for integration when his leisure time activities are considered. In contrast, the mother may hold completely to Italian language use and social interactions, feeling that she is unable to get involved in the work or cultural activities of the host society. She employs the separation strategy having virtually all her personal, social and cultural life with the Italian world. In further contrast the teenage daughter

is annoyed by hearing the Italian language in the home, by having only Italian food served by her mother, and by being required to spend most of her leisure time with her extended Italian family. Instead she much prefers the assimilation option: to speak English, participate in her school activities, and generally be with her Canadian age mates. Finally, the son does not want particularly to recognize or accept his Italian heritage ('What use is it here in my new country?') but is rejected by his school-mates because he speaks with an Italian accent and often shows no inter-est in local concerns such as hockey. He feels trapped between his two possible identity groups, neither accepting or being accepted by them. As a result he retreats into the social and behavioural sink of marginaliza-tion, experiencing social and academic difficulties and eventually coming into conflict with his parents.

Berry (1990, pp. 245–6)

This quote also illustrates a very important point about acculturative strat-egy, that the acculturation experienced may not be the type preferred by the individual. The son wants to be accepted, but is not, by his new culture; instead he is rejected. This moves him from a preferred option of assimilation to one of marginalisation. More recently Berry has developed the framework to take account of an important third dimension – the acculturation attitudes of the – usually much more powerful – receiving society. As illustrated in Figure 2.2, the same two choices concerning identification with 'own' or 'other' identity produces four dichotomised options (which again are in reality located along continua). When the dominant receiving society seeks assimilation, this 'mixing in' to the receiving society is termed the 'melting pot' (or 'pressure cooker', in extremes!). When the dominant group seeks separation from immigrants this constitutes their segregation. When the dominant group seeks to marginalise the migrant group, by not wishing them to identify with either their heritage culture or the receiving culture, this is termed 'exclusion'. Finally, when the receiving society seeks to become a culturally diverse society and recognise the cultural heritage of immigrants while also promoting their own cultural heritage, this is termed 'multiculturalism'.

Although the majority of research inspired by Berry's acculturation frame-work has addressed the migrant's acculturation strategies, there is a relative paucity of research on the acculturation strategies of receiving societies. As these latter strategies may constitute important situational determinants of migrants' behaviour, this imbalance needs to be redressed urgently. It is important to emphasise that, although the framework was developed with regard to the situation of immigrants, it can also act as a useful way of con-ceptualising the experiences of refugees, sojourners, diplomats and others. Echoing the interplay between the dimensions of heritage culture and involve-ment recipient culture, Kalin and Berry (1995) have suggested that cultural identity may also be construed as arising out of ethnic identity and civic identity. It is important to note that the two-dimensional model of acculturation developed by Berry and his colleagues has been challenged and continues to be a matter of lively debate (see, for example, Berry & Sam, 2003; Rudmin, 2003).

Health and acculturation

Especially interesting from the point of view of health professionals is that Berry also suggests that the four different types of acculturation have implications for physical, psychological and social aspects of health, through the experience of 'acculturative stress'. Cultural norms for authority, civility and welfare may break down. Individuals' sense of uncertainty and confusion may result in identity confusion and associated symptoms of distress. In fact Berry and Kim (1988), reviewing the literature on acculturative stress and mental health, have identified a hierarchy of acculturation strategies: marginalisation is considered the most stressful, followed by separation, which is also associated with high levels of stress. Assimilation leads to intermediate levels of stress, with integration having the lowest levels of stress associated with it (Berry, 1994; Ward et al., 2001).

As we note in detail in Chapter 5, physical health differs across cultures in several respects. For example one study examined coronary heart disease (CHD) in middle-aged (white) men in Framingham, Massachusetts, Honolulu (Japanese–Americans) and Puerto Rico. Twice as many men died from CHD in Massachusetts as in Puerto Rico and four times as many as in Honolulu. In all three places cholesterol and blood pressure were related to the incidence of CHD. However, cigarette smoking and weight were not equal risk factors for all three groups (Gordon et al., 1974). In reviewing subsequent research in this area, Ilola (1990) suggests that the changes in lifestyle and diet that immigrants experience may increase or decrease the chance of developing certain chronic diseases. In another study that attempted to link 'pace of life' with CHD across cultures, researchers were surprised to find that Japan, which had the fastest pace of life, also had the lowest death rate from CHD (Levine & Bartlett, 1984). Such a finding questions a common assumption that stress is related to CHD.

However, to complicate matters, Japan does have one of the world's highest mortality rates for stroke. This may be an example of how the experience of stress is expressed in different ways – not just mentally but physically too – in different cultures. Ilola also reviewed research that found that Japanese men who migrate to the USA increase their risk of developing CHD, but reduce their likelihood of dying from a stroke. Such studies present us with valuable insights into health and illness. People who change cultures represent a potentially revealing natural experiment: they bring with them their genetic endowment evolved in one environment and often adopt new lifestyles, diets, attitudes, etc. for coping in a different environment. In doing so they offer

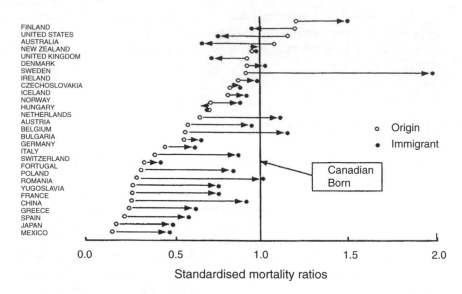

Figure 2.3   Coronary heart disease, Canadian male immigrants, 1969–73.
Source: Kliewer, E.V. (1992)

researchers a unique perspective in trying to understand the contribution of genetics and environment to health and illness.

Figure 2.3 represents the standard mortality ratios for CHD for men immigrating to Canada between 1969 and 1973 and compares them with the rates in the countries from which the emigrants originated. Although these are rather old data it very clearly illustrates how immigrants tend to regress to the mean of the receiving country. Although there are some exceptions, generally migrants into Canada during these years increased their likelihood of death from CHD, relative to what was likely had they stayed in their own country. In the case of Irish migrants this change was very dramatic and in fact far exceeded the Canadian rate. More recently, research on Irish emigrants in the UK has found that the incidence of CHD remains above that in the resident UK population, not just for first-generation emigrants (which is commonly found) but also among second- and even third-generation emigrants (see Chapter 5). Clearly not all migrant groups have the same political or social experience of the country into which they migrate. It has been argued that the Irish in Britain have a number of factors that distinguish them as a cultural group, e.g. that they constitute an 'invisible minority' (because they are white), they often do not need to integrate to the same extent as other migrants because their 'home' is so close, and the recent 'troubles' between the Irish and the British, particularly in Northern Ireland, constitute a charged context for their integration into British culture (Curran, Bunting & MacLachlan, 2002). Perhaps these factors are related to the unusual health characteristics of Irish migrants to Britain.

I have only briefly described some stressful and damaging aspects of moving between cultures because this issue is dealt with in more detail in Chapters 4 and 5. However, it is important to acknowledge that migration, and the adoption of new lifestyles and diets, as well as many other types of transition, need not necessarily be stressful experiences that interfere with health; in fact, they can be quite positive experiences. However, before moving on from Berry's acculturation model it is important to note that 'acculturation is not everything'. Lazarus (1997) has argued that migrants, for example, experience a range of stressful demands that have more to do with changing contexts than changing cultures. So, Lazarus and Folkman (1984) see their own 'stress-coping' model accounting for such factors as loss of social support, the need to find new employment, etc., as an equally valid account of migrants' experience. Of course, the stress-coping and acculturation accounts interact, the cultural backdrop constructing the meaning of stress-coping difficulties, and perhaps the ways in which these occur and the resources that may be accessible for dealing with them. The general point is, however, that perhaps, at times, migration can be over-culturalised (Ryan, 2005) and that culture may therefore be 'over-cooked' as the primary analytical perspective. It should also be noted that 'cultural identity' may be nested within ethnic, civic and/or national identities (Berry, 2005).

Cultural or cross-cultural?

Over the last 20 years there has been a lively debate about 'How universal is human behaviour?'. The crux of this debate is whether some aspects of the human psyche are common to all peoples, irrespective of age, gender, class, culture, location, etc. In some respects the assertion that human behaviour is universal is commendable because it embraces the 'we are all the same and therefore equal' philosophy. Underpinning this argument is the idea that wherever people are, and in whatever cultures, there are certain basic problems of human living that they must confront. This is undoubtedly true when we consider such needs as food, water and shelter. However, it is also suggested that there may be 'universal' needs of a more psychological nature. One such suggestion is that how we relate to authority, to our own self and to conflict situations is a universal dilemma, i.e. problems that must be confronted by every person (Inkeles, 1969).

The search for psychological universals is sometimes seen as a particularly scientific pursuit:

> Perhaps the most important objective of science is to discover universals, and in attempting to become a science, social psychology is in search of universal principles that can explain and predict the behaviour of individuals in all societies.
>
> Moghaddam, Taylor & Wright (1993, p. 43)

The notion that cultural differences in behaviour reflect different attempts to solve similar (universal) problems is certainly appealing. One of its corollaries is that different behaviours have the same underlying cause. Some psychologists are so committed to this idea that their search for 'universals' precludes the possibility that they may be wrong! Smith and Bond (1993) suggest that cross-cultural researchers respond to inconsistent results in two ways: (1) they sort out the studies that show the same results in different cultures and infer universal processes from them, and (2) they consider the studies that do not show the same results and suggest ways in which the variations suggest universals that may not be immediately apparent. Thus, either way – whether or not a finding replicates across cultures – universalism is the conclusion!

Another approach to studying people in different cultures has been to forget about the idea of comparison as such. Here one tries to understand the meaning of behaviour within its own cultural context, rather than by referring to a concept abstracted from other cultures. In this sense people are studied in their own culture, in their own right. To contrast this approach with the previous one, it could be thought of as 'we are all different and therefore equal'! Here, 'equal' means that we should resist the temptation to understand the meaning of a behaviour occurring in another cultural context, by translating the behaviour into our own (more 'natural') terms.

By analogy, an apple and an orange may have similar needs (light and water). They may both represent attempted solutions, by different types of trees, to the problem of reproduction. But an apple is not an orange. Even so, we could describe an apple as the apple tree's equivalent of an orange! We could further build on their similarities to convince ourselves that they are nothing more than different responses to similar problems. Let us try and ground this in a clinical example. Brain-fag (brain fatigue) syndrome is found in several African cultures (Prince, 1987). It is most often found in very academically able students from very rural backgrounds, and is characterised by headaches, crawling sensations in the brain, blurred vision and various other symptoms. Its effect is to prevent students from studying. For the practitioner with some knowledge of culture's influence on health, it is 'easy' to see brain fag as the somatisation of a psychological conflict (say between modern and traditional beliefs), which would be more likely to express itself as 'depression' in the western world. Furthermore, amitriptyline hydrochloride appears to be effective in removing the symptoms of depression, for some people, and it also appears to be successful in removing the symptoms of brain fag, for some people. The practitioner may therefore conclude that brain fag is really 'just' depression. But is it? If brain fag is depression then why is it *not* depression? Why is depression not brain fag and why are they different, if they are really the same? In short, why is an apple not an orange? The fact that apples and oranges both respond to the same fertiliser does not detract from their 'appleness' or 'orangeness'.

I think I have taken the fruity analogy far enough. Trying to understand the processes involved in brain fag by referring them to another problem, which is possibly more familiar, such as depression, is also trying to remove the cultural context of the problem. Illness and distress, be it anxiety or Alzheimer's disease, come about for a reason. In this sense the experience of illness and distress can be said to have a 'meaning' ascribed to it by society. If we believe that human problems have a 'meaning', then attempting to translate the problem into a more familiar clinical/cultural language can lose much of the meaning. Meaning can be present in the cause, experience, expression and treatment of a problem. As culture is a medium of communication, we cannot hope to understand problems presented in different cultures by stripping them of their meaning. We return in greater detail to this issue when we consider the similar and more familiar comparison between depression and neurasthenia in Chapter 4. For now the key point is that *cross-cultural analysis should always be grounded in prior cultural analysis*, so that we are aware of the degree of comparability in what is being compared across cultural settings. This echoes Berry's (2005) view, which is that 'the central position of cross-cultural psychology is that no individual behaviour can be understood without understanding the cultural context in which it developed' (p. 5).

Different understandings of health and illness

In accord with our discussion in Chapter 1, Landrine and Klonoff (1992, p. 267) have argued that health psychologists must give more recognition to anthropological studies in considering how people think about health:

> The major contribution of anthropology to knowledge of health-related schemas is that the health beliefs of professionals and laypersons alike are structured and informed by a cultural context from which they cannot be separated and without which they cannot be fully understood. . . . White Americans tend to view illness as . . . an episodic, intrapersonal deviation caused by micro level, natural, etiological agents such as genes, viruses, bacteria, and stress. Thus, many White American laypersons and professionals may assume that illness can be described and treated without reference to family, community or the gods.

This could be considered to be the westernised view of illness and it is important to see this view as a cultural construction rather than the one and only truth.

In 1980 Murdock published his world survey of beliefs about illness in 189 different cultures. He distinguished between 'natural' beliefs and 'supernatural' beliefs (of course such a terminology presupposes a fundamental difference between such beliefs as well as reflecting a cultural understanding of what is 'natural'). He found that theories of 'natural' causation (including infection, stress, organic deterioration, accident and 'overt human aggression') were far outnumbered by theories of supernatural causation. Supernatural causation was broken down into three categories. 'Mystical causation' refers to illness caused by some act or experience of the individual as opposed to the involvement of some other person or supernatural being. This category includes fate ('the ascription of illness to astrological influences, individual predestination, or personified ill luck' – Murdock, 1980, p. 17), ominous sensations (including dreams, sights and sounds), contagion (coming into contact with a 'polluting person', such as a menstruating women) and mystical retribution (violating a taboo, where the violation itself directly causes illness, in contrast to it being caused by an offended spirit or god).

The second category of 'animistic causation' refers to illness caused by a personalised supernatural being such as a soul, ghost, spirit or god. Included in this category are soul loss (the departure of the soul from the body) and spirit aggression ('the direct hostile, arbitrary, or punitive action of some malevolent or affronted supernatural being' – Murdock, 1980, p. 20). The final category of 'magical causation' ascribes an individual's illness to another person, or persons, who use magic in a malicious way. Envy or a feeling of effrontery usually motivates this. Sorcery and witchcraft come under this heading. Murdock's distinction between the two is that any person could attempt sorcery, whereas witchcraft is performed only by those who are witches, with 'a special power and propensity for evil' (Murdock, 1980, p. 21).

In addition to developing this classification of supernatural theories of illness, Murdock rated the prominence of these causes across the cultures that he studied. The four most common across the 189 cultures were (in descending order) spirit aggression, sorcery, mystical retribution and witchcraft. Table 2.1 shows the percentage of cultures, from a particular geographical region, in which these four types of belief were rated as being either the predominant or a significant cause of illness. As can be seen in Table 2.1 these theories of illness are not evenly distributed across the regions surveyed. Murdock provides a fascinating analysis of these results, putting forward an appealing argument that accounts for the distribution of theories in terms of the psychosocial structure of different cultures. For the purpose of this book, however, his point is a simple one: 'supernatural' theories of illness are more common than 'natural' theories and they differ in their popularity across cultures.

Table 2.1   Percentage of societies studied showing predominant or significant evidence of popular theories of illness in different geographical regions.

	Sub-Saharan Africa (%)	Circum Mediterranean (%)	East Asia (%)	Insular Pacific (%)	North America (%)	South America (%)
Spirit aggression	70	96	100	92	63	91
Sorcery	57	23	26	52	83	68
Mystical retribution	48	8	21	36	46	9
Witchcraft	35	62	0	4	8	0

Based on Murdock (1980).

Dimensions of culture

As long ago as 1935 Dollard was grappling with the problem of how clinicians ought to incorporate an awareness of culture into their practice. Dollard describes the individual seeking help as a palpable, concrete and real entity. The immediacy of the individual stands out against the abstractness and generalities of his or her culture. Thus Dollard notes that the individual always remains 'figure' while the culture is 'ground'. In other words the individual is seen as the foreground and the cultural context as the background. The difficulty is to appreciate the contribution of each at the same time. I like to think of this problem as being similar to that of a reversing figure, where only the foreground or background can be focused on at one time, but both exist together and depend on each other in order to define their own existence. What we really need therefore is a way to see both – foreground and background – at once. The illusion is that only one – foreground or background – can be focused on at a time.

One interesting line of research in this regard has been to look for psychological dimensions that may be endorsed, to a greater or lesser extent, across different cultures. We have already considered Murdock's classification of beliefs in the causes of illness. The way that Murdock breaks down his categories can be simplified statistically. In an attempt to develop a questionnaire sensitive to different ways of explaining mental distress, Eisenbruch (1990), who has been critical of the dimensions suggested by Murdock, asked people to indicate the extent to which they agreed with the various categories given by Murdock. Their answers tended to cluster together, so that agreement with a certain cause was associated with endorsing some categories, but not others. Through the use of some complex statistics, the way in which people answered could be simplified into two dimensions (see Eisenbruch, 1990).

Without going into the detail of these dimensions I want to make the point that complex ideas about the causes of illness can be simplified empirically, to yield a small number of underlying dimensions. The essence of this approach is that, by knowing where somebody 'stands' on a particular dimension, it is possible to infer his or her answers to other questions. To return to the debate on 'universalism', a particular belief may not be universal but it may lie at some point along a dimension that has wide relevance. However, crucially for us, not only will cultures vary across some dimensions, but so too will individuals within a particular culture. An individual's rating on culturally salient dimensions will reflect the impact that his or her culture has had on him or her, with regard to that dimension. Thus, a German culture may not endorse the idea of mystical causation of illness, but the opinion of an individual German may not be that of the 'average' German. Individuals therefore have their own opinions about certain dimensions, within the context of their culture.

The notion of a 'cultural character' does, however, seem to be very appealing, especially to psychologists who effectively seem to want to 'individualise' the character of a collective group, e.g. Triandis (1990) has used the term 'cultural syndromes' to refer to beliefs, behaviours and norms that constitute a discernable pattern in one culture, distinguishable from that in another culture. Personally, I do not like the term 'cultural syndromes' because, in the context of health and illness, it has the (admittedly unintended) implication of disease or disorder. However, associated with this 'syndromal' approach is one that seeks to compare many cultures along only a few dimensions.

Hofstede's dimensions

Let us consider the most influential of those studies that seek empirically to identify psychological dimensions relevant across many cultures. Hofstede (1980) reported the results of a survey conducted in 50 countries around the world. The survey had the advantage of all the respondents working for the same company – IBM – thereby reducing one possible source of variation in their responses (that accounted for by their work environment) not directly related to culture. Once again Hofstede statistically analysed the data to try to identify any underlying themes, or patterns, present for the whole sample. He identified four dimensions and subsequently appreciated the presence of a fifth dimension (through examining the relationship between his own data and that of other researchers, particularly Bond's data). The five dimensions so identified were: power/distance (from small to large), collectivism–individualism, femininity–masculinity, uncertainty avoidance (from weak to strong) and time orientation (from short term to long term). In acknowledgement of the influence that Hofstede's dimensions have had we now consider them in some detail although the interpretation of these dimension remains problematic and controversial.

The low power/distance–high power/distance dimension

The first dimension of power/distance is defined as:

> ... the extent to which the less powerful members of institutions and organizations within a country expect and accept that power is distributed unequally. 'Institutions' are the basic elements of society like the family, school and the community; 'organizations' are the places where people work.

> Hofstede (1991, p. 28)

This dimension is concerned with how inequality is dealt with by society. Some social (or emotional) distance may separate people of different rank in the sense that a subordinate may not feel free to approach or interact with a boss. If this is the case – high power/distance – a certain distance is expected between people of different rank. The dimension can be seen to be primarily concerned with dependence relationships. In low power/distance societies there will be interdependence between different ranks (e.g. through consultation), whereas in high power distance societies subordinates are more dependent on their bosses, perhaps fearing the consequences of questioning or contradicting a decision made by them. Hofstede also provides an index by ranking countries for each of his dimensions. In the case of power/distance, Malaysia, Guatemala and Panama had the highest power/distance ranking, whereas Austria, Israel and Denmark had the lowest ranking (smallest power/distance).

The individualism–collectivism dimension

Hofstede describes individualism as pertaining to 'societies in which the ties between individuals are loose: everybody is expected to look after himself or herself and his or her immediate family', whereas collectivism describes 'societies in which people from birth onwards are integrated into strong, cohesive groups, which throughout people's lifetime continue to protect them in exchange for unquestioning loyalty' (Hofstede, 1991, p. 51). Thus individualism–collectivism refers to the extent to which you act, think and exist as an individual (including your relationships as a parent, spouse or child) or as a member of a much larger social group (including extended family and community members). According to Hofstede those who value 'personal time', 'freedom' and 'challenge' exemplify individualism. Alternatively those who value 'training', 'physical conditions' and 'use of skills' reflect collectivism. Samples from the USA, Australia and the UK scored the strongest on individualism, whereas the samples from Panama, Ecuador and Guatemala most strongly endorsed collectivism.

The low uncertainty avoidance–high uncertainty avoidance dimension

This dimension concerns 'the extent to which the members of a culture feel threatened by uncertain or unknown situations. This feeling is, among other things, expressed through nervous stress and in a need for predictability' (Hofstede, 1991, p. 113). People who are high on uncertainty avoidance are attracted to strict codes of behaviour and believe in absolute truths; they will dislike unstructured situations and ambiguous outcomes. High uncertainty avoidance is characterised by the notion: 'what is different, is dangerous'. Hofstede suggests that cultures that are high in uncertainty avoidance are characterised by active, aggressive, emotional, compulsive, security-seeking and intolerant individuals. By contrast he describes people from low uncertainty avoidance cultures as being contemplative, less aggressive, unemotional, relaxed, accepting of personal risk and relatively tolerant. Singapore, Jamaica and Denmark had the lowest uncertainty avoidance scores, whereas Greece, Portugal and Guatemala were the highest scoring countries.

The masculinity–femininity dimension

This is perhaps the most troublesome dimension and for that reason difficult to understand. The basis for labelling the dimension 'masculinity' was that men differed much more on the attributes of this dimension than did women. This was true across cultures. Masculine cultures are those that show the greatest *distinction* between men and women. In feminine cultures the roles of men and women appear to be less distinguished and more overlapping. This dimension might therefore be more accurately described as a dimension of androgyny, reflecting the extent to which there is a difference between the roles adopted by men and women. According to Hofstede, in masculine cultures men are expected to be assertive, ambitious, competitive, striving for material success, and respecting the 'big', the 'strong' and the 'fast'. In masculine cultures women are expected to 'serve and to care for the non-material quality of life, for children and for the weak' (Hofstede, 1986, p. 308). At the other end of the dimension are feminine cultures in which men need not be ambitious or competitive, and they may respect the 'small', the 'weak' and the 'slow'. In sum masculine cultures are those in which there is a greater difference between men and women, whereas in feminine cultures there is less of a difference. Hofstede stresses that he does not advocate such differences but that his terms simply reflect differences in the responses of men and women in different cultures: 'It's not me, it's my data!' Now, you may wonder, which countries fall at the poles of this strange dimension? Japan, Austria and Venezuela were found to be the most masculine cultures, with Sweden, Norway and the Netherlands being the most feminine cultures.

The short-term orientation–long-term orientation dimension

This is the dimension derived from the Chinese values survey (see Bond, 1988, 1991). As the items in this survey were made up by Chinese as opposed to 'western minds', this extra dimension, Hofstede argues, reflects a psychological dimension that is not easy for 'western minds' to grasp. Initially Bond described this dimension as Confucian dynamism because it related to the teachings of Confucius. Hofstede claims: 'In practical terms, it refers to a long-term versus short-term orientation in life' (15, p. 164). He describes the short-term pole of the dimension thus: 'fostering of virtues related to the past and present, in particular respect for tradition, preservation of "face", and fulfilling social obligations' (Hofstede, 1991, pp. 262–3). Preservation of 'face' (i.e. 'face saving') refers to maintaining a person's position of respect. The long-term end of the dimension 'stands for the fostering of virtues orientated towards future rewards, in particular perseverance and thrift' (Hofstede, 1991, p. 261). The 'top scoring' long-term orientation country is China, followed by Hong Kong, Taiwan and Japan. The shortest-term oriented scores were for Pakistan, Nigeria and the Philippines.

Before proceeding we should acknowledge that, despite being an impressively large study, Hofstede's research has a number of important limitations. Most fundamentally there has been controversy over his naming of the factors arising out of his statistical analysis. It can be argued that the names given by Hofstede relate more to ideas familiar to the general public (such as the differences between men and women) or to researchers (such as individualism and collectivism) than they do to the statistical results of his data analysis. This is a crucial point because, if the dimensions we use to understand cultural variation are a misinterpretation (or at least an idiosyncratic interpretation) of the available data, then they will surely mislead us. However, in Hofstede's defence it must be said that the interpretation of data (especially with regard to factor analysis) is to some extent subjective. Hofstede's work remains perhaps the most comprehensive study of its kind and a potentially enlightening piece of opportunistic research.

Without doubt the most influential of the dimensions identified by Hofstede has been the individualism–collectivism (I-C) dimension. This dimension manifests itself at the personal level (how people define themselves), at the interpersonal or relational level (the sort of relationships people prefer) and at the societal or institutional level (relationships between individuals and groups, particularly their relationship with authority) (Ward et al., 2001). It may not of course be necessary to assume that individualism and collectivism are polar opposites; in fact, they may both be used by the same people in different contexts. More recent research has also suggested that there may be more than one way to be collectivist or individualist. Triandis and Gelfand (1998) describe vertical and horizontal, collectivism and individualism, where 'vertical' emphasises hierarchy (people differ) and 'horizontal' emphasises equality (people are similar). So, for example, in horizontal individualistic cultures (such as Norway or Sweden) people want to be distinctive but do not necessarily strive for achievement, whereas in vertical individualist cultures (such as the USA, the UK, southern Europe) people want to be the best. In horizontal collectivist cultures (such as in an Israeli kibbutz) people see themselves as similar to others, as having common goals, being interdependent and sociable, but they do not easily submit to authority. In vertical collectivist cultures (such as many east Asian cultures) people emphasise the integrity of the in-group, are willing to sacrifice personal goals, and support in-group–out-group competitiveness. It has been suggested that the typologies described above are also related to different political ideologies. If so, we might expect people from horizontal individualistic cultures to value 'equality and freedom' whereas those from vertical individualistic cultures would value 'freedom but not equality' (Gelfand & Holcombe, 1998). Furthermore, we might expect that such differences will be of relevance to people's belief regarding whether health should be seen as a human right, with equal access to healthcare for all. In Chapter 9 we consider this further but for now we return to other applications of Hofstede's dimensions.

Applying Hofstede's dimensions

The original four dimensions derived by Hofstede have been applied independently to the contexts of teaching and psychotherapy. It is useful to see how these apparently abstract dimensions can be applied to practical settings. In another publication Hofstede himself (1986) illustrated how the four dimensions were relevant to the educational context. Believing the teacher–pupil relationship to be an 'archetypal role pair' occurring in all cultures, he discussed how the four dimensions interact with this relationship, e.g. in collectivist cultures pupils speak in class only when they are addressed directly by the teacher, whereas in individualist cultures they will speak up more readily in response to a general invitation from the teacher. In small power/distance cultures, when conflicts arise between teachers and pupils, parents are expected to side with the pupil. However, in large power/distance cultures parents would be expected to side with the teacher. In weak uncertainty avoidance cultures it is all right for a teacher to say, 'I don't know', whereas in strong uncertainty avoidance cultures teachers are expected to have all the answers. Finally, in feminine cultures pupils admire friendliness in a teacher whereas in masculine cultures they admire brilliance (see Hofstede, 1986, for a more detailed discussion of this). Hofstede thus suggests some ways in which his rather abstract dimensions have clear practical implications in everyday life.

Draguns (1990) has undertaken a similar venture with regard to the sort of psychotherapeutic relationship suggested by each of the dimensions. He suggests that individualist cultures favour insight-oriented therapy and seek distant 'professional' therapeutic relationships, and that themes of guilt, alienation and loneliness are emphasised in therapy. Collectivist cultures, on the other hand, would have closer, more personal and expressive therapeutic relationships, with a paternalistic or more directive–nurturing stance being adopted by the therapist. Draguns suggests that the alleviation of suffering rather than self-understanding would be the target of therapy. Cultures high on uncertainty avoidance would seek the 'scientific' biological approach to mental distress, with psychotherapy being seen as messy, unpredictable and inefficient. By contrast low uncertainty avoidance cultures would encourage a plethora of psychotherapeutic approaches, with fads in therapeutic style coming and going. The high power distance cultures would emphasise the expert role of the therapist, with therapy focusing on behaviour change, compliance with the therapist's instructions and adjustment to social expectations. Low power distance cultures would encourage self-growth, group work and patient support groups and movements. Finally, masculine cultures expect the therapist to advocate responsibility, conformity and adjustment on behalf of the patient, rather than the patient's own aspirations. Once again guilt would be a major theme in therapy. Feminine cultures would expect the therapist to side with the client against social demands, emphasising expressiveness, creativity and empathy. In feminine cultures Draguns suggests that the focus would be on anxiety rather than guilt.

Draguns's analysis also illustrates how Hofstede's dimensions can be made concrete by focusing on their application to specific issues. Indeed by doing this Hofstede's dimensions have been made the back bone of 'culture-centred counselling' which is reviewed in Chapter 6. There is also support for the idea that certain psychological dimensions may be relevant across cultures and that these are related to health. Bond's research was motivated by the reasonable belief that cultures differ in what they value or believe to be important (Bond, 1988, 1991). Students from each of 23 countries (but note that countries are not synonymous with cultures) indicated the extent to which they felt that different values (e.g. 'moderation', 'reciprocation') were important. First of all these data were collapsed together and analysed to find patterns in how the students responded. Once again two dimensions came out. Each of the countries were then assessed in terms of where their averages fell on these dimensions. Perhaps surprisingly, scores on these dimensions were significantly related to death rates from a number of illnesses including ulcers, circulatory diseases and cancer. I consider these interesting findings in more detail in Chapter 5. However, at this point I return to the problem of finding an individual in the mass of statistical summations and averages.

The fallacy of averages

This sort of large-scale research, spanning thousands of people and many cultures, as described above, has produced some fascinating results and spurred on intriguing speculation. These data may be very useful at the level of policy making but they have their limitations at the level of the individual presenting their problems to the community practitioner. These studies tell us about the norm, or the average, in a given culture. They are therefore a form of what we might call 'statistical stereotyping', i.e. they simplify (or reduce) the variation between people of the same culture. However, few people would be comfortable assuming the role of the statistically average Indian, Scot or Spaniard. Although we recognise, and may take some comfort from, our similarity to other people in our own culture, we are also acutely aware of how we differ from those people with whom we have most in common. Our self-identity demands such awareness because without it we would be prisoners of our own culture.

Each person represents an amalgam of differing cultural experiences, to which they may give more or less credence than others do, and these experiences may relate to their health and welfare to different extents. Each individual represents a unique interplay between culture and health. The challenge for the clinician might appear to be to decipher the extent to which somebody's distress (physical and/or psychological) is an expression of a cultural context. But this is not the problem at all! For in deciphering we are only translating a foreigner's experiences into our own – cultural – terms. We have already noted that culture is a medium of communication. Instead of stripping the client of the ability to communicate we must embellish their attempts to do so. The clinician must therefore find a way of understanding the patient's problems, in the terms that the patient experiences them. Fortunately, this is not as difficult as it may seem.

Pluralism in health

It is very important not to make a dichotomy out of the 'natural' and the 'supernatural' causes of illness. These causes can and do coexist in the minds of client and practitioner alike. In Malawi we have conducted a series of studies into the cause, risk reduction and treatment of a variety of conditions (malaria, schistosomiasis, epilepsy and psychiatric symptomatology), and have consistently found evidence for an ability to tolerate apparently 'contradictory' or at least competing explanations of illness (MacLachlan & Carr, 1994a). This ability for 'cognitive tolerance' is relevant to health provision not only in 'less developed' countries but also in 'more developed' and industrialised countries. This is because 'supernatural' beliefs also abound in 'developed' countries. A substantial body of research attests to the presence of such beliefs among Americans who originate from Africa, Haiti, Italy, Mexico, Puerto Rico, China and Japan, and among the Native Americans themselves (Landrine & Klonoff, 1992). It is already the case that minority ethnic groups within the USA have established traditional healing services within their communities. Reviewing the effects of immigration on the health services in south Florida, DeSantis and Halberstein noted that 'Virtually every type of traditional healer as well as complete pharmacopoeias of the health cultures in their country of origin are available to south Florida immigrant groups' (1992, p. 226). The role of traditional health services and traditional healers is not restricted to traditional illnesses either; they may also have a role to play in combating 'modern' afflictions such as AIDS (MacLachlan & Carr, 1994b).

Another obvious example of the coexistence of 'natural' and 'supernatural' theories of illness is when we attribute the cause or cure of an illness not just to physical or mental factors but also to spiritual influences. In many western societies people sometimes explain illness and misfortune as 'God's will'. Consequently people will pray – to their God – for the recovery of a sick friend or relative. Although we may think of 'natural' and 'supernatural' causes of illness as being quite distinct, this need not be the case. We have reported a study of the explanations, which psychiatric patients gave for their admission to Zomba Mental Hospital in Malawi (MacLachlan, Nyando & Nyirenda, 1995). Attributing admission to traditional factors was the most common explanation, followed by physical and psychological reasons. However, sometimes an explanation included more than one of these factors, e.g. one patient explained his admission thus: 'I was working very hard and getting quite tired. . . . I had dizzy spells and my heart would jump and beat very fast . . . because of the success I had achieved, other people were jealous and put a spell on me' (p. 10). This quotation includes the psychological idea of stress, the physical notion of cardiac arrhythmias and the belief in magical causation through sorcery or witchcraft.

The reality of working across cultures as community practitioners is that we will encounter understandings of illness and health that are quite different from our own. Sometimes our clients will adopt theories quite different from our own, and at other times they may adopt more than one type of theory to explain their suffering. To understand the suffering we need to appreciate the cultural context in which it is being communicated. We also need to hold back from automatically accepting assumptions that are a product of our own cultural communication and upbringing. We must address the problem of how we can 'think through', not only our client's culture, but also our own. The need for this is illustrated in the following case study, which is based on Sachs' (1983) book exploring how the Swedish health service responded to the health needs of Turkish immigrants.

Case study: evil eye or bacteria?

Mrs Mehmet, from Kulu in Turkey, has recently come to Sweden where her husband has secured a well-paid job. After several visits to her house by a health visitor Mrs Mehmet has been persuaded to take her children to a 'well child clinic'. The doctor, dressed in jeans and a T-shirt, welcomes Mrs Mehmet by shaking her hand and asking, 'How are you?' Because the translator feels that it is unnecessary to translate this common greeting, the doctor gets no reply from Mrs Mehmet and proceeds to examine her 6-year-old son, Yusuf. The young boy, cautious of the doctor, is encouraged by his mother to comply with the translated requests. While Yusuf is being examined Mrs Mehmet tends to her 9-month-old baby girl, Gulay, wrapped tightly in a large blanket, and resting on her lap.

The doctor asks Mrs Mehmet various questions about her son's health and she replies to them by addressing her answers to the translator. The doctor asks, 'How is his health?' and Mrs Mehmet replies 'Good?' 'Does he eat well?' asks the doctor, and Mrs Mehmet replies, 'Not so well; it would be good to get some medicine so that he can eat better.' 'Does he sleep well?' 'Yes, fine.' The doctor shines a small torch into Yusuf's ears and nose. He then examines his throat, using a spatula to hold down his tongue. He looks at his back and runs his hands down the boy's legs, grimacing to himself. Finally, he lowers Yusuf's underpants to inspect his genitals.

The doctor sits down behind his desk and starts to write out a referral slip. As he writes, he appears to speak to his pen, and says 'Basically your son is in good health but I would like to refer him to a specialist in Stockholm for a second opinion about his legs which appear a little bent to me.'

'OK let's have a look at your baby then,' says the doctor as he gets up from behind his desk and moves towards Mrs Mehmet and Gulay. However, Mrs Mehmet hesitates, appears anxious and tells the translator that she is just here for Yusuf. The translator tells Mrs Mehmet that since she has brought both children to the clinic she must let the doctor examine both. Uncomfortably, Mrs Mehmet allows the doctor slowly to unwrap her baby, revealing a tiny skeletal motionless body. The doctor cups Gulay's fragile head in his big hands, examines Gulay's neck and ears, and tests various reflexes, while rapidly firing off questions to the translator. The mother says that her Gulay has always been that way and that she nurses the baby herself. The doctor, beginning to appear frustrated, asks 'Why haven't you taken her to a doctor before now?'

Mrs Mehmet starts to wrap the blankets around Gulay again, explaining to the translator that there is little point in taking her daughter to doctors because they would not understand what is wrong with her. Meanwhile the doctor, suspecting chronic diarrhoea and fluid loss as well as an upper respiratory infection, and fearing meningitis, announces, 'This baby needs immediate hospitalisation!' He explains to Mrs Mehmet that she must take her baby to the hospital today and that he will telephone the hospital so that they know to expect her. He draws out a rough map of how she can get to the hospital from the clinic and recommends that she goes right away. Mrs Mehmet smiles gratefully and thanks the doctor as she gets up and leaves his office with Yusuf close by her side. They go straight home. They do not go to the hospital as instructed by the doctor.

The encounter between Mrs Mehmet and a Swedish doctor reflects what we have described as 'cross-cultural misattribution'. Swedish and Turkish cultures have different ways of explaining illness. This means that different actions will be motivated as a consequence of the experience of illness. The Swedish doctor wanted to admit Mrs Mehmet's baby daughter to hospital because he observed that she was underweight and had diarrhoea; he suspected that she had also developed a respiratory tract infection and meningitis. He attributed her symptoms to being caused by bacteria.

Mrs Mehmet had for some time been aware of the worrying condition of her baby, but she attributed the same symptoms to 'evil eye'. Furthermore, she believed that, because the Swedish health system does not account for evil eye, it could not help to cure Gulay's illness. Mrs Mehmet is, however, familiar with the problem of evil eye and knows that only certain healers in Turkey can cure it. She has therefore been planning a trip back to Kulu for some time. Her belief is that her baby daughter is the victim of an evil force, which is sometimes passed to children soon after birth. The evil eye – 'nazar' in Turkey – is a notion common to many different cultures, generally referring to the evil glance, which a jealous or envious person casts in the direction of the person they envy. The glance has the effect of transmitting illness or bad luck to its recipient. It is believed any person can transmit nazar at any time. There are various ways of protecting against nazar, of driving it out of the victim and of locating the person who transmitted the evil eye (Sachs, 1983).

Of course, none of these readily relates to a Swedish conception of illness, and many Turkish people who live in Sweden continue to turn to their traditional ways of dealing with illness and adversity in time of need. These traditions are able to provide something that the modern Swedish system cannot: they provide an effective medium for communication and social regulation among the Turkish immigrants. If the Swedish doctor believes that he has a contribution to make to the health of Mrs Mehmet's baby daughter, then he is going to have to understand what it is that Mrs Mehmet values in her own understanding of her child's illness. We now consider a technique, which I have develop, that can assist in doing this.

The problem portrait technique

According to Chambers' *Twentieth Century Dictionary* a portrait is 'the likeness of a real person'; it is also 'a vivid description in words'. The problem portrait technique (PPT) seeks to convey a likeness of a person's presenting problems through both words and images. First of all we will consider the use of this technique with words. The PPT is simply one way of trying to understand a person's inner experience.

The problem portrait begins with the person's description of his or her own distress, be it a broken leg, a broken marriage or a broken heart. Figure 2.4 shows the conceptual outline of a problem portrait for a Chinese immigrant to Britain who has been living in London for 2 years. Mr Lim presented to his GP with a continuous need to go to the toilet, watery faeces and loss of bowel control. The GP classifies Mr Lim's problem as irritable bowel syndrome. However, in describing the problem Mr Lim used the term 'digestive problems' and it is therefore Mr Lim's own terminology that goes at the centre of the portrait. If a portrait is a 'vivid description in words' they must be the words of the beholder!

Causes

Perhaps the first obvious question is how and/or why has the problem occurred? What is the cause of the problem? The problem portrait is intended to give an impression of the ecocultural context in which the person is living and in which the problem occurs. This means that we need to know the range of causes, which possibly relate to the problem at hand. First, as is good clinical practice, Mr Lim is asked for his own ideas about the cause of his problem.

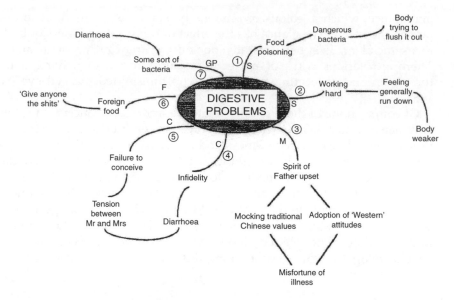

Figure 2.4   The Problem Portrait Technique illustrating different causes identified by Mr Lim for his 'digestive problems'. S, self; M, mother; C, China; F, friend; GP, most GPs.

Mr Lim says that he believes that he has some form of slow-acting food poisoning and that there may be some dangerous bacteria inside his stomach, which his body is continually trying to rid itself of, or 'flush out'.

When asked what else might cause the diarrhoea Mr Lim suggests that he has been working very hard and feels generally run down. He speculates 'somehow this can make my body weaker'.

When asked for other causes Mr Lim cannot think of any. Now this may be true, but it might also reflect his judgement of the social situation: that this is not the appropriate place to mention other possible causes. Perhaps he feels the context – the often rather exacting relationship that exists between British doctors and their patients – does not give him permission to discuss other explanatory models of his problem. If asked 'How might other people in your family explain the cause of a problem such as this?', he may give exactly the same answer. However, the slight distancing – from his personal views – that is implied by the question might liberate him to talk about factors that he felt uncomfortable mentioning in his own right. For instance, Mr Lim may tell us that his mother believes that it is the spirit of his dead father, unhappy with Mr Lim's mocking of traditional Chinese values and his adoption of many western attitudes, that has brought about his misfortune.

In order to distance alternative causes further – away from the family – we could ask Mr Lim 'How might other people, either in Britain or in China, explain the cause of something like digestive problems?' Mr Lim may feel that this gives him permission to talk about beliefs, which he may possibly be uncomfortable with. This could be because he does not want to be seen to endorse them, but at the same time cannot altogether dismiss them. Other people may feel a lot freer to discuss cultural beliefs in which case such coaxing, or facilitation, would not be necessary. Mr Lim describes the belief, common among people from his region of China, that diarrhoea may result from infidelity, or the bad feeling that has arisen between himself and his wife because of their failure to conceive a child.

Mr Lim should also be asked about views that he has heard from 'significant others', i.e. from people who are in some way important to him. For example, he may tell us that a work colleague told him that 'that foreign muck you eat would give anybody the shits!'. Now Mr Lim may not agree with this view but nevertheless it could still influence him.

Clearly the list of causes can be long and their excavation requires careful and sensitive interviewing. For some people, explanations for their problems, which arise though consideration of their ecocultural framework, will be easily discussed. In terms of a 'clinician as archaeologist' analogy, their 'social artefacts' are buried just below the surface. Yet for others their social constructions of reality may be much further below the surface, lodged in various strata of uncertainties or unwillingness to speak about things that you and I may not understand and may possibly even ridicule.

To conclude the investigation of possible causes and to appreciate something of Mr Lim's expectations of the consultation he is asked: 'What do you think that most GPs in London would say about the cause of your problem?' (Note that Mr Lim is not being asked to predict what his own GP is going to say – again referring to 'most GPs' retains some 'distance'.) Mr Lim responds by saying that most GPs would suggest some sort of bacteria as the cause. This gives us a range of possible alternative causes to work with. The PPT presents the clinician with a complex outline of causal factors that a more conventional approach to assessment would have overlooked. However, those tempted towards a 'simpler' form of assessment – identifying the 'main' or 'real' cause – will simply be operating out of ignorance. If such complexity exists it is always better to know about it, even if it does not make your job any easier!

For each cause given, it is important that the clinician understands its rationale. It may be that asking for immediate explanation of a cause could make the person defensive, feeling the request for more information to be a demand for justification. Just think of it: most middle class, white, British GPs are unlikely to ask for an explanation of the rationale behind a bacterial cause, but quite likely to ask for an explanation of how infertility can cause diarrhoea. It may therefore be better to come back to requests for the rationale of causes unless, of course, they are spontaneously offered. Such requests for the rationale of certain beliefs can therefore be used as a way of legitimising beliefs that the patient holds but is unsure of expressing. Alternative beliefs are often genuinely intriguing and simply expressing interest in an open and non-judgemental fashion is all that is required of the clinician.

Measurement

Although we now have a sort of 'word map', or picture, of the ecocultural context in which Mr Lim is experiencing his problems, we have yet to identify what is 'figure' (foreground) and what is 'ground' (background) from his own perspective. The ease with which he discusses different causal beliefs may be no indication of this. We can, however, now ask Mr Lim to rate the causes that he has mentioned. This could be done in many ways but the recommended way is illustrated in Figure 2.5. A brief description of each cause is written at the end of lines radiating from a circle. Each of these lines is the same length. Each line now becomes a scale of measurement (a visual analogue scale) wherein the strength of belief in each possible cause can be rated. The further one moves along the radiating arms, away from the centre, the stronger is one's belief in that particular causal factor. For instance, in Figure 2.5 'infidelity' has been more strongly rated as a cause of digestive problems

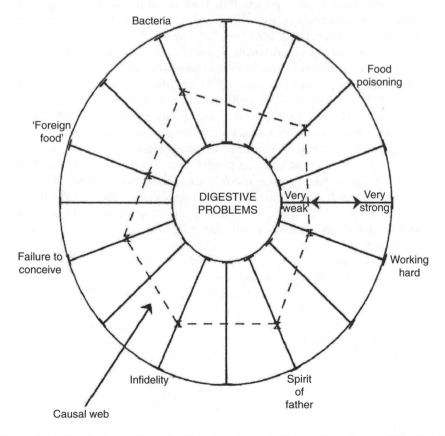

Figure 2.5   The Problem Portrait Technique for Mr Lim's 'digestive problems' with the strength of different causal factors rated along visual analogue scales.

than has 'working hard'. In each case it is of course Mr Lim who decides where the 'X' should be placed on the line in order to reflect his feeling about it. As in Figure 2.5 the scale may be made clearer by the use of statements 'anchoring' each end of the radiating lines.

Mr Lim could now rate each of the beliefs described previously. In doing this we can get an impression of how his own beliefs stand in relation to (his perception of) the beliefs of family members, other people in his community in Britain, people in China and significant others. We can also establish some measure of how tolerant of different beliefs Mr Lim is. If each of the lines radiating from the centre is made the same length (say, 5 cm) then where the 'X' is placed on each line constitutes a relative ranking of the different causal factors. However, most importantly this ranking is not presented in a linear context but in the context of multiple comparisons. There are significant advantages of these attributes of measurement when it comes to statistical analysis. Statistical analysis will not be necessary for the majority of clinicians, however, who simply wish to use the PPT to gain an impression of the range of causal factors and their relative importance.

Mr Lim can be asked to rate his own beliefs not only in the causes of his problem but also in each of their 'consequential treatments'. He could also be asked to rate what he judges to be the beliefs of his cultural community (or indeed any other party of interest) on these scales. The comparison of Mr Lim's own beliefs with his estimation of his cultural community's beliefs can help us to understand not the extent to which but how his own perception of his cultural background is influencing his own beliefs.

Consequences

We might expect that beliefs in different causes are associated with certain beliefs regarding the appropriate treatment for the problem, e.g. the consequence of Mr Lim believing in a bacterial cause may be that he perceives the problem to be beyond his immediate control, and remediable only through the prescription of the correct medication by the GP. The consequence of the 'hard work and making the body weaker' cause is, on the other hand, that Mr Lim may be able to alleviate his problem through changing his own behaviour to reduce the stress that he is experiencing, and therefore making his body 'stronger'. Mr Lim may also change his behaviour in order to appease the spirit of his father or ancestors who might have been offended by his behaviour. Another consequence of the 'father's spirit' belief may be that his problem is best treated by offering some form of symbolic sacrifice and/or prayers to his father's spirit. The 'social transgression' or 'infidelity' or 'infertility' causal beliefs may each infer different ways of putting the problem to rights, probably through traditional cultural practices, ceremonies or rituals.

The treatments described above may be referred to as 'consequential treatments' because they reflect treatments suggested as a consequence of believing in a particular cause. The treatment actually employed can be referred to as the 'actual treatment'. Thus the treatment, which is explicitly chosen, may subsume some, but not all, of the 'consequential treatments'. Indeed it is quite conceivable that the 'actual treatment' is incompatible with some of the 'consequential treatments'. However, it may also be the case that, despite a strong belief in a particular cause of a problem, a person may chose a treatment that does not appear to be a 'consequential treatment' for their strongest causal belief. An example of this would be where a person believed that an illness was caused by a spell being put on them, but that the best treatment to remove the illness is pharmacological rather than one involving a spell of protection. Of course, it could equally work the other way around where, although somebody believes in a biological cause to their illness, they put greatest hope in prayers, rather than in drugs.

We have now developed Mr Lim's problem portrait to centre on his own definition of his distress (or presenting complaint). Radiating from this are various explanations for these problems as expressed by Mr Lim through his own beliefs, those of his family, other members of his community and culture, close friends and Mr Lim's expectations of the sort of explanation that his GP is likely to opt for. Arising from these causal beliefs are variations implications for how the problem should be treated and we have given these the term 'consequential treatments'. Figure 2.6 subsumes Figure 2.5 and illustrates how Mr Lim's belief in the strength of 'consequential treatments' can be similarly illustrated. For the case of both causes and treatments a 'web', or map, can be constructed as a qualitative reflection of the relative strength of Mr Lim's beliefs. Such a map adds images to the words used in the PPT and these images can help to illustrate the extent to which beliefs in causes and beliefs in treatments overlap.

What I have described here is the 'Rolls Royce' version of the PPT. Sometimes it will be possible to use the technique in its entirety, whereas at other times simplifications and perhaps dilutions of it will be necessary. Constraints of language, translation and time, to mention just a few, may prohibit the power of the technique. However, whether the version you use is the 'Rolls Royce' or the 'Mini', the orientation adopted through using the technique should enhance the quality of clinical assessment and therefore the efficacy of the treatment.

Conclusion: what can we know?

One conclusion is that if we study one illness or problem in many different cultures it is as if we see the problem from many different angles. It is sometimes thought that by taking away the cultural 'noise' we can reveal the true nature of the illness or problem outside its cultural context. This 'sterilising' view sees the cross-cultural perspective affording us with a sort of psychological X-ray, penetrating more deeply to a common bedrock of human processes. Culture in this scenario is a problem to be overcome, a social con-

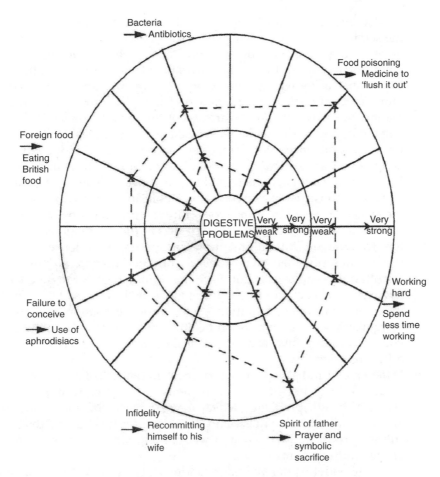

Figure 2.6   The Problem Portrait Technique incorporating causal factors and consequential treatments identified by Mr Lim for his 'digestive problems'.

struction to be deconstructed and outwitted, something that clouds the essential objective truth. An alternative view developed here is that different cultures create different causes, experiences, expressions and consequences of suffering, be it physical and/or mental. A complaint makes no sense in a cultural vacuum, because its meaning cannot be accurately communicated.

Guidelines for professional practice

1. A society's culture can be likened to an individual's memory. Understanding how collective identity and individual identity interact is of primary importance for health practitioners. Although certain personality dimensions may be salient across cultures, it is important to appreci-

ate that different cultures construct different understandings of just what the self is.

2. Stereotyping, in-group identification and prejudice against out-group members may result from exposure to people of a different culture. Clinicians must acknowledge that their helping role does not make them immune from such reactions and that they too can behave in a racist manner towards patients. Awareness of this, and acknowledgement of it when it happens, should be recognised as a key clinical skill.

3. Cross-cultural encounters are often uncomfortable and confusing for people even when disease or suffering is nothing to do with their reasons for meeting. Highly competent clinicians have human frailties, anxieties and confusions, just like anyone else. Clinicians may try to work through the anxiety aroused by some cross-cultural encounters by imposing their own structure. However, what is needed in these situations is *less* structure (compared with within-culture encounters) in order to 'free up' the client to describe their own problem from their own perspective.

4. Acculturative stress can result from the coming together of peoples of different cultural backgrounds. Clinicians should be aware of the effects that different forms of acculturation – integration, separation, assimilation or marginalisation – may have on health. It is also important to remember that the acculturative experience of members of the same family may differ considerably.

5. Different cultural groups may respond differently to similar stressors and be at risk for different sorts of ailments. It is therefore important to be aware of health problems, which may be particular to certain cultural groups, and to be able to explain the reason for this both to the minority cultural group and to the majority cultural group who may control many of the health resources.

6. There are widely different understandings of disease and disorder and the meanings ascribed to them across cultures. The biomedical model is, on a worldwide scale, a minority view. Clinicians should try to elicit the model, which their client uses to understand their own problem.

7. Although large-scale cross-cultural studies have identified psychological dimensions that can be used to characterise different cultures, and these dimensions have been very influential in cross-cultural psychology, the dimensions do not necessarily apply to individuals. Furthermore, there is a danger of treating individuals as 'cultural dopes' by assuming that they comply with a statistically derived stereotype of their culture. The individual must always be seen as the 'foreground' and the context in which they live – including their culture – as the 'background'.

8. Of the dimensions identified by Hofstede's multi-nation IBM study, the individualism–collectivism dimension has been the most influential. There may, however, be more than one way of being a collectivist or an individualist. Vertical and horizontal types of individualism and collectivism have been described and these dimensions may be relevant to the

sort of beliefs people hold about whether equal provision for health is a human right.

9. Many people are able to cope with more than one explanation of their problems. Perhaps because they have invested so much of their own time in their professional training, many health professionals may be intolerant of explanations that do not coincide with the models into which they have been socialised (trained). Health professionals need to adopt a more pluralistic approach to health practice. They could, for example, include traditional or alternative healers, who their client may also be attending, in discussions about that individual's treatment. If a client is motivated to get an alternative and additional treatment from somebody else, that practitioner may well have a useful alternative view of the person. This view should be sought out.

10. Being more tolerant of other explanations for disorder and disease may be uncomfortable for clinicians if they see this as challenging their own legitimacy. However, different practitioners may have equally legitimate, but incomplete, perspectives. Is there any one profession or approach that can claim a monopoly on a holistic approach?

11. The problem portrait technique is offered as a technique to help clinicians appreciate the many influences that may inform a client's understanding of their problem. It can be used to measure and weigh up these different influences and to relate them to the client's belief in different treatment options. Clinicians should use the technique in a flexible manner in order to facilitate the process of 'finding out' rather than to reach a predetermined treatment goal. The technique may be especially useful for identifying alternative treatments that could be used simultaneously.

12. Clinicians working across cultures should not try to strip away the confounding effects of culture in order to understand their clients better, but to explore how their clients use their culture as a medium of communication through which to express their suffering.

CHAPTER 3

Cultures and their syndromes

It has already been emphasised that many major cities are now home to a great range of cultural groups and, as such, the ailments presented to clinicians are much more diverse than ever before, at least in urban areas. A French community nurse at the beginning of the twenty-first century may encounter forms of suffering known to only specialists in tropical medicine at the turn of the last century. In the USA it has been predicted that, by the year 2025, 35% of the population will be from a cultural minority group and this cultural plurality will 'test numerous assumptions ingrained in all fields' (Miranda & Fraser, 2002).

It is easy to alienate oneself from the baffling array of 'foreign disorders', seeing them, for instance, as the 'cultural baggage' of immigrants. One way in which this alienation can unintentionally occur is through our assumptions about what does and what does not constitute a 'culture-bound syndrome'. In this chapter we consider to what extent any, or all, forms of suffering can be considered 'culture bound'. We pay specific attention to understanding the social function of human suffering. We also look at the extent to which culture 'exploits' universal phenomena, on the one hand, and the extent to which it sculptures forms of suffering out of the social and environmental fabric that different cultures provide, on the other. Miranda and Fraser (2002, p. 424) have argued that cultures establish complex relationships between illness, myth and ritual: 'Myth sets the stage for the ritual to address the illness.' By turning this form of analysis on European peoples too we consider to what extent western disorders are bounded by western cultures. The chapter ends with some guidelines on how to think through the role of culture in the causes, experience, expression and consequence of human suffering.

Santa Claus: more than just good fun

When we consider the diversity of beliefs across different cultures it is important to look at the consequences of the beliefs within the culture in which they are held. If we think of cultural beliefs as part of a broader process of communication within that culture we can begin to understand what functions are served by a particular belief system. Consider, for instance, the popular western belief in Santa Claus. This is an interesting belief for many reasons.

Children tend to be the strongest believers, and are encouraged in their belief by adults. Although adults tend not to believe in Santa Claus, they often behave as though they do and will even act out his role in order to perpetuate the myth. Children who have themselves discovered that Santa is not 'real' will often go along with the notion in order to retain the magic of the myth for younger children.

What is the function of the Santa Claus myth? Let us consider just one interpretation. As already mentioned, children may be educated, or socialised, into believing in Santa Claus. We understand him to be a cheerful old man with a large white beard who will give us presents, at Christmas time, if we are good. Santa Claus, apart from being good fun or perhaps because he is good fun, can also be seen as having a social regulatory function on children growing up. Through Santa they may learn to respect older people, see them as kind and be encouraged to behave according to certain rules or norms, in order to be rewarded. These ideas – among others – are communicated to us through the vehicle of Santa Claus. If we get the message, we get the present!

It is not, of course, the case that the idea of Santa is part of some devious plot to control little children (although many such plots doubtless exist!), but instead that the notion of Santa Claus has been used (selected) across many generations (of parents) because it has some beneficial social spin offs, as well as being good fun. The social function of Santa is also apparent in our choice of him being old, bearded and plump. We have not chosen to endorse alternative images of Santa. He is not presented as a reformed alcoholic or a miniskirted blonde in stiletto heels. Either of these figures could just as easily be the bearer of gifts to our children in reward for their good behaviour. However, they are not. Santa Claus cultures do not want to communicate those messages. It can therefore be seen that the myth of Santa is not an arbitrary idea, it has not just been chosen at random for its 'feel good' factor.

At least some of the beliefs that a society encourages its members to adopt can be seen to have a regulatory function for the society. I have focused on the idea of Santa Claus as just one example of a general principle and given only one interpretation of the Santa Claus myth. Sorry if I am the first to break the news to you! Other ideas – God, nuclear explosions and prisoners on 'death row' – can also be analysed in terms of their having a social function and a social construction. However, it often seems easier to analyse the social function of a myth than the social function of a reality. Perhaps this is because, if we know something to be a myth, we can ask 'What is the function of this idea?' based on the assumption that if the idea did not have a function it would not continue to exist.

Something that is a reality can also serve a social function. Real events may take on 'mythical' significance. Cancer, AIDS and heart disease are all illnesses around which myths have built up. Indeed the greater the basis of an idea in reality, e.g. that AIDS is incurable, the stronger a vehicle it may be to transmit ideas that are myths: 'AIDS is a punishment from God for promiscuity.' Although one possible regulatory function of this belief – to reduce promiscuity – may be rather obvious, many health beliefs have more subtle functions.

Culture bound or concept bound?

Before we consider two of the classic 'culture-bound syndromes' let us consider in more detail the term 'culture bound'. Specifically let us from the outset acknowledge the ethnocentricity of the term 'culture bound'. Essentially this term is used to describe disorders or illnesses with which the people making the classification are not familiar, e.g. Margaret Clark has described the problem of 'latido' in a community of Mexican–Americans. Latido is characterised by significant weakness, abdominal pulsations and emaciation brought on by the victim being unable to eat. As this array of symptoms is not familiar to us, and yet occurs in sufficient clusters to be called a syndrome, it is described as a condition found within the bounds of another culture.

If we stop and think about it for a moment we realise that some of the conditions that we may accept as universal (or 'non-culture bound'), e.g. anorexia nervosa or obesity, may simply be bound by our own culture. Once again looking across cultures may allow us to view our own culture in clearer perspective. It may also lead us to review our concept of some syndromes being 'culture bound' and others being 'un-culture bound', or universal.

There is without doubt something intuitively appealing about the 'dramatic exotica' (Simons, 1985) that culture-bound syndromes represent. It is important not to view these problems in a voyeuristic fashion, but to see beyond the 'colourful display' and understand the social meaning and function of the disorder. After all, a Martian who happened to be looking in on your house on Christmas Eve could come away with a rather bizarre impression of human behaviour, unless it understood the context in which the bearded man in the red costume was hanging (handling!) a stocking above a little girl's bed!

If our cultural constructions are so crucial but also so subtle for our understanding of what things mean, how can the nuances of culturally constructed disorders be accommodated within a universal diagnostic system? In the fourth edition of the *Diagnostic and Statistical Manual of Mental Disorders* (DSM-IV – American Psychiatric Association or APA, 1994, p. 844):

> The term culture-bound syndrome denotes recurrent, locally specific patterns of aberrant behaviour and troubling experience that may or may not be linked to a specific DSM-IV diagnostic category. Many of these patterns are indigenously considered 'illness', or at least afflictions and most have local names.

Thus culture-bound syndromes in the DSM-IV are characterised as 'localized, folk diagnostic criteria', and these appear to be presented as being in some sense 'lesser' than the professional criteria used in the DSM-IV. Andary et al.

(2003) note that, in effect, the APA is claiming that DSM categories can be found universally and are not restricted to particular cultural groups. As we see in this chapter such an assertion is untrue.

The DSM-IV recommends that local idioms of distress be 'translated' into 'matching' categories of disorder, although rightly Andary, Stock and Klimidis (2003, p. 8) question the appropriateness of this approach:

> Should the clinician work on the basis of an 'artificial' (DSM) syndrome that poorly fits the experience of the client, or should the clinician try and capture the client's experience by yielding towards a diagnosis that is meaningful within the client's culture?

The two syndromes that we will consider in some detail, koro and latah, have been chosen to illustrate particular points. In describing koro I pay particular attention to demonstrating how apparently bizarre behaviour can be understood to have both an *order* and a *function*, when presented in the context of salient cultural beliefs. The second syndrome, latah, helps to illustrate the intricacies of debates concerning the ways in which 'culture-bound syndromes' are related to culture. To understand and assist people who present problems that are foreign to us, it is important to be aware of these two issues.

Koro

Koro is a condition where people believe that their sexual organs are shrinking. It is believed to be a fatal condition and occurs mostly in southern China and south-east Asia (Cheng, 1994, 1996). Although it usually occurs in isolated cases, epidemics of koro may also occur. It is, of course, natural to try to understand new problems by classifying them into more familiar ways of seeing the world. Thus, koro, in terms of western diagnostic criteria, has been subsumed as a variant of dissociative disorder, somatoform disorder, panic disorder and even psychosis.

Koro is most commonly associated only with males through their fear of penis shrinkage. In fact, although it is much less common in females, it is also found in women as a fear of retracting nipples, breasts or labia. For both sexes the fear of shrinkage is associated with the fear of imminent death, the shrinkage being only a precursor to this. Cheng (1994, pp. 7–8) gives a vivid description of the onset of koro:

> Usually, the malady begins with a feeling on the part of the victim that his or her sex organ is shrinking. Believing that the condition is critical, the victim becomes extremely anxious, doing whatever he or she can to stop the sex organ from further retracting and crying vigorously for help. A man may be seen holding his penis, 'anchoring' it with some clamping device, or tying the penis with a piece of string. Similarly a woman may be seen grabbing her own breasts, pulling her nipples, or even

having iron pins inserted through the nipples, all to prevent the retraction of the respective organs.

The process of rescuing the organs may look highly absurd to an outsider, even to a Chinese. Imagine someone shouting for help and at the same time pulling his or her genital, thus exposing it, in public. The victim's relatives and neighbours will rush to 'help out' because they too believe that the condition can be fatal. . . . In fact, many so called 'patients' were diagnosed with Koro not because they themselves had initiated the complaint, but because other people around them had misinterpreted signs of discomfort to mean Koro and performed the rescue. . . . For example, a bride was thought to have Koro on the wedding day because she appeared pale and weak. The rescue effort continued for a while until she yelled out that she was not experiencing breast shrinkage.

Such behaviour may indeed seem absurd to us. Does it still seem absurd if we consider its sociocultural context? Attempts to rescue a person suspected of having koro are so strenuous because a person with koro is seen as a dying person. Everybody of the same sex as the victim (the social norm is that only members of the same sex can attempt to rescue a victim) in the vicinity will rush to help the person suspected of having koro. Their efforts will continue until everyone becomes exhausted and anxiety about the victim's imminent death subsides.

To diagnose this condition purely in terms of its symptoms – suspected organ shrinkage, pale complexion, shivering, hyperventilation, palpitations, sweating, fainting, etc. – would be quite insufficient. We can meaningfully classify it only if we understand it. Cheng's (1994) study of koro found that it is most common among adolescent males who are single, poorly educated and lacking (alternative) sexual knowledge, and had a strong belief in the notion of koro. From the perspective of this book, koro is an especially interesting phenomenon because, as Cheng argues, it cannot be understood from the perspective of the individual's (psycho)pathology, but rather as an expression of a *community's* anxiety.

Cheng provides us with information on the cultural context in which koro occurs. The notion of sexual restraint is prominent in Chinese cultures. The amount of semen that a man can produce is understood to be limited. It is considered a man's 'vital energy' and must therefore be used economically; sexual intercourse resulting in ejaculation should occur only when the women is ovulating. The notion that death can result from a depletion of semen may be an important background factor in koro, because it relates sexuality to death.

A second thread to this complex fabric of understanding the sociocultural context of koro comes from the Chinese folklore of the 'fox spirit' which can seduce people, sap their 'vital energy' and thereby make them weak. The 'fox spirit' is able to shrink tissue and this provides a direct link, in folklore, to koro. It does not, however, explain the social function of koro.

A community may come to expect or experience misfortune in, for instance, its agricultural production or the health of its members. The 'fox spirit', it is believed, roams the world in search of victims. When things are not going well this may be taken as an indication that the 'fox spirit' has visited a community. A fortune-teller's prediction of its visitation will create considerable uncertainty and anxiety. The community becomes hypervigilant to detect the first arrival of the 'fox spirit'. Cheng suggests that the failure to identify any objective signs of a ghost heightens tension to such a degree that victimisation becomes an inevitable outlet for the community's anxiety.

An individual's behaviour may lead others to 'realise' that the person is suffering from a koro attack. On the other hand, an individual himself may suspect a koro attack is beginning (cold sensations or insect bites in the genital area, which can temporarily reduce the size of the genitalia, along with weakness or sickness, may be interpreted as the onset of an attack). Through the identification of a victim the anxiety of the whole community may be relieved. As people rush to help rescue the victim, the failure of the victim's genitalia to truly retract is taken as evidence that the 'fox spirit' has been exorcised and moved on. The community is thus saved, tension reduced and effort may be turned to overcoming other problems, be they health or crop production. Once the spirit has visited a community and moved on it should not return for some time.

The above is only one interpretation of the koro syndrome and a simplified one at that. Nevertheless is does stand to illustrate how koro can be understood in terms of the sociocultural context in which it occurs. In this context it is an *ordered* and *functional* phenomenon: it occurs in a particular way that makes sense (order) and it has a purpose (function). Koro is a vehicle through which the community can communicate its anxiety and engineer its own cure. Naturally, individual members of the community may not interpret koro in this manner. To them it will be a frightening reality to be avoided at all costs – a visitation of death to be escaped.

Kirmayer and Santhanam (2001), suggest that in koro:

> as with other epidemics of hysteria, social stresses create widespread feelings of vulnerability in a population or group, and combine with individual vulnerabilities to anxiety to give rise to symptoms that follow *culturally available symptom schemas*. (p. 257, italics added)

These 'symptom schema', it has been argued, are not stable phenomena but, like culture itself, are continually changing ways of patterning meaning in life. Kirmayer and Santhanam (2001, p. 266) also stress that seeing hysteria as 'social communication, interaction and positioning can go further to explain the clinical phenomena than purely psychological or physiological explanations that ignore the social matrix of experience'.

When individuals steeped in one social matrix attempt to communicate the meaning of their experience to a clinician steeped in another social matrix, the challenge for the clinician is to hold back from assuming a cure and learn about its cause and function. Only through such an approach can the concerns of the patient be truly relieved. It has been assumed by many western clinicians that the longer minority cultural groups stay in western countries the less they will present problems arising from their own cultural heritage. It is now becoming clear that this is not the case. People define themselves in relation to their family, friends and communities. These are the vehicles of culture. It is now recognised that tolerance towards ethnic differences is to be valued and encouraged. Social legislation across the European Community, the USA, Australia and other traditionally western countries explicitly states this. Many clinicians may need to adapt their perspective on health and culture if they are to be of service to the array of people within their own communities. Koro demonstrates how understanding the cultural context demystifies certain behaviours. Before considering how latah also illustrates this point, let us just briefly note the occurrence of koro elsewhere and under somewhat different circumstances.

Earleywine (2001) recently reported three cases of cannabis-induced koro in a sample of 70 men who responded to a survey on negative reactions to cannabis use. Interestingly, all three white respondents had learnt about cannabis-induced koro before experiencing it themselves. Furthermore, they had each used cannabis in either a novel setting or an atypical manner, and Earleywine suggests that all three had an anxiety reaction to cannabis that may have preceded their experience of penile contraction. All three also altered their drug consumption after the experience. The role of prior knowledge and therefore possible expectation, combined with an anxiety-provoking experience, indicate some similarities with Cheng's description of the causal mechanisms in south-east Asia. Two of the three cases reported by Earleywine also conveyed dissatisfaction with their genitals, which may, given the above circumstances, have triggered a koro-type panic reaction. Finally, a further case of koro, reported in an Eastern European asylum seeker in Ireland, was apparently completely successfully treated with fluoxetine (Kennedy & McDonough, 2002). Although presumably the experience of asylum seeking is not without distress (see Chapter 4), it is interesting to note that the authors describe this occurrence of koro as a culture-bound syndrome in a 'non-culture bound context' (see also Chowdhury, 1998).

Latah

Latah is another syndrome found in Malaysia and Indonesia. It is characterised by an exaggerated startle response to a surprising event. This response may take the from of throwing or dropping an object which was being held and the utterance of rude words, such as 'puki!' ('cunt!'), 'butol!' ('prick!') or 'buntut!' ('ass!') (Simons, 1985, p. 43). The startled person may also, apparently automatically, carry out instructions given by somebody, or mimic the words or movements of someone, who is close at the time of the startle. The spectators of such behaviour are usually amused by it and this may lead someone who is known to have latah to be intentionally startled (perhaps several times a day) in order to amuse others.

Latah may develop into a life-long condition regardless of whether its onset is abrupt or gradual. It is found in both men and women, being most common in middle-aged women of low social status. Although common in some families, it also occurs in people who have no relative with latah. Simons (1985, p. 81) gives the following account of latah offered by a Malaysian man, who has latah himself:

At first one is merely startled. One sees a centipede or snake or a coconut leaf falls, and one is startled. Then someone sees this happen. Later when he sees me again perhaps he'll poke me in the ribs. After a while something can happen. Take an ordinary person like Betsy here – if she's startled – Whenever you see her you startle her with a poke in the ribs. After a while she'll get very frustrated! She'll say whatever comes out. If you tell her to dance, she'll dance. If you startle her with a poke in the ribs whenever you see her, she'll do this too [demonstrates]. That's what its like.

In her study of latah, Geertz (1968) contrasted the behaviour with the Malayo-Indonesian social norms of order, self-control and courtesy. Taking it in its cultural context she emphasised how the behaviour of someone with latah contravenes and challenges the norms of the society in which it occurs. By exhibiting behaviour which reflects an apparent lack of orderliness and absence of self-control and the exact opposite of courteous behaviour, a Malayo-Indonesian can be seen as singling herself out from other members of the culture. There could be many motivations for drawing such attention to oneself. A common interpretation has been that marginalised members of the society may behave in this way to protest against how they are being treated. The person who becomes a latah is therefore 'using' the syndrome (perhaps unconsciously) to communicate their protest.

We use the term 'culture-bound syndrome' to refer to a cluster of behaviours that occur together only in certain sociocultural contexts. We mean that the condition is not found universally. However, an interesting feature of latah is that apparently similar behaviours have been reported in culturally diverse and geographically distant parts of the world, as well as in Malaysia and Indonesia. Latah-like conditions have also been reported, albeit rarely, in Japan, South Africa and the USA.

This appears to present us with a paradox: How can a syndrome be both 'culture bound' and found all over the world? Two different answers to this question reflect the confusion that can visit any practitioner confronting a condition with which he or she is unfamiliar. The first explanation is that latah represents a universal psychophysiological startle response (Simons, 1985): in some cultures this naturally occurring behaviour has been elaborated into stereotypical ways of responding to being startled, among some people who are 'hyper-startlers'. Thus according to this view all societies have 'hyper-startlers' although the behaviour associated with the startlers (e.g. swearing, jumping, hyper-suggestibility) may vary across cultures. Startle behaviour may also be ignored or 'encouraged' to different extents, depending on what sort of attention and how much attention is given to it.

A second explanation is to look on latah not as a universal neurophysiological event shaped by culture, but as a 'performance' relating to social norms (Kenny, 1985). This is not to deny that anybody can be startled, or that some people react more than others. This explanation says that the form that startled behaviour takes is determined, not by neurophysiological events, but by the norms of the society in which a person lives. How better can a Malay–Indonesian individual demonstrate his or her difference from other people than by contravening the social norms of order, self-control and courtesy through latah behaviour?

Thus the second argument says that latah will coexist in different societies and cultures if the condition can perform a social function in each of those cultures. Different cultures may have different forms of latah depending on what functions are performed by it and on how the messages are best conveyed. Kenny (1985, p. 72) writes: 'The body is a symbol. Its appearance and actions point beyond itself to an inner world, but also beyond itself to a total life situation. The body expresses a state of being . . .'.

Thus two specialists in the field of culture-bound disorders come up with two apparently similar, but actually quite different, interpretations of latah. One is that it is a universal condition, with a neurophysiological basis, shaped by different cultural contexts. The other says that it is not a neurophysiological 'condition' any more than sneezing is and its expression is purely the result of the social function that it can serve within a culture. The reason why such an apparently small distinction is clinically important is that one may be taken as suggesting that it is a 'real' condition whereas the other suggests that it is a social construction and perhaps somehow less 'real'. It is to elucidate this point that we have gone into latah in some depth. Whatever explanation one favours it should be remembered that the patients' distressing experiences of latah are *their own reality*.

Where do culture-bound syndromes come from?

Thus far we have considered only two 'culture-bound disorders', but hundreds must exist. Hughes (1985) has provided a glossary of some of them:

- 'Bebainan', found in Bali, where a person may suddenly break into tears and attempt to run away from their present situation. They will try to fight off anybody who tries to stop them. Ultimately they collapse with exhaustion and subsequently have no memory of these events.
- 'Inarun' is a condition found among the Yoruba of Nigeria. It is characterised by weakness and burning or itching of the body, skin rashes, dimness of vision, impotence, deadness of feet and paralysis of the legs. Psychotic behaviour may also be displayed.

- 'Quajimaillituq' is found among the Eskimos of the Hudson's Bay region of Canada. This is a condition of periodic hyperactivity, paranoid preoccupations, making up of new words, compulsivity and performing antisocial acts.
- 'Tabacazo' is found in Chile and describes agitation and despair, and aggression in association with a loss of consciousness.

When we talk of 'culture-bound disorders' it seems that we are usually referring to problems found in Asia, Africa, the Arctic regions or South America, i.e. they are rarely disorders of people of European origin. Although there are a large number of 'Hispanic' disorders, many of them derive from peoples indigenous to South America, rather than from the Spanish influence itself. Of course some of these 'culture-bound disorders' have not only been 'discovered' by Europeans but also possibly caused by them, e.g. Kirmayer and Santhanam (2001, citing Dick, 1995) noted that prototypical cases of *pibloktoq* (Arctic hysteria), found among the Inuit women of Greenland, were first recorded during a voyage of Admiral Peary. The condition was characterised by women running wild across tundra/ice, tearing off their own clothes, eating excrement and raving incoherently. As might be expected, such an intriguing condition encountered much anthropological curiosity and a raft of proposed mechanism for its occurrence, including, shamanistic practices, neurotic conflicts, nutritional deficiencies (hypocalcaemia) and toxicity (hypervitaminosis) (see Simons, 1985).

However, Dick's (1995) review of all published accounts of *pibloktoq* suggests that the initial cases arose in the context of sexual exploitation and abuse of the Inuit women by Admiral Peary's men. Thus, the social context of the behaviour again makes it understandable as a response to interpersonal violence and abuse, and may be seen as a means of social protest and defence in the face of an intercultural encounter with a much more powerful group (Kirmayer & Santhanam, 2001). Also, presumably such behaviour would have made the women a less attractive 'prospect' for rape to Peary's men. Dick's (1995) research nicely illustrates the value of 'an interrogation of the cultural or professional presuppositions of the scientists studying such phenomena' (p. 9). Dick (1995, p. 23) concludes that *pibloktoq*:

> did not constitute a specific disorder but rather encompassed a multiplicity of behaviours associated with Inuhuit [sic] psychological distress ... that were largely confined to the early twentieth century, and often precipitated by the stresses of early contact with Euro-Americans.

Perhaps Europeans and North Americans not only have contributed to the production of culture-bound syndromes elsewhere, but actually have some of their own too. If we looked at culture-bound syndromes from a different cultural perspective perhaps European peoples would also appear to have some bizarre behaviours. A glossary of syndromes bounded by western culture, or people of European origin, might include some of the following:

- 'Anorexia nervosa' is usually found among adolescent females who starve themselves of food, sometimes to the point of death. As well as exhibiting extreme weight loss, amenorrhoea is common. Some sufferers also develop a distorted perception of their own body shape.
- 'Type A behaviour' is most commonly exhibited by adult males, as they struggle against perceived time pressure to achieve as many goals as possible. Often behaving aggressively and competitively towards others, they are also very impatient and concerned with 'deadlines'.
- 'Obesity' is characterised by eating beyond the requirements of bodily function, resulting in excessive weight gain. This may be associated with reduced mobility, complaints of physical discomfort, disorders of mood and apparent inability to 'lose' the weight gained.
- 'Agoraphobia' is a fear of leaving a restricted area, usually one's home, in case something dreadful happens. Mood disturbance and moments of panic are also common. The disorder is especially prevalent among 'housewives' who spend a lot of time inside the family home.
- 'Kleptomania' is a condition where people steal goods from a shop when they are, in fact, quite capable of paying for them. This problem is usually found among financially well off, middle-aged women.
- 'Exhibitionism' or 'flashing' (usually) involves men dramatically displaying their genitals in public for brief periods of time, apparently with the intention of shocking somebody close by, usually a member of the opposite sex.

In the above descriptions I have deliberately simplified and extracted particularly striking aspects of some disorders commonly found in European cultures. Each of the disorders is a good deal more complex than suggested by these potted descriptions. They also make a good deal more sense, given the sociocultural–cultural context, than 'foreigners' might imagine. However, I have described them in the above form because this is reminiscent of the language used to describe many (non-European) 'culture-bound syndromes'. Let us explore further the culture 'boundedness' of eating disorders by considering some relevant research on anorexia nervosa.

Are eating disorders culture-bound syndromes?

The debate concerning whether media and 'modern culture' reflects or creates the desire for slimmer bodies continues (see MacLachlan, 2004). However, the extreme nature of such modern imagery was nicely conveyed in a study by Rintala and Mutajoki (1992). They analysed the size, shape and proportions of 'female' mannequins in clothes shop windows. Although noting that they had become progressively thinner over the previous 80 years and were now virtually anorexic, they also estimated their likely ability to (theoretically) menstruate, given their bodily appearance. The percentage body weight needed as fat in order for a woman to start menstruating is 17%, and for her to have a regular cycle 22% is required. As the mannequin forms fell below this, Rintala and Mutajoki concluded that women shaped like modern mannequins probably could not menstruate because of being underweight.

It is intriguing to note that eating disorders have become *more* frequently reported within some immigrant groups in western countries. Indeed one report from England (Mumford & Whitehouse, 1988) found that there were significantly more cases of eating disorder among Asian schoolgirls than among 'white' schoolgirls. Most of the Asian girls in this study were born and educated in England. Thus, the increase in the prevalence of different eating disorders – obesity, anorexia nervosa, bulimia nervosa – is not necessarily the same across different cultural groups, even within the country.

We might well ask 'Why should anorexia nervosa be a culture bound syndrome?' Khandelwal, Sharan and Saxena (1995) suggest that people in western societies are very concerned with body weight and shape, and that there is aesthetic preference for thinness in women. Certain aspirations, e.g. to become a dancer, are likely to coincide with an emphasis on thinness. An example of this is research showing that there is a higher risk of anorexia nervosa in those dance schools that put greater pressure on their pupils to succeed (Garner & Garfinkle, 1980). Other literature cites over-dependence and at the same time hostility towards very protective parents as being characteristic of anorexia nervosa. My own work with people with anorexia has impressed upon me how they may use their intake of food to demonstrate (to themselves) control over an often transitional life situation fraught with emotional challenges and demands, which they perceive to be beyond their control.

Thus, from a cultural perspective the experience of anorexia nervosa among young women may be accounted for by the expectations of a western society that is ambivalent about the maturing of its daughters. These concerns are internalised by the person with anorexia. Yet we may be so imbedded in our own culture that this is hard to grasp. Other systems of child rearing differ considerably from those in the west. The very concept of adolescence would not be recognised in some other cultures; indeed it has been argued that adolescence is primarily an issue for western cultures. Elsewhere children may pass straight into the state of 'adulthood' often after their initiation at the age of 13 or 14. They assume the roles and responsibilities of adults immediately. From their perspective the slow 'letting go' of the parents and the 'building in maturity' of the youngster are no doubt curious.

If anorexia nervosa is a disorder of western maturation it is hardly surprising that people in other cultures do not (have the need to) experience it. However, when members of 'foreign' cultural groups have become part of western societies, such disorders do become more common. Such disorders may then have a reason for being, and indeed their higher rates may in some cases represent their use as an expression of the dynamics between different cultures, e.g. an Asian girl who develops an 'English disorder' could be interpreted as demonstrating her identity with England and rejecting her Asian ancestry. In this way 'culture-bound disorders' may be used to 'manage' the demanding interplay between different cultural traditions. If this is indeed true further research might find an important relationship between different patterns of acculturation and the sort of disorders that people develop.

Gordon (2001, p. 1) claims that 'eating disorders are unique among psychiatric disorders in the degree to which social and cultural factors influence their epidemiology, development and perhaps their aetiology'. As I have noted elsewhere (MacLachlan, 2004), Gordon emphasises the rapid acceleration in reports of anorexia from the 1960s through to late 1980s, and also the appearance of the previously unknown condition of bulimia, in the late 1970s, to a position of greater prominence than anorexia, in only a few years by the mid-1980s. This 'modern epidemic' of eating disorders, it is suggested, reflects a number of societal forces in the west, such as: the rise of the consumer economy with its concomitant emphasis on achieving individual satisfaction, often at the expense of more collective goals; increasing fragmentation of the family and intergenerational conflict; and changes in traditional gender roles (Gordon, 2000).

For many women in the latter part of the twentieth century, the possibilities and expectations for high performance and personal achievement often contradicted traditional demands for dependency and submissiveness, resulting in self doubt that, for some, has been channelled into the cult of the physical, and of the less curvaceous (and traditionally feminine) woman's body. Gordon (2001, p. 3) suggests that 'the contradictions and transitions in female identity represent the most profound basis of eating disorders throughout history and across cultures'. If this is true, how do different 'cultural vocabularies' express such conflict through the symptoms of eating disorders?

Although once considered a culture-bound disorder, anorexia nervosa is now recognised in many non-western countries, perhaps because they have recently undergone rapid industrialisation and experienced facets of globalisation. Gordon (2001) notes that almost all the countries that had reported instances of eating disorders before 1990 were European or North American (with the exception of Japan and Chile) whereas countries reporting eating disorders since 1990 include Hong Kong, mainland China, South Korea, Singapore, South Africa, Nigeria, Mexico, Argentina and Italy. However, it is instructive to consider cases of anorexia nervosa in Hong Kong because these differed from the typical western cases in several important ways: most were from lower socioeconomic levels (as opposed to the middle classes); patients often interpreted their inability to eat as gastric problems (as in bloating) rather than a fear of getting fatter; and most of them did not experience body image distortions, or express body image concerns. This may lead you to wonder if the 'anorexia nervosa' diagnostic label is appropriate for such a different body experience (see Chapter 4). The research that Gordon cites was primarily conducted by Sing Lee; however, his later research did show a developing concern with body image, even though plumpness is understood to be a sign of health in traditional Chinese culture. This might suggest the interplay of modernist and consumerist forces with more traditionalist forces.

In 1999 Lee and Lee reported a study explicitly designed to explore these relationships. They compared eating attitudes among secondary school pupils in Hong Kong (highly westernised), Shenzhen (an increasingly westernised city in mainland China) and the Chinese province of Hunan (relatively untouched by western media and fashion trends). Despite students in Hunan having the highest body mass index (BMI) they showed the lowest desire to lose weight. Gordon (2001, p. 11) suggests that one theme uniting the 'new' countries where eating disorders have been reported is that 'they are either highly developed economies (such as Hong Kong or Singapore) or they are witnessing rapid market changes and their associated impact on the status of women'.

The symbolic meaning of anorexia nervosa has been much debated. Nasser (1999) has linked it to the increasing popularity among some Moslem women, particularly in the Middle East, of wearing a veil. Nasser argues that one must look beyond the notion of reactivation of tradition or an Islamic revival, or western stereotypes of veil wearing. She sees the voluntary adoption of the veil by educated working women as a kind of 'veiled resistance' (see also Nasser, 2001) to the experience of conflicting gender roles. Nasser notes a similarity between anorexia and veiling in terms of them both being a means of reproducing the self through hiding or evading, or of negating the body. In each case the body 'appears to disappear'.

Both veiling and anorexia may be seen as attempts to establish boundaries around the self through what is perceived as a morally elevated position that encompasses purity and superiority: 'Each woman pursues her externally different but psychologically analogous and culturally approved objective with fanatical and compulsive devotion' (Nasser, 1999 p. 176), intertwining self-control with self-discipline, with self-denial, with self-validation.

We have not fully answered the question of whether or not eating disorders are culture bound? Recently, Keel and Klump (2003) addressed this question through three types of data: a quantitative meta-analysis of changes in the incidence rates since the formal recognition of anorexia nervosa and bulimia nervosa; a qualitative summary of historical evidence of eating disorders before their formal recognition; and an evaluation of the presence of these disorders in non-western cultures.

Comparing incidence rates for anorexia nervosa, Keel and Klump found a 'modest' but statistically highly significant increase in the disorder over time and noted that this coincided with increasing idealisation of thinness. Their *historical* review concluded that, if the core feature of anorexia nervosa 'is taken to be an intentional yet non-volitional self-starvation, then evidence of AN [anorexia nervosa] appears to trace back to early medieval times' (Keel & Klump, 2003, p. 754). Their *cross-cultural* review of evidence of anorexia nervosa concludes that 'excluding the criteria of weight concerns, AN appears to represent a similar proportion of the general and psychiatric populations in several Western and non-Western nations' (p. 755). These conclusions are not, however, compelling because they represent a 'cafeteria-style' definition of anorexia nervosa. The historical overview essentially traces the history of a specific symptom, whereas the cross-cultural comparison suggests equivalence of several symptoms, although excluding weight concerns, which 'may be a culturally bound phenomenon, restricted to sociocultural contexts that idealize thinness and denigrate fatness' (p. 755).

Applying the same methodologies to bulimia nervosa Keel and Klump (2003) note that there is evidence of 'changing rates of BN [bulimia nervosa] during the latter half of the twentieth century, however, the causes of these changes are unclear' (p. 759). Regarding their *historical* review Keel and Klump state that 'our attempts to find evidence of BN in earlier historical periods were largely unsuccessful' (p. 761), yet they note that the majority of historical cases of binge eating represent binge-eating disorder (there was a lack of compensatory behaviour, e.g. purging) or anorexia nervosa – binge–purge subtype, because of the presence of low weight. Their argument is that it is not BN, it is 'BN-like' but without the associated symptoms. The *cross-cultural* review found 'no studies reporting the presence of BN in an individual with no exposure to Western ideals' (p. 761). On the basis of these complex and necessarily uncertain data, Keel and Klump conclude, on rather dubious grounds, I think, that although *bulimia nervosa* is a culture-bound syndrome, *anorexia nervosa is not*.

Keel and Klump (2003, p. 764) go on to argue that there is substantial evidence of genetic influences on the development of both anorexia and bulimia nervosa, but that 'The genetic diathesis of BN may exhibit more pathoplasticity cross-culturally than the genetic diathesis of AN.' In other words, although a genetic disposition is a factor in both disorders, there is greater variation in the manner in which this is expressed in bulimia nervosa. I have gone into Keel and Klump's scholarly review in some detail, because I do not feel that the data that they have methodically amassed unambiguously support their conclusions. Also their rationale is quite suspect in arguing, for instance, that 'In cultures in which the thin ideal is ubiquitous, these kinds of environmental factors are held relatively constant across individuals and thus cannot account for individual differences in eating disorder development' (p. 763). As we have previously noted, people are not 'cultural dopes'; the same 'dose' of culture has quite different effects on different individuals. Individuals interact reflexively with the social matrix of which they are a part.

Cultural forms and functions of disorder

A classic adage in architecture is that 'form should not give way to function', i.e. the way something looks should not be primarily determined by what it has to do. The aesthetic value of an object is important, not just its use. This distinction between form and function may be useful for understanding 'culture-bound syndromes'. The 'form', in this context, is the way in which a problem is presented – self-starvation, stealing unwanted goods, fearing genital shrinkage, reacting with extreme startle. The 'function', again in our context, refers to what the event can achieve within the cultural context where it is present. Thus restating this architectural adage one might say that 'form serves function'. In that different cultures require things to be done in different ways to achieve the same ends, form may well have to give way to function. Indeed it is often where form fails to give way to (our understanding of how things) function that we define a condition as being bound outside our own culture.

It has been argued that all disorder is related to cultural factors and that, by implication, some cultures 'encourage' some sorts of disorder whereas other cultures 'encourage' different forms of disorder. Weisz et al. (1987) set out to examine how the cultures in which children were brought up were related to the sorts of disorders that children develop. They considered two alternative models:

1. The suppression–facilitation model suggests that cultures facilitate the development of some behaviours through rewarding children for them, and suppress the development of other behaviours through punishing them, or failing to reward them. This model suggests that the problem behaviours presented by children in the clinic will be similar to those behaviours that are culturally encouraged, except that they will performed to an excessive extent.
2. An alternative model, the adult distress threshold model, suggests that problem behaviours presented in the clinic will, in contrast, be those that are discouraged, because parents are less tolerant of them.

Weisz et al. compared children referred to clinics in Thailand and the USA. They characterised the Thai culture as emphasising peacefulness and non-aggression, and the importance of being polite, modest and deferential towards others. Parents in Thai culture were seen as being intolerant of under-controlled, aggressive and disrespectful behaviour. Consistent with the suppression–facilitation model they found that Thai children referred to clinics tended to exhibit over-controlled behaviours, such as inhibition, anxiety and fearfulness. Weisz et al. characterised American culture as being more tolerant of aggressiveness, encouraging self-expression, independence and assertiveness. Once again, consistent with the suppression–facilitation model, they found that children referred to clinics in the USA tended to exhibit under-controlled behaviours, such as aggression, impulsivity and distractibility. This research therefore suggests the very important point that culture influences the exhibition of disorder, not only through symbolism, but also through behavioural mechanisms. The characteristics (form) of disorder reflect the functioning values of society.

Analysing health through culture

Despite the seemingly vast array of forms of suffering that are found across different cultures, there are in fact a finite number of ways in which we can express our distress. Classification of different forms of suffering is an attempt to simplify their complexity. Yet an appropriate classification may give great

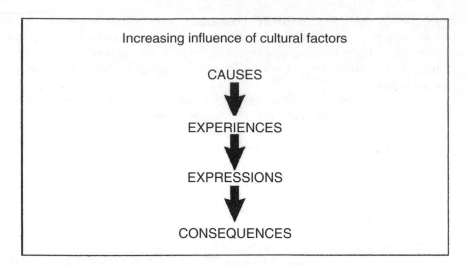

Figure 3.1   Levels of suffering.

conceptual insights to the nature of suffering. It is argued here that the term 'culture-bound syndrome' is something of a misnomer. Presumably all suffering is to some extent influenced by the context in which it occurs. However, the use of the term 'culture-bound syndrome' could be taken to suggest that some forms of suffering are influenced by culture whereas others are not. The value of the culture-bound approach is that it turns our attention to the contextual factors that may play a role in human suffering. We should embrace the benefits of this approach by applying it to all types of suffering, whatever their cultural or geographical origins (Hughes, 1985).

Figure 3.1 shows four levels through which culture may influence suffering. First, there is the *causal* level, i.e. the agent responsible for bringing about the suffering. Such causal factors could include infection, bewitchment, reinforcement and stress, to mention just a few. Clearly people's beliefs about the cause of a problem will be influenced by sociocultural factors. The practitioner must also appreciate the extent to which their own beliefs are shaped by such factors. Whatever working hypotheses are used to describe the cause of suffering, the clinician needs to appreciate the extent to which different hypothetical causes are influenced by culture.

The next level at which culture may influence suffering is at the level of *experience*. Thus, the way in which we know that we are suffering may be influenced by our physical environment and the people around us. This level is concerned with the form of suffering. A Chinese person may suffer from stress through somatisation – developing aches and pains – whereas a German person might suffer from stress through cognitisation – focusing on the negative aspects of life and having a poor self-concept. Here somatisation and cognitisation may be different forms of suffering, brought on by similar circumstances. It is through the experience of physical aches and pains or through the experience of negativity and poor self-concept that a person knows that he or she is suffering.

The next level is concerned with the *expression* of suffering. This can be taken at two levels: one is the private level that constitutes the content of the suffering – which parts of the body have the aches and pains, or what are the negative thoughts actually about. The other is more public and concerns how such suffering is displayed. One display of negativity might be to withdraw into a corner to avoid contact with other people. Another form of negativity could be to tell other people about all the problems and pessimism that the person harbours. As well as individual differences, cultures also differ in their norms for the expression of suffering. In some cultures people cry openly and hysterically at funerals whereas in other cultures people are very stoical.

Finally, the fourth level concerns the *consequences* of suffering, which may be very different in different cultures. At one extreme, recall the bride who people believed was undergoing a koro attack, and the subsequent efforts to 'rescue' her and alleviate her suffering. At the other extreme must be the 'bystander apathy' effect, a social psychological phenomenon often exhibited in urban areas of the west, where a person who is obviously suffering (perhaps even being mugged) is ignored by those close by. More generally the expression of suffering may attract sympathy, pity, help, frustration, anger, etc. Each of these reactions will be influenced by the sociocultural meaning of suffering.

Perhaps the key question to understanding a culture's influence on welfare and suffering is this: 'Is suffering a product of the culture or does it exist independently of it?' Volumes of research literature attest to the important impact that culture has in shaping the causes, experiences, expressions and consequences of suffering. Yet it is also undeniable that some suffering is beyond the bounds of culture, e.g. the contraction of meningitis in an infant will result in predictable symptoms whether it occurs in Dublin, Delhi or Durban. A gunshot wound in the thigh will have certain similar features whether it occurs in Belfast, Berlin or Bombay. One could, of course, argue that certain forms of suffering (e.g. gunshot wounds) are found more frequently in some places than in others, and relate this to environmental and/or cultural factors. This is a valid argument but beyond the scope of the present chapter.

From the perspective of the clinician it is important to recognise that some forms of suffering will not be attributable to culture, at least at the objective causal level. Subjective causes are obviously related to culture. I would suggest that as one moves along the chain – cause–experience–expression–consequence – at each step culture makes a progressively greater contribution to the person's suffering. This sequence of suffering is therefore a useful way for the clinician to think through the interplay between culture and suffering.

Guidelines for professional practice

1. A person's beliefs about illness may reflect social myths and social desirability within his or her culture. The social functions of illness can be

expected to influence not only the beliefs of the lay public, but the beliefs of health professionals too. Clinicians should consider what social functions are served by their own ways of working.

2. Although the idea of 'culture-bound syndromes' is well established it may lead clinicians to assume that most syndromes ('non-culture-bound syndromes') are uninfluenced by the culture in which they are expressed. This would be a dangerous assumption and often reflects the erroneous belief that 'our own' syndromes are not influenced by our culture. All syndromes are, at least to some extent, influenced by their cultural context. So, too, is the way in which clinicians respond to them.

3. Accepting the cultural embeddedness of many 'culture-bound syndromes' is problematic for multi-axial classifications of disease that seek to be universally applicable. Such breadth of applicability would undoubtedly be advantageous in terms of identifying the incidence, prevalence and health service needs for a range of disorders across countries. However, the idea that local idioms of distress should be 'translated' into 'matching' categories of disorder in a universal diagnostic system is misguided, because it loses the context of their meaning.

4. The 'exotic' nature of many 'culture-bound syndromes' can deflect the clinician from analysing their social meaning and function. The clinician should avoid discounting apparently bizarre conditions and investigate them in terms of their order and function.

5. The problems that an individual presents with may be a reflection of more than their own state of well-being; they may, for instance, also reflect anxiety within their wider community. In such a case the individual who presents the problem may be a social scapegoat, as in the case of koro. It is therefore important to look beyond the client to his or her community and culture.

6. Some theorists see the human body as a symbol that can be moulded by culture into different types of suffering. Other theorists believe that there are some basic and universal bodily experiences and that the extent to which, and manner by which, these experiences are expressed is influenced by culture. The important point for the clinicians to remember is that neither of these accounts diminishes the genuineness of their client's experience of suffering.

7. 'Culture-bound syndromes' do not come from somewhere else. Many European and North American conditions are equally influenced by culture. Understanding the cultural construction of disorders common to one's own people can be difficult because it calls for the clinician to fight against his or her ethnocentricity and see his or her own culture as one among many.

8. Sometimes indigenous 'culture-bound syndromes' can be seen to increase in incidence among immigrant groups. This should not be taken as indicating that a syndrome is not 'culture bound', but may instead reflect the acculturation of the immigrant group, such that some of its members express their problems though local cultural idioms.

9. Recent analysis of historical records concerning the 'culture-bound syndrome' *pibloktoq* suggests that it arose in response to sexual exploitation and abuse of Inuit women by Admiral Peary's men. There is thus a danger that 'local' responses to oppression and exploitation may be interpreted as pathology, when in fact they are more to do with a struggle for survival and identity amidst a more powerful and denigrating group.

10. Eating disorders are an area that has attracted a good deal of research from a cultural perspective. Largely it seems to be the case that eating disorders are more common in more westernised parts of the world. Although some have argued that there is more evidence of cultural factors shaping eating disorders in bulimia nervosa than in anorexia nervosa, both of these (overlapping) conditions are likely to be influenced by cultural pressures within and between cultures.

11. Suffering can be described at the levels of causes, experiences, expressions and consequences. On average, culture will have a progressively greater influence the further down this chain one travels.

CHAPTER 4

Culture and mental health

This chapter builds on our review of culture-bound syndromes in the preceding chapter. If, as Shweder (1991) suggests, culture and mind 'make each other up' we might expect not only that different cultures make up different minds, but also that different cultures make up different disorders of mind. Yet if, in a post-modern sense, we need the 'abnormal' to define what is 'normal' (Foucault, 1990), it is also possible to argue that 'madness' is more universally similar, whereas normality is more culturally distinctive.

We begin this chapter by considering problems with diagnosing, or classifying, or perhaps simply *identifying*, mental health problems in different cultures. We then look in some detail at one of these – depression – and to what extent and in what form it may be said to occur in different parts of the world. The complexities of understanding depression across cultures can be taken as a model for analysing many different mental health problems. We note particular aspects of suicide and personality disorders that also make them important experiences to understand from a cultural perspective. Migrant groups encounter a broad range of stressors as part of their transition. These may lead to mental or physical problems, or both. Indeed the dichotomy I have drawn between mental and physical health is itself a culturally biased one, and in many cultures would be taken as quite arbitrary. This distinction is therefore made only for the convenience of dividing our discussion up. The final section considers how stress is embodied in physical problems, which is developed further in Chapter 5.

Cultural complexities are daily beamed into our sitting rooms so that we are presented with the anguish, fear and suffering of people struggling to come to terms with the meaning of their existence, either 'here' at 'home' or further afield. Cross-cultural services for mental health have never been more important, or as inescapable, as they are now. In this chapter we explore and debunk some old myths, highlight some recent innovations in research and provide the clinician with an informed context in which to (co)operate.

Identifying mental health problems

We have already noted, in Chapter 3, that according to the American Psychiatric Association culture-bound syndromes are 'localised, folk diagnostic criteria', whereas, in contrast, those disorders found in the fourth edition of the *Diagnostic and Statistical Manual for Mental Health* (DSM-IV – APA, 1994) are to be found universally. Chapter 3 has highlighted how the DSM recommendation that local idioms of distress be 'translated' into 'matching' categories of disorder is at best simplistic and naive. What of the universality of the contents of DSM? Might they be Euro-American 'folk' categories, examples of what Kleinman (1980) has referred to as the 'category fallacy': where the diagnostic categories of one culture are applied to another culture, in which they lack meaning, coherence or validity.

Andary, Stolk and Klimidis (2003) have argued that the international studies of depression and schizophrenia, conducted by the World Health Organization (WHO) throughout the 1960s, 1970s and 1980s, constitute a category fallacy on a grand scale. These studies sought evidence for the existence of conditions that would match predetermined western diagnostic criteria, in cultures and contexts quite different from those in which these criteria were developed. The existence of such patterns of disorder (without investigation of supplementary or alternative cultural constructions of disorder) has been largely taken to indicate their universality.

Andary et al. (2003) note that, although the WHO have claimed similar rates of florid schizophrenia across countries, there were in fact quite significant differences in a broadly defined schizophrenic syndrome – ranging from 4.2 per 10,000 in rural India to 1.6 per 10,000 in Denmark. Furthermore, the onset and remission of this 'same' disorder varied between more and less industrialised countries. There was a higher proportion of people in 'developing countries' (now increasingly referred to as 'low-income' countries) who had an acute onset (51 vs 28%), and who experienced a single psychotic episode, followed by complete remission, in comparison to those in 'more developed' countries. Andary et al. note that the subdiagnosis of schizophrenia also differed: with acute and catatonic schizophrenia more frequently being diagnosed in 'developing countries' (40 vs 10%, and 10 vs 1%, respectively) and paranoid schizophrenia more frequently being diagnosed in 'developed' countries (34 vs 23%). Symptom profiles also differed, with auditory hallucinations being more prominent in 'developing' countries and depressed mood being more prominent in 'developed' countries. Finally, those in 'developing' countries had better outcomes (at 2 years of follow-up) than those in 'developed' countries. Andary et al. (2003, pp. 14–15) conclude: 'when rates, onset, symptoms, course and recovery are shown to differ in studies not designed to reveal these differences, it seems reasonable to question whether the disorders are the same'. As an added complexity, Bhugra et al. (2000) also reported differences in criteria and route of admission, and in schizophrenic symptoms, in a sample of African–Caribbean individuals diagnosed with schizophrenia in London compared with Trinidad, as well as higher associated unemployment rates in London. Thus, culture and context confound a simple 'universalist' concept of schizophrenia.

It would be possible to give a sort of epidemiological audit of the incidence and prevalence of a spectrum of mental disorders across different cultures.

Such information might well be useful if it truly reflected the health service needs of different cultural groups. However, one difficulty here is that epidemiological data are inevitably generated from a particular perspective, a particular way of classifying mental well-being and mental disorder, as illustrated above. Nowhere are the intricacies of this problem more clearly demonstrated than in the case of depression. I therefore use the case of depression to explore in some detail the complexities of comparing mental health across cultures.

Depression

Depression has been described as 'the common cold of psychopathology'. Indeed it is a relatively common form of distress experienced to some extent by most westernised people at some time in their life. Statistical estimates vary, however; on average western studies have found an incidence rate (the percentage of people who experience the condition at a given time) of between 9 and 20% for significant symptoms of depression (e.g. Boyd & Weissman, 1981), and that women are twice as likely to experience clinical depression compared with men. Depression also appears to be more frequently identified now than it was 50 years ago, perhaps up to 10 times more. This increase in depression in the west may be accounted for by factors such as the decline of religion, changes in community environments, more frequent uprooting of individuals and families from one locale to another, disintegration of family structures and the increased social isolation of some people (Sartorius, 1987).

Most of the existing statistics on depression refer only to those who experience depression to a severity sufficient to warrant a diagnosis of clinical depression. The depressed mood that most people experience is, thankfully, not of great severity and lacks many of the other features that define depression of clinical severity. So what are the characteristics of depression of clinical severity?

The two most prominent western systems of classification have an inherent assumption that their criteria may be globally applied to give valid and reliable diagnoses. These two classification systems are the DSM (APA, 1994) and the *International Classification of Diseases*, (ICD – WHO, 1988?). For many conditions there is very little difference between the criteria used in each of the two systems. As depression is one of the conditions on which there seems to be strong convergence, let us look at only one of these systems for a definition of depression.

The DSM-IV (and its revised form) recognises several different sorts (or subtypes) of depression, including dysthymia, adjustment disorder with depressed mood, major depressive disorder, cyclothymia, bipolar disorder (manic depression), and mood disorders associated with other primary problems such as substance abuse or a serious medical condition. Major depressive disorder is the condition that I want to concentrate on because more cross-cultural research has been done on this type than on any other type of psychological/psychiatric disorder. According to the DSM an episode of major depressive disorder ('depression' from here on) is said to exist when a person experiences either markedly depressed mood or a marked loss of interest in pleasurable activities for most of the day, every day, for at least 2 weeks. In addition to this, the person must simultaneously experience at least four or more of the following symptoms:

- Significant weight loss (when not dieting) or weight gain, or a decrease or increase in appetite
- Under-sleeping (insomnia) or over-sleeping (hypersomnia)
- Slowing down (psychomotor retardation) or speeding up (psychomotor agitation) of mental and physical activity; fatigue or loss of energy
- Feelings of worthlessness or excessive or inappropriate guilt
- Diminished ability to think or concentrate or indecisiveness; and recurrent thoughts of death or suicide.

Kleinman (1980) has suggested that the way in which people experience distress – such as depression – varies across cultures and at different times within the same culture. He uses the word 'illness' (as many people do) to refer to a person's experience of a disease. Most of the diseases that affect the body are not observed at their source of action. Instead it is the consequences of the disease's actions – the rash, the limp, the lethargy, etc. – that is observed. This 'illness behaviour' includes our physical and mental responses to a disease. For the moment it is the psychological component of this response to disease that is of interest to us. A key point in Kleinman's argument is that illness behaviour is the result of an underlying disease process and that this disease process may be expressed in different forms of illness behaviour.

Now, at first inspection this distinction between disease and illness seems a very useful one because it helps us to account for the admittedly vast array of symptoms associated with a diagnosis (of the disease) depression. According to the diagnostic criteria described above, two people may be depressed, but their experience of being depressed may be quite different, e.g. one person may have depressed mood, weight loss, poor appetite, difficulty sleeping and behave in a very slow and withdrawn manner, but another person, with the same diagnosis, may not experience depressed mood at all, but instead may show a loss of interest or pleasure in many different activities, gain weight, feel constantly hungry, over-sleep and appear very agitated. However, according to the DSM criteria the very different 'illness behaviours' are explained by the presence of the same underlying disease process. This understanding of depression has its critics, and I am one of them. In psychological terms it is better to think of people as suffering *with* or *through* (see MacLachlan, 2004, for a discussion of this in terms of embodiment) what they are experiencing – early morning wakening, low self-esteem, depressed mood, etc. – not *from* something else. In terms of the DSM and the ICD, however, people are usually suffering from something else, an underlying disease entity, not through their immediate experience.

Table 4.1   Different types of causes for depression.

Domain	Factors
Biomedical	Organ pathology
	Physiological impairment
	Hormone imbalance
Moral	Transgression
	Sin
	Karma
Sociopolitical	Oppression
	Injustice
	Loss
Interpersonal	Envy
	Hatred
	Sorcery
Psychological	Anger
	Desire
	Intrapsychic conflict
	Defence

Based on Shweder (1991).

The experience of depression within an individual can vary over time – commonly referred to as the disease course – and, as already noted, it can vary between individuals of the same culture – commonly referred to as a disease syndrome. Kleinman's suggestion that depression can also vary across cultures and across different historical epochs is quite consistent with a biological view of depression. He has also studied a condition known as neurasthenia. This condition, commonly reported in China, is characterised by a lack of energy and physical complaints such as a sore stomach. Kleinman has suggested that, although depression and neurasthenia are different illness experiences, they are both products of the same underlying disease processes – depression. In other words, neurasthenia is the Chinese version of western depression.

Shweder (1991) suggests that this interpretation 'privileges' a biological understanding of how depression occurs. He points out a range of factors that can theoretically cause depression, including biological ones. Table 4.1 illustrates the different factors in what he calls biomedical, moral, sociopolitical, interpersonal and psychological 'causal ontologies'. Now things become complicated. Kleinman believes that the ultimate cause of depression and neurasthenia is the same, and concerns the experiences of defeat, loss, vexation and oppression by local hierarchies of power. Such 'sociopolitical' experiences produce a biological disease process. However, the way in which this disease is expressed is influenced by the culture within which one lives.

Some forms of suffering – because they can be understood to provide a message, a communication – are more acceptable than others. In North America, for instance, there is a great emphasis on individualism, competitiveness, slogging it out in the market place, achieving, personal growth, real-ising one's own (amazing) potential, etc. There is also a great emphasis on 'letting it out', on the right of the individual openly to express what she or he feels. This allows for the expression of depression as a demonstration of the individual's disillusionment with not 'succeeding'. On the other hand, in China, or so it can be argued, depression is not the 'right' form of suffering. In China demoralisation and hopelessness may be stigmatised as losing faith in the political ideals of 'the system'. Such a public display of disengagement is not welcome. Instead a variety of symptoms consistent with fatigue, being physically run down and being exhausted by the pressures of work may be seen as an acceptable reason for failure.

In summary, Kleinman (1980) is suggesting that depression and neurasthe-nia have similar sociopolitical origins, which produce a similar biological disease process that expresses itself differently in North America and China because the different cultural conditions favour different forms of expression. Once again this seems to be a perfectly reasonable argument. However, Shweder (1991) makes the perfectly reasonable criticism that there is no need to say that the Chinese's neurasthenia is somatised depression. We might just as well say that North American depression is emotionalised neurasthenia and that neurasthenia is the underlying disease process, not depression. However, Shweder questions the value of talking about disease processes at all. For him, the concepts of 'illness' and 'disease' do not add any value to our understanding of the relationship between neurasthenia and depression. Although these two conditions may have similar origins in sociopolitical adversity, we are able to distinguish between the two forms of suffering. If there is therefore no need to think in terms of a biological 'middle man', there is no need for either neurasthenia or depression to be the primary disorder.

How acceptable you find this conclusion will no doubt depend on your own professional (subcultural) training. However, you may still ask 'does it really matter?'. Well, yes it does. If Mr Lim presents symptoms of neurasthenia in my Dublin clinic and I interpret him as 'really suffering from depression', my interpretation of his condition may be radically different from his experience of his condition. Turn it the other way round: if you go to the doctor in Beijing and she tells you that you are not really depressed as such, but that you are really suffering from stomach problems, you are unlikely to feel understood (and you may wonder if you took a wrong turn somewhere along the hospi-tal's maze of corridors)!

Does it really matter in terms of treatment? This may well depend on your method of treatment. If it involves prescribing 'antidepressant' medication then (paradoxically) Mr Lim may be happier having that for his neurasthenia than many westerners would be having it for their depression. Incidentally, even if the same medication is effective for both conditions, it does not nec-essarily mean that they share the same cause (I may take an aspirin for a headache and a toothache, but it does not mean that I have a hole in my cranium corresponding to the hole in my tooth). Returning to Mr Lim's neurasthenia, if I think he is 'really depressed' and try out Beck's cognitive therapy on a man who does not report any cognitive symptoms of depression, I may only worsen his problems. The reason for the distinction between neurasthenia and depression being so important and for the practitioner acknowledging it is that in doing so we are acknowledging the person's experience of their own suffering. We are not imposing our culturally myopic perspective on another human being in order to treat a problem that we know about, even if it is not the problem that they have 'got'. In short, we are being clinically practical, not hegemonically, theoretical.

Diagnosis

Again, does it really matter if they are so similar in any case? Yes it does, because they are not necessarily so similar after all. If the DSM criteria are used to classify Chinese neurasthenics a good proportion of them do not fulfil the criteria for depression. Also a good proportion of North American depressives do not fulfil the Chinese criteria for neurasthenia. Thus, their distressing experiences are different. We can join them together only by assuming a biological syndromal model of depression, worldwide. This idea is that everybody suffers from the same things that we do, except that they express it differently. The idea that neurasthenia is 'masked depression' subsumes the experience of somatisation under depression. It gives primary importance to the depression.

This assumed primacy of depression over somatic symptoms has been explored in Banglagore, India. Weiss, Raguram and Channabasavanna (1995) sought to explore the interrelationship of depressive, anxious and somatoform experiences, not only from the western diagnostic perspective of the DSM classification system, but also from the perspective of the individual's own illness experience. Their study used established structured interview schedules to glean both types of information from their interviewees who were all presenting for the first time at the psychiatric outpatient clinic in Banglagore. When the same 'symptom' presentation was interpreted by the patient and by the DSM system, in general patients preferred to describe their problems in terms of somatic symptoms whereas the DSM system described them in terms of depression.

It is important to point out that the experience of somatic symptoms is also common in European and North American contexts. Indeed 'somatization disorder' is a recognised diagnostic category in the DSM classification system. Such a diagnosis is made when people report somatic distress without any evidence of organic cause. A recent study of somatisation in primary care settings in Spain reported that almost 10% of people presenting a new episode of illness to a primary care clinic, and approximately one-third of people who presented psychological problems that were severe enough to be classified as 'psychiatric cases', fulfilled the criteria for somatisation (Garcia-Campayo et al., 1996; Lobo et al., 1996). Table 4.2 gives the frequency of somatic symptoms most commonly reported in 147 Spanish somatisers. Backache, dizziness

Table 4.2 Most frequent somatic symptoms in Spanish somatisers ($n = 147$).

Somatic symptoms	Percentage
Back pain	71.4
Dizziness	65.3
Pain in extremities	60.5
Bloating (gassy)	52.3
Shortness of breath	50.3
Palpitations	49.6
Joint pain	45.5
Chest pain	44.2
Nausea (other than motion sickness)	43.5
Amnesia	39.4
Abdominal pain	37.4
Intolerance of different foods	24.4
Diarrhoea	23.1
Difficulty swallowing	21.7
Painful menstruation[a]	21.4
Blurred vision	20.4
Paralysis or muscle weakness	20.4
Excessive menstrual bleeding[a]	18.6
Sexual indifference	17.6
Trouble walking	17.0
Irregular menstrual periods[a]	15.8
Vomiting (other than during pregnancy)	14.9
Pain during urination	14.2
Loss of voice	11.5
Urinary retention	10.2

[a] Only in women.
Reproduced from Lobo et al. (1996). (With permission.)

and pains in extremities were cited by over 60% of somatisers. Table 4.2 illustrates a wide range of somatic distress including problems that may not often be associated with this diagnosis, including diarrhoea, vomiting, trouble walking and urinary retention. Most of these somatising patients fulfilled the criteria for the DSM diagnoses of depression or anxiety.

The Spanish investigators subdivided their 'psychiatric' sample into 'somatisers' (described above) and 'psychologisers', of whom there were 46. Thus, three times as many 'psychiatric' patients were rated as 'somatisers' rather than 'psychologisers'. The most frequent diagnosis made for 'somatisers' was generalised anxiety disorder, whereas for 'psychologisers' it was major depression. Table 4.3 shows the DSM diagnoses given to the whole sample. As can be seen here there is substantial overlap between these two groups and the diagnostic categories used. The most dramatic contrast is for the diagnosis of dysthymia, which refers to a chronic (at least 2 years), although less severe, form of depression than major depressive disorder. In the dysthymic category there was a ratio of 10:1 between 'somatisers' and 'psychologisers'.

Table 4.3   DSM-IV diagnosis (APA, 1994) in Spanish somatisers and psychologisers.

Diagnosis (DSM-IV)	Somatisers $n = 147$	Psychologisers $n = 46$
	No. (%)	No. (%)
Generalised anxiety disorder	32 (21.7)	12 (26.0)
Depressive disorder NOS	23 (15.6)	11 (23.9)
Major depression	22 (14.9)	13 (28.2)
Dysthymia	21 (14.2)	2 (4.3)
Somatisation disorder	14 (9.5)	–
Adjustment disorder	12 (8.1)	5 (10.8)
Undifferentiated somatoform disorder	7 (4.7)	–
Panic disorder/agoraphobia	3 (2.0)	–
Others	13 (8.8)	3 (6.5)

NOS: not otherwise stated.
Reproduced from Garcia-Campayo et al. (1996). (With permission.)

Such results, and many others similar results, illustrate the complexity of understanding and categorising the distress that people present to practitioners. Indeed we do not need to go to China to find that many people presenting physical problems receive a diagnosis of depression. We do not need to go to China to ask about similarities and differences of the underlying nature of presenting complaints. These dilemmas are on our own doorstep. As is often the case in cross-cultural psychology, comparisons between cultures can also sharpen the focus on one's own culture. Our own cultural assumptions often blind us to our own complexities. This is hardly surprising because assumptions are often simplifications to make the world more manageable. In short, we do not stereotype only other cultures, we also stereotype our own. Wherever you come from your people are pretty complicated too!

In the west, people are so versed in the notion of psychosomatic problems (where the psychic is primary and the soma secondary) that even contemplating the somatopsychic (where the soma is primary and the psychic secondary) is hard going. As a psychologist, even writing the very word 'somatopsychic' makes me feel awkward. Furthermore, although we use diagnostic systems to try to simplify the phenomena that we encounter, these systems are so much a product of our cultural and professional (subcultural) thinking, that they may veil the true experience of an individual's suffering.

Weiss et al. (1995), commenting on their results, write:

These limitations of the diagnostic system identified here appear to reside more with the professional construction of categories than with the inability of patients and professionals to comprehend each other's concepts of distress and disorder. . . . Personal meanings and other aspects of phenomenological and subjective experience should be incorporated into psychiatric evaluation and practice . . . facilitating an empathic clinical alliance and enabling a therapist to work with patients' beliefs over the course of treatment . . .

Weiss et al. (1995, p. 358)

Thus, whatever the presenting complaint, the belief system of the person who 'owns' the complaint has to be the medium through which you work. The context of the presentation – not an abstract diagnostic system – is what gives the complaint meaning. Without taking the context into account, clinically we can misinterpret the meaning of somatic complaints as the 'masked' presence of cognitive distortions, low self-esteem, and low mood, etc. In a recent review of the literature on somatisation, neurasthenia and depression in China, Parker, Gladstone and Tsee Chee (2001) concluded that the 'Chinese do tend to deny depression or express it somatically', a conclusion all the more remarkable for their acknowledgement that the literature is fraught with interpretative difficulties caused by:

. . . the heterogeneity of people described as ' the Chinese' and due to factors affecting collection of data, including issues of illness definition, sampling and case finding; differences in help seeking behaviour; idiomatic expression of emotional distress; and the stigma of mental illness.

Parker et al. (2001, p. 857)

Lee (2001) claims that the *Chinese Classification of Mental Disorders* (CCMD) instrument has resolved differences between international classification systems and Chinese 'culture-related' disorders. However, in an article curiously entitled 'From diversity to unity: The classification of mental disorder in 21st century China', Lee concludes that 'Personality disorders are not common diagnoses or popular research topics in China because personality disorders are perceived as *moral rather than medical problems*' (Lee, 2001, p. 429, italics added). Now, does that sound familiar?

Lessons from the developing world

Psychology as a discipline is strongly associated with Euro-American thinking. However, psychology as an activity exists in all human beings and indeed, even in the so-called 'lower' species of animals. Psychology is a universal activity. Unless we were all to some extent psychologists, communication would be impossible. There can be little doubt that, for instance, Asian, African and South American psychologies are every bit as complex and sophisticated as the (false) amalgam of Euro-American psychology. Although alternative psychologies do have a voice in western societies, they tend to be marginalised. Most of the 'psychological traffic' is in one direction, from

Europe and America outwards towards the less industrialised (low income or 'developing') countries. This has resulted in a degree of psychological colonisation, where foreign peoples are encouraged to think that the Euro-American way of thinking is the right way of thinking. Such a position is an effrontery to the thousands of indigenous psychologies that have existed for generations. It is to be hoped that, apart from nurturing aspects of our own psychologies, each of us can also learn something from different ways of being in the world. Within this spirit Schumaker (1996) has recently set out to explore some of the lessons that the 'less developed' countries may have for the 'more developed' countries, especially regarding an understanding of depression. As we will seen, there is much to learn.

Two of the most prominent models of psychopathology in the west – the cognitively based psychological model and the biologically based medical model – both locate the origin of psychopathology in the individual. In essence, because these individualist models do not take cultural factors into account, they assume universalism: that every individual, given appropriate cognitive/biological conditions, is at risk of becoming depressed. We have already explored the complexities of understanding the possibility of depression being expressed in different ways in different cultures. However, Schumaker (1996) explores the intriguing possibility of cultures that are free of all symptoms associated with depression, including somatic symptoms.

The Kaluli of New Guinea have no word in their language for 'depression' and do not recognise the western description of depression. Is it possible that some aspects of Kaluli culture – of their way of living in the world – protect against depression? One striking feature of the culture appears to be a propensity to get angry, with social displays of anger being encouraged and used to rank the status of a person. Among the Kaluli it is good to get angry because it stimulates attempts at compensation. According to the principle of social reciprocity a person who is angered deserves to have things 'made up' to them. Being angry is therefore a good way to get what you want. It does not induce antagonism or grudges. The Kaluli reaction to anger is therefore significantly different from that in western cultures.

An interesting psychoanalytic explanation of depression is that it represents the results of anger towards another person being turned inward, on the self. So, for example, the loss of a loved one may produce not only feelings of great sadness but also feelings of desertion. Usually it is not acceptable to be angry with the person who has died and so, rather than displaying this anger, and because it cannot simply disappear, it is turned against the self, perhaps being experienced as guilt and self-depreciation and leading to depression. Might it then be the case that the Kaluli do not get depressed because they live in a society in which anger need not be turned inward upon the self, but can instead be projected outward in a socially sanctioned display? Indeed this might be the case. Often such conclusions are drawn on comparisons between western culture and another culture. However, spreading the cross-cultural comparison net wider proves to be even more informative.

The Toraja of Indonesia is another culture in which depression does not appear to be experienced. However, among the Toraja it is not good to display anger. Anger is shameful and dangerous and may result in punishment from supernatural forces, resulting in physical and mental suffering. It is not just the social expression of anger that is to be avoided; one should not feel anger, even if it goes unexpressed. This seems to eliminate the expression of anger as the sole responsible cause for the Kaluli's freedom from depression. Schumaker argues that what distinguishes how many western cultures deal with anger. from how Toraja culture deals with it is that although anger is clearly undesirable in Toraja culture it is not relegated to the 'social unconscious' as it is in many western cultures. In other words the Toraja see anger as an expected reaction to certain situations and as an issue to be dealt with, to be worked through. Western societies, it is argued, do not afford the same inevitability to anger. Rather than individuals being encouraged to deal with angry feelings, they are expected not to work through them but to tuck them away, to hide them, to banish them. It is this banishment of emotion from social discourse, which constitutes the anger being turned inward, that may be associated with depression in many western cultures.

The apparent non-occurrence of depression in the Kaluli and Toraja and countless other cultures challenges assumptions about the universality of this form of suffering. It is particularly a problem for the biological model that assumes that a particular disease process will inevitably result in a corresponding disease experience. It is less of a problem for psychosocial models of depression because these models do at least allow for the malleability of psychosocial processes. However, there is still a problem here. Quite understandably, Schumaker (1994), writing from Australia, attempts to understand the occurrence or non-occurrence of depression across diverse cultures by reference to the psychoanalytic formulation of anger turned inward. Although this is clearly a western concept it is also true that we can only work on problems for which we have the tools available. Schumaker should not be criticised for putting these tools – concepts – to use in unravelling this intriguing mystery of why some cultures experience 'depression' and others do not.

It will be terribly difficult to identify one factor, such as the internalisation of anger, that accounts for the varied experience of depression across cultures. Cultures are 'package holidays' for life. There is a whole lot thrown in and these many factors will probably interact in unique ways in their different social and geographical contexts. This should not stop us searching for factors salient to human health and welfare, but it should encourage us to broaden our net to multifactorial causes. For the practitioner working across cultures, some understanding of the process of interaction between variables is going to be a more achievable goal than identifying the salient content of causation across many cultures. Depression has exemplified many of the complexities of understanding mental distress in the context of culture. We now turn to consider cultural differences in a related problem – suicide – and then review the relationship between the social and the cultural in personality disorder.

Suicide

According to Berman (1997, p. 6):

> ... culture is the nutrient medium within which the organism is culti-
> vated. Suicidality grows, as well, when that culture is pathological. ...
> Suicidal behaviour can be designed to protect, to rescue the self from oth-
> erwise certain annihilation.

Suicide is both individualised and pathologised. Western psychology and
psychiatry, by focusing their attention on the individual, have constructed
suicide as being the deviant act of a disturbed, dysfunctional or ill mind.
However, when multicultural perspectives on suicide are examined, it
becomes clear that culture may act either as a *protective factor* or as one that
increases risk in already-vulnerable groups – a *facilitating factor*. I consider here
two cultural groups in the USA who occupy opposite extremes with regard
to their incidence of suicide: whereas one has the highest rate of suicide and
the other the lowest, they are both minority groups, marginalised by 'mainstream' American society (see also Range et al., 1999; Smyth, MacLachlan &
Clare, 2003).

Contrasting African–American and Native American suicide

Suicide is the only condition in which the African–American population
exhibit lower rates than their European–American counterparts (Allen &
Farley, 1986) in spite of the fact that this group are often economically and
socially disadvantaged. Among African–Americans there is a similar gender
discrepancy as found in other cultural groups, with a male:female ratio of
about 4:1. The greatest at-risk period is between the ages of 25 and 34 years,
and the most common case of suicide has been found to be that of a young
man using a gun, or some other high-lethality means. Suicidal behaviour in
the African–American population is surrounded by distinct sociocultural,
political and economic issues. Mental health status is not the only factor to
consider, and that these other elements may be more salient is noteworthy.

African–American culture may serve to protect against suicide in several
ways. Early et al. (1993) argue that religion in this group provides steadfast
support to families and strengthens social integration. Also, suicide is seen
as an 'unpardonable sin', alien not only to their religion but also to
African–Americans as a whole. Furthermore, African–Americans are also
more likely than those of European extraction to live in multigenerational
groupings, and this offers the possibility of elderly suicide being reduced, as
elderly people can feel that they continue to make a valuable and meaningful contribution to their family and their community. Range et al. (1999)
further suggest that the characteristics of the African–American population

require some move away from traditional, western, individualised, psycho-logical approaches, and perhaps a greater inclusion of the extended family in 'clinical' interventions.

Native American groups (or First Nations, i.e. 'we were here first!') are often impoverished and have a high incidence of alcohol dependence: both prob-lems recognised as independent risk factors for suicide, which is higher in this group than for any other on mainland North America, especially in the 15- to 24-year-old category (EchoHawk, 1997). One of the main concerns with regard to the suicide rate of the various Native American groups is the impact that the process of acculturation has had. Faced with the problems of tribal relo-cation and deregulation of tribal life, maladaptive forms of coping have emerged. Furthermore, in the absence of a formal rite of passage (further reflecting imposed changes on the structure of tribal life) signalling the move from childhood to adolescence, consumption of alcohol may begin at a very early age, with Range et al. (1999) suggesting that, in some tribes, children as young as six have been seen to participate in tribal drinking sessions.

Despite the apparently clear links between substance use and suicidal behaviour, Novins et al. (1999) argue that a more complex view of this rela-tionship is needed if a more accurate picture is to be obtained. In comparing the Pueblo, Southwest and Northwest tribal groups (specific names were not mentioned in the study for reasons of confidentiality) the best explanation of the link between substance use (e.g. alcohol) and suicide was that it made people more likely to act on suicidal thoughts. In short, alcohol does not *cause* people to have suicidal thoughts or behave in a suicidal manner, but for those who already hold such thoughts, the consumption of alcohol may make them more likely to act (i.e. it may reduce inhibition for suicide).

About a third of Native Americans live on reservations, another third live in urban settings with the remaining third living between reservation and urban areas. When suicide is considered among the tribes, reports range from 150 per 100,000 to zero per 100,000, depending on the tribe and source of sta-tistics. The male:female ratio has been recorded at a high of 12:1, with lethal means frequently being favoured by males (55.2% of male suicides in this group use firearms, with a further 40% adopting the method of hanging). Reflecting this, Range et al. (1999) offer the typical profile of a Native American suicide as being that of a young, single male who kills himself at home with a firearm after a drinking session. Further to this, when three tribes (the Navajo, Apache and Pueblos) were compared it was the Apache who were seen to have the highest rate of suicide and the lowest level of intratribal (i.e. within their own tribe) social integration, thus further pointing to the role of social and cultural factors in the experience of suicide.

Elements of acculturation such as western education, religious conversion, legislation, language barriers and being moved from native lands to reserva-tions can all be seen to have contributed to the suicide problem. If a culture orders and gives meaning to life experiences, the dismantling of that culture may result in a disordered and personally meaningless world. Traditional safeguards that protected against suicide, such as interdependence, clear role orientation and traditional tribal structure, are no longer typical. In contrast, modern tribal structure is characterised by chaotic family structures, divorce, alcoholism and child neglect, meaning that Native American cultures (as they are today) play a more negative role than before and in this way are seen to be linked to suicide (EchoHawk, 1997).

Six variables in particular have been recognised as being of importance in predicting the likelihood of suicide in Native American peoples (Dizmang et al., 1974):

1. Having more than one significant caretaker before the age of 15
2. Primary caretakers with numerous arrests
3. Two or more losses by divorce or desertion during childhood
4. Being arrested by the age of 15
5. One or more arrests in the 12 months before death
6. Attendance at a boarding school before ninth grade.

Thus, by the process of culture change and the resultant effects of acculturation, what was once a unique and strong culture is now plagued by suicide (but see Chapter 6). In EchoHawk's own words, 'indigenous clients must be allowed to grieve and talk about their feelings of historical trauma, alienation and poor sense of identity' (1997, p. 66) if the positive culture of the past is to be reclaimed, re-established and re-awakened. Suicide and mental health problems are not of course restricted to any one country or historical record; similar themes recur elsewhere.

Cultural evolution, anomie and suicide

Beautrais (2000) shows that New Zealand/Aotearoa has experienced a steady increase in the rate of youth suicide over the period 1977–96 from 20.3 per 100,000 to 39.5 per 100,000 (it is important to note that, during this same period, female rates of suicide remained steady as is the general international pattern in nations dominated by male suicide). Of the 3.6 million people of New Zealand, 400,000 are Maori. Historically there has been a low suicide rate among the Maori and therefore it may be of value to understand the underlying cultural construction of suicide. Death in the Maori language is translated as *mate*. There is no specific translation for suicide as English speakers would understand it, with the closest approximation being the word *whakamomori*, which does not imply death directly but a loss of alternatives so overwhelming that death is the result. The root of the word *mori* means distress, helplessness, unfulfilled desire, broken attachment, etc., perhaps linguistically representing a more holistic view and more accurately reflecting the psychological experience that we know often precedes suicide.

In traditional Maori culture there are recognised circumstances in which self-inflicted death is seen as 'acceptable'. Among these is the sudden loss of some significant other, intolerable loss of status, overwhelming insult, and personal failure to perform in some valued domain or a belief that some pow-

erful magic has been performed against the person. Traditional Maori morality is determined by elements such as honour, respect, status, politically
imposed restrictions and supernatural events. Death is seen as a natural part
of life (with no great fear or dread attached to it). In death, one does not escape
the concerns of life, or indeed contact with family. Dead ancestors play a very
important role in Maori life and may be evoked at any time to help the living.
The newly dead person has to answer to the ancestors and account for his or
her own deeds. In this sense, a 'wrongful' suicide would have to be accounted
for, which also acts as a deterrent. Thus death is not seen as an escape and, as
such, this begs the question: 'What would be the point of suicide?' Langford
et al. (1998) argue that these beliefs may have contributed to the historically
low suicide rate of the Maori culture. Another very important part of the traditional Maori culture was the concept of family or *whanau*, who were the
agents of socialisation (Ritchie & Ritchie, 1979). However, as with the Native
American societies, rapid social change and the stripping of cultural icons and
practices, seem to have created a context in which suicidal behaviour
has flourished in a society that was once culturally more resiliant.

Culture change across time may be considered as a form of cultural evolution, or 'temporal acculturation' (see Chapter 1), and it has been argued that
this may produce an increased likelihood of suicide as a result of a falling
away of traditional support and coping mechanisms, and an increased sense
of anomie. Durkheim's seminal work *Le Suicide* (1897/1952) appeared at a
time when knowing about the world was dominated by the positivist perspective – the push to discovery of ultimate truths and basic facts. The same
methodologies that had proved so successful with the natural sciences could,
it was argued, be applied to questions of humanity (such as suicide) and
produce equally certain 'solutions' to the problems of humanity. At this time
there were two general schools of thought on suicide (Taylor, 1982). The first
thought of suicide as a form of inherited madness, whereas the second (which
used comparative studies of official suicide rates) explained its occurrence in
terms of various environmental factors. Both viewed suicide as an individual
act and presented humankind as being quite uninvolved in their own fate –
either madness or circumstance took over and determined the nature of their
actions. On this point and with regard to future investigations of suicide,
Morselli (1903) asserted that:

> The old philosophy of individualism had given to suicide the character
> of liberty and spontaneity, but now it became necessary to study it no
> longer as the expression of individual and independent faculties, but cer-
> tainly as a social phenomenon allied with all the other racial forces.

> Morselli (1903)

Durkheim argued for social and cultural forces to be given primary importance in understanding suicide. The degree of integration and regulation that
the individual experienced as a result of the type of society and culture in
which he or she lived were seen to influence the likelihood of him or her contemplating the act of suicide. Durkheim understood that people were born

into sociocultural contexts that may be organised in different ways, but all of which hold a reality thoroughly independent of the individual. Societal elements such as religious denomination and economic development were therefore of concern and each society was seen to have a certain capacity for suicide related to its structure at any given time (Durkheim, 1897/1952).

Durkheim (1897/1952) delineated four types of suicide: egoistic, anomic, altruistic and mixed. Egoistic suicide resulted from a lack of integration of the individual into the society of which they are a part. Anomic suicide was presented as resulting from the state of (the then) 'modern' economies, the idea being that when any drastic change is experienced (such as a sudden increase in wealth) individual's horizons may be broadened beyond what they can endure, and with the diminishing traditional support structures suicide becomes more probable. So-called 'altruistic suicide', as it was conceived by Durkheim, continues to be seen in the form of suicide bombers and others who choose to end their lives for a 'higher purpose'. This type of suicide relates to the taking of one's own life for a 'cause', such as political affiliation or religious sacrifice, rather than reasons of personal circumstance. Thus, even in the nineteenth century, there were various ways in which cultural beliefs could be considered to be related to suicide, often the sort of ideas that we may attribute to a more recent era.

Returning to Durkheim's idea of anomic suicide, different historical epochs, although characteristic of the same 'national' culture, usually constitute very different social environments, or cultures, e.g. the Irish psyche has been shaped by the experience of colonialism, civil war, terrorism, Catholicism and being a small island on the fringes of Europe. At the same time, as Ireland has distinguished itself through literary and artistic fame, the Irish have also been stereotyped as heavy drinkers, lawless, violent and sexually repressed (Halliday & Coyle, 1994). What happens to the impressions people have of themselves and others and to their cultural values when they experience rapid socioeconomic change? Willis et al. (2002) argue that the rising rate of suicide among young African-Americans is associated with their experience of the 'post-modern' society, a society characterised by institutional deconstruction, decreased collectivism, increased normlessness and helplessness, and an increased personal risk for stress. Willis et al. (2002, p. 907) state: 'post-modernity characteristically loosens the bonds between the individual and society, thereby increasing vulnerability to depression, related pathologies . . . and suicide'.

Inglehart and Baker (2000) examined three waves of the World Values Survey (1981–82, 1990–91 and 1995–88), encompassing 65 societies on 6 continents, and apparently representative of three-quarters of the world population. They argue that the results provide strong evidence for both massive cultural change and the persistence of distinctive traditional values (Inglehart & Baker, 2000, p. 49):

A history of Protestant or Orthodox or Islamic or Confucian traditions gives rise to cultural zones with distinctive value systems that persist after controlling for the effects of economic development. Economic development tends to push societies in a common direction, but rather than converging, they seem to move on parallel trajectories shaped by their cultural heritages. We doubt that the forces of modernization will produce a homogenized world culture in the foreseeable future.

This would suggest that it is not simply a matter of 'out with the old and in with the new', but of people finding a way to combine the old with the new. In the case of the Irish 'Celtic Tiger', internationalisation and globalisation seem to have interacted with internal change and resulted in unprecedented immigration, increasing secularisation, economic prosperity and liberalisation of social attitudes (MacLachlan & O'Connell, 2000; O'Connell, 2001). This Ireland can surely be distinguished form the Ireland of even just a decade ago (traditional, conservative, devout and often unemployed). As such, this transition is somewhat similar to that which people experience when they move from one culture to another, across geographical boundaries. Adaptation to such change may be termed 'temporal acculturation', i.e. culture change, over time, within the same society.

MacLachlan et al. (2004) investigated how Irish people have acculturated from the traditional Ireland to the 'Celtic Tiger' Ireland. As an innovation to Berry's framework however, we also allowed for an 'uncertain' or 'cultural ambivalence' classification, where participants gave mid-range responses to their desire to identify with the culture of 'old Ireland' and to the culture of 'new Ireland'. Of over 700 respondents, 88% agreed that there had been a 'big change in Irish culture over the past 10 years' leading us to the conclusion that temporal acculturation was more than an abstract theoretical concept – it was a lived experience for the vast majority of our sample. Importantly, however, it was those people who exhibited some degree of uncertainty or ambivalence who also experienced the poorest mental health. While either state of being thoroughly caught up in 'Celtic Tiger' Ireland or rejecting it in favour of a remembered traditional Ireland may not be the optimal situation, in terms of psychological adjustment, well-being and functioning, having *any* strong feeling towards these changes was relatively better than being uncertain; it is this uncertainty, lack of clarity and sense of nebulousness that appeared to be most problematic.

Brendan Kennelly's poem, *Now* (2001), asks 'In Ireland now, why so many Young men kill themselves?' This is indeed a most timely question. Figure 4.1 plots male and female suicide against gross national product (GNP) and gross domestic product (GDP) over a 20-year period in Ireland. The resulting relationships are plain and startling to see. There is a particularly strong relationship between male suicides (with most of these being accounted for by young men, particularly more recently) and increased economic growth, as indexed by GNP, with an associated correlation of $r = 0.82$. Thus changes in the Irish economy, which have surely been a hallmark of the 'Celtic Tiger', are clearly associated with changes in the rate of suicide, particularly among young men.

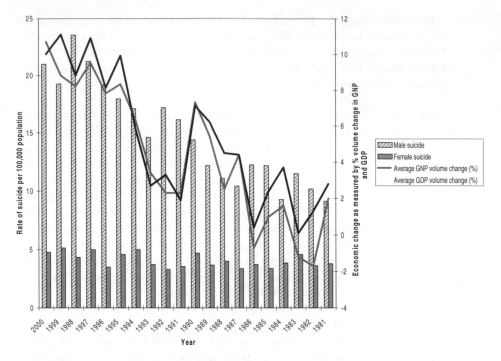

Figure 4.1   Annual male and female suicides per 100,000 in the Republic of Ireland against economic growth over 20 years (reproduced from MacLachlan, 2003).

Elsewhere we have gone into some detail to explain this current surge in young male suicide in Ireland (see Smyth, MacLachlan & Clare, 2003). We have argued that an interplay of various influences, at the levels of globalisation (e.g. materialism, individualism, male identity), Irish society (e.g. high rate of alcohol consumption, the tradition for men not to express their emotions openly) and local communities (e.g. a reduction in the availability of social support mechanisms), as well as family (e.g. a history of abuse) and individual factors (e.g. help-seeking behaviour) have effectively created paths along which individuals are drawn, which result in experiences of hopelessness, depression, isolation, etc. which in turn lead to suicide. If our findings are indeed a reflection of the process of rapid 'modernisation' in Ireland, they seem to resonate across three centuries to the original insights and provocative suggestions of Durkheim – that social and cultural factors are primary in understanding suicide. The fact that this suggestion is still provocative today suggests that our thinking has evolved more slowly than our economic growth. Another way in which mental health is patterned by cultural variations within society is with regard to cultural minorities and migrants, and it is to these major areas of interest that we now turn.

Cultural minority mental health

Group densities

In recent years there has been a great deal of concern expressed about the high rates of mental disorder in cultural (or ethnic) minority groups. In both studies of admission to psychiatric facilities and of 'psychiatric case' prevalence in the community, cultural minorities have been over-represented in comparison to members of their host culture. Culture is only one of a range of factors that have been associated with a higher rate of mental disturbance. For instance, Brown and his colleagues, working mostly in London, have illuminated a range of 'risk factors' for mental disorder. These factors include social class, employment status, gender, social support, personal history and situational demands, e.g. in their classic book *The Social Origins of Depression*, Brown and Harris (1978) reported that women who had experienced the death of their own mother before the age of 11, who did not have an intimate relationship with their partner and who were at home caring for three or more young children, were more likely to develop depression of clinical severity than women who had not experienced these psychosocial stressors. Research of this sort drew attention to the neglected influence that social contexts can have on mental functioning (see also Chapter 9).

This sort of analysis also encouraged researchers to identify sociocultural factors that may be responsible for the observed high rates of mental disorder in cultural minority groups. However, membership of a cultural minority group is not simply a cultural phenomenon. It is often the case that the most socially and economically disadvantaged groups in a society are those that have most recently immigrated into the country. Such groups are often expected to join the 'bottom of the pile' and work their way up – something like an 'acculturation apprenticeship', where it is expected that you will have it rough to begin with, but that, in time – with effort – things will come good in the end. The multiplicity of social and economic factors implicated in cultural minority status has made it difficult to identify the extent to which being a member of a minority culture group is, in and of itself, a stress factor related to mental disorder. However, an analysis of cultural minority group densities offers the clinician a social psychological framework for understanding mental health in the community.

Halpern (1993) has shown how previously contradictory research can be accommodated within his theory of group densities. First of all, let us consider some of the contradictory research findings. As an overall group Black Americans tend to have higher first admission rates to psychiatric facilities than do White Americans, as an overall group. However, if we look within each of these groups something very interesting becomes apparent. Whites with the highest rates of admission are those who live in primarily black areas. Previously this finding had been explained in terms of 'social drift': that poorer white people, who could only afford to live in the poorer areas of cities, experienced the social and economic difficulties of living in poor areas, and that this resulted in increased social stress, which produced higher than average (for white people) rates of admission. These white people had 'drifted' down to the lowest socioeconomic sector of society, where, because of the immigrant history of the USA, they were now in the minority. An alternative, but related, explanation was in terms of 'selection': other things being equal, the poor and/or people from minority cultures were more likely to be admitted to a psychiatric institution because clinicians were more willing to admit them than they were to admit middle-class or more 'successful' people.

However, within the black group the highest rates of admission were among those who lived in areas where black individuals were in the minority. Thus black people living in middle-class, white American, 'good' areas had higher admission rates than black people living in the more deprived areas. Given the superior services and facilities enjoyed by predominantly white communities in the USA, downward 'social drift' could obviously not be the explanation for their higher morbidity relative to their white co-residents. Nor could 'selection' be the explanation, for why would middle-class black people be 'selected' for admission over poorer black people.

Further research on other cultural groups has shown that the larger the number of people in a minority cultural group living within a given area, the lower the psychiatric admission rate for minority cultural group members in that area. This suggests that living in a neighbourhood that encourages an unfamiliar lifestyle, culture and language is a risk factor for the development of mental disorder. Of course categorising people as black or white and assuming that all black and all white people identify with their own ethnic culture are gross simplifications. Furthermore, as cultural minorities become more established in 'good' areas, the assumed monocultural white ethos of these communities will presumably diminish. However, throughout the world, and especially the world's major cities, we continue to find areas that are synonymous with one cultural group or another, e.g. most major cities of the western world now have Chinese, French, Indian and Italian districts. There now appears to be good evidence that people who live in communities characterised by a large number of members of their own cultural group experience a feeling of 'fitting in'.

What prevents the negative effects of cultural isolation appears not to be the absolute number of other members of your cultural group, but their number relative to other groups. Interestingly the high rates of admission to psychiatric facilities found in British African–Caribbean individuals are not so characteristic of Indian and Pakistani communities in Britain. Halpern (1993) reviews research suggesting that this can be accounted for by the differing tendencies of these groups to 'cluster'. Apparently, a geographical analysis of immigrant settlement in Britain reveals that Asians have tended to cluster more than West Indians. Such segregation may help to protect the members of Asian communities from direct prejudice and provide them with social support that operates through culturally familiar customs.

As described in Chapter 1 social psychology emphasises how an individual personally gains from being an accepted member of a group. Individuals may define themselves with reference to their cultural group, feel empowered by being a member of that group and evaluate themselves in relation to other people within the group. If members of a cultural group live far apart geographically (low density) they may become less able to identify with membership of it. Other factors, interests or demands will impinge on their experience of life. Their sense of a cultural community will dissipate and they may become less able to deal with their problems. In this way, both geographically and psychologically, their loss of a sense of community may predispose them to mental disorder. Also, possibly related to this is Bhugra's (2003) interesting and perhaps unexpected finding from his review of the literature on migration and depression: using language as a proxy measure of acculturation, 'acculturated individuals' are more likely to be depressed, than those with poorer 'host' language skills (see also Chapter 2).

More recent research has broadly supported Halpern's original findings (Smaje, 1995; Neeleman & Wessely, 1999; Halpern & Nazroo, 2000) although not in every case (see Karlsen, Nazroo & Stephenson, 2002). Naturally the effect may not be the same for each ethnic group in every socioeconomic and political context. Thus Halpern's (1993, p. 605) conclusion that 'to dwell amongst members of the same perceived group offers some kind of perceived psychological advantage' requires further research to delineate limits to its legitimate generalisation, but it should remain central to the clinician's endeavours to create health through the strengthening of community resources.

Personality disorder

Cultures are the products of different ways of 'being' in the world. They describe the ways in which groups of people experience, think, feel and behave. Within cultures, at the level of the individual, there are also different ways of experiencing, thinking, feeling and behaving. These individual differences form the basis of individuals' personalities. It is the variation of personalities within a culture that makes stereotyping an erroneous method of dealing with people. Yet it is undeniable that cultures differ in what characterises their customary behaviour. A widely accepted notion within personality theory is that childhood experiences influence subsequent personality development. It is therefore reasonable to assume that cultural variations in family life and gender role, for example, will have an influence on the sort of personalities that develop, in order to adapt to the customary requirements of their culture. In short, different cultures place different expectations on individuals and make different allowances for individuals.

Culture has a strong influence on the construction of a self-concept, because by comparing ourselves with other people we are able to 'describe' ourselves: 'I am sensitive like Mary', 'I have a bad temper, much worse than Jimmy's', and 'I am not as attractive as Liz.' Culture not only helps us place ourselves in relation to other people and/or ideas, it also delineates what is good or bad, mad or sad. Culture conveys certain expectations of normative behaviour: it defines normality and abnormality. It is in this sense that cultural differences are especially salient for personality disorders. Alarcon and Foulks (1995, p. 6) have suggested that a personality disorder 'reflects difficulties in how an individual behaves and is perceived to behave by others in the social field, and this, of necessity, brings into play cultural values related to what is expected, valued, and devalued in a person'. If personality disorders concern failing to adapt to, or function in, certain situation then they are clearly related to culture. Deviance from the culturally expected, or 'normal', personality may define disorder and dysfunction. Awareness of this has led to a concern for 'culturally contextualising' behaviour: understanding it in its cultural context.

The prevailing understanding of personality disorders is based on a western understanding of behaviour, which promotes active, autonomous and self-reliant behaviour. The western conception of the 'ideal person' probably also incorporates the Protestant work ethic, the accumulation of wealth, scientific rationality, etc. Such values contribute to definitions of people who are on the margins of a culture, people who have personality disorders. Alarcon and Foulks (1995) describe how many of the traits included in contemporary psychiatric diagnoses may be considered quite appropriate in other cultures. In Table 4.4 I have extracted material from their review to give some idea of culturally appropriate behaviours that could be clinically misleading and therefore misclassified as indicating a personality disorder. When reading Table 4.4 it is important to remember that DSM-IV is a product of the American Psychiatric Association, so it reflects American (often white, middle-class, Anglo-American) views of behaviours that are not common or desired in that (sub)culture.

A few of the examples in Table 4.4 deserve further comment. The possibly traumatic experience of migration and acculturation may lead to behaviours that others interpret as signs of paranoid, schizoid, antisocial or avoidant personality disorder. This is saying nothing more than that some immigrants do not know or have not adopted the culturally acceptable ways of behaving, as implied by DSM-IV. Ethnic groups who are 'settled' into mainstream society, and yet retain aspects of their original cultural identity, also run the risk of being misunderstood. Wrist slashing among Native and Asian Americans would be a good example of this. In some Native American cultures this behaviour is a method of achieving bonding. The closest approximation to this behaviour in mainstream American culture occurs as suicidal behaviour often associated with aggression and is therefore associated with borderline personality disorder.

Table 4.4 Culturally normative behaviours that may be clinically misleading and misclassified as personality disorder (PD) according to DSM-IV criteria (APA, 1994).

Examples of behaviour	Cultures/contexts in which it is normative	DSM-IV diagnosis
Secretive, mistrustful, self-protective	Arabs, Mediterraneans, Eastern Europeans, immigrants	Paranoid PD
Social isolation, indifference to society, communicative deficits	Rural-to-urban and international migration	Schizoid PD
Peculiar ideation, appearance, 'speaking in tongues'	Evangelical religions, Native Americans, Hispanics	Schizotypal PD
Displays of tension, conflict, antagonism, dysphoria	Welfare activists in deprived communities, immigrants from 'oppressed countries'	Antisocial PD
Suicidal-like behaviour such as wrist-slashing	Native and Asian Americans and Arabs	Borderline PD
Emotionality, seductiveness, self-centredness, dramatic, hypersociability, somatisation	Mediterraneans and people of Latin descent	Histrionic PD
Flamboyance, self-importance, self-aggrandisement	Ethnic groups of Latin descent	Narcissistic PD
Distrust of officialdom, poor self-efficacy, demoralisation, oversensitivity, suppression of affect	Oppressed or minority groups especially Asian, Filipino and Hispanic immigrants	Avoidant PD
Passivity, deferential, faith in authority figures and elders	Traditional Asians and Arctic groups	Dependent PD
Strong work ethic, intolerance, inflexibility, judgemental	Scholars, scientists, priests, Japanese	Obsessive–compulsive PD

Based on Alarcon and Foulks' (1995) literature review.

As a final comment on Table 4.4 it is important to emphasise how some apparently pro-social (positive) behaviours can also fall foul of psychiatric classification, e.g. the behaviour of an Italian woman who is extremely sociable, dramatic and seductive (prosocial?) could be interpreted as symptomatic of histrionic personality disorder. Putting it another way, I know a number of women who would feel their holidays were completely wasted if Italian men did not behave in this manner! Personality disorders are about misbehaving in certain contexts, they are about not knowing of or abiding by certain social norms. Let us make no mistake, this difficulty can reflect great mental distress and require appropriate intervention to alleviate an individual's suffering. It is therefore all the more important not to confuse behaviours characteristic of some cultures or contexts with the diagnosis of western suffering. To do so dilutes the validity of true personality disorder and affronts the life styles of people from non-western cultures.

Transition mental health

I have tried to emphasise the importance of keeping the individual characteristics of people in the foreground while acknowledging the broader social and cultural factors as the context in which individuals operate. It is important not to stereotype an individual by over-identifying him or her with a particular cultural persona. In the same way we must avoid making easy assumptions about people who can be easily grouped together, e.g. 'refugees', 'elderly people', 'handicapped people', etc. Yet it is also important to acknowledge that, to the extent that people share common problems or situations, an awareness of these can be helpful in understanding their health needs. The aim here is only to touch on certain issues relevant to clinical practice in order to create awareness and hopefully motivate further reading, reflection and research, so that clinicians can explore those issues in their own practice.

Transition refers to change. The changes that accompany resettlement can be many and varied. An *emigrant* is somebody who leaves a place where they have been settled; an *immigrant* is somebody who arrives to resettle in a new place. Thus the same individual will be both an emigrant and an immigrant, depending on whether they are coming or going. This process of change is referred to as migration.

Migration

Contemporary migrations are on a scale and diversity previously unknown. The World Bank has estimated that the number of international migrants now exceeds 100 million and migration is now recognised as a global challenge. The urbanisation of many cultures has come about as a result of economic and industrial pressure to centralise resources. With the mechanisation of agricultural production and the decreasing proportion of many countries' GNP, which is constituted by agriculture, there has been a decline in rural populations. Thus within many countries there has been, and continues to be, a major migration from rural to urban areas. International migration is also now occurring on an unprecedented scale, with the proportion of people living outside their country of birth now approaching 2%. This migration of course occurs for many different reasons but is, in most cases, in one direction.

Each quarter of each year the UN's Refugee Agency, UNHCR, reports on applications for asylum, worldwide. In the first quarter of 2005 (January–March) 81,900 asylum applications were submitted in 36 countries, on which they report (see www.unhcr.ch/statistics). As shown in Figure 4.2, this represents a decline in asylum applications, a continuation of the trend over the last 3 years. France, which received 19% of all asylum applications, submitted during the first quarter of 2005, was the most popular country for asylum seekers, followed by the USA, with 17%, and then the UK, with 10%.

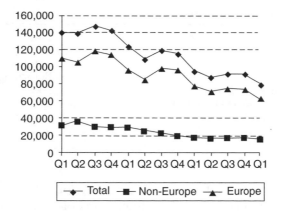

Figure 4.2   Asylum requests submitted in industrialised countries in the First Quarter (Q1) 2002, through to the Q1 2005.
Reproduced from *Asylum Levels and Trends in Industrialized Countries – First Quarter 2005*, UNHCR, Geneva.

Serbia and Montenegro was the leading country of origin of asylum seekers (5,100), followed by the Russian Federation (4,900), China (4,700), Turkey (3,700), Iraq (2,900), Georgia (2,600), Haiti (2,600), Nigeria (2,400), the Democratic Republic of Congo (2,400) and Iran (2,200). The dominant movement is from eastern Europe and the former Soviet Union into western Europe and North America.

Patterns of migration reflect changes in the economic, political, social and cultural relationships between different peoples. However, the combinations of poverty, rapid population growth and environmental damage (e.g. soil erosion) often create instability, resulting in the outpouring of people. Although once immigrants were viewed as extra workers for a thriving economy, now they may be viewed as a threat to the security and well-being of local workers and to the recipient society at large. Also, previously many migrants were men, but now women and children form a substantial proportion of migrants. This has heightened the role of gender in migration. Although both men and women migrants often experience 'downward occupational mobility' (working at a lower level than they were trained for in their own country) this effect appears to be much stronger for women. Women have also had to confront the dilemmas that radically different cultural expectations of their role, in their 'home' country and their host country, may present. At another extreme, people from industrially rich countries may emigrate to poorer countries in search of a better life. In Hawaii, the 'coconuts and bananas syndrome' refers to the expectation among some migrants that life there will be easier, simpler, with luscious foods dropping into their outstretched hands from nearby trees!

Whatever the reasons for migration, some of the experiences of transition will be shared by different groups. Table 4.5 summarises some of these common themes, as described by Westermeyer (1989) in his book on refugees

Table 4.5   Changes associated with migration.

Attitudes/values/beliefs/mores	Laws/regulations/legal status
Recreational activities	Loyalties
Circadian rhythms	Religious practices
Communication	Returning home
Delayed culture conflicts	Social network loss
Developmental/life cycle changes	Social roles
Ecological changes	Vocational changes

After Westermeyer (1989).

and migrants, some of which are more obvious than others. For instance, 'delayed cultural conflict' refers to those people who may have successfully adjusted to life in a different culture on a day-to-day basis, but who again experience conflict at irregular events such as funerals, weddings, childbirth, etc. Such events may embody quite different symbolic meanings in different cultures. 'Life cycle changes' may result in intergenerational conflicts, e.g. immigrant children, as a result of their more rapid language acquisition and possibly easier entry into a new culture, may serve as translators and socialisers for their parents and grandparents. Such role reversal may be stressful for all those concerned. 'Loyalties' to past commitments and to the demands of the present may be in conflict. One rather abstract example of this is if, in order to become a national of a new country, one has to renounce citizenship of one's country of origin. 'Returning home' may be an unexpectedly stressful experience for some emigrants. Often they themselves have changed and others may find it difficult to slot them back into what was once their familiar social network.

In one study, which we entitled "Returning Strangers", Cornish, Peltzer and MacLachlan (1999) explored the experiences of young refugees who had 'returned' to Malawi, even though they had never actually lived there: many of their parents, who were Jehovah's witnesses, had been forced to flee the country up to 30 years earlier because of President Banda's oppressive regime. The children had been born in Zambia, Zimbabwe or Tanzania. Many of the children reported being disappointed in Malawi (not living up their idealised expectations) and yet still cherished its significance as a 'homeland'. They experienced confusion between their sense of national and cultural identity, further contributed to through feelings of isolation and, in some cases, by animosity from their parents' former neighbours, who did not want to return lands and possessions taken from the children's families when they had to flee. Furthermore, some local people held negative views about Jehovah's witnesses, thus making it difficult for them to 're-integrate' and necessitating a process of 're-acculturation'. Ager (1999) suggests that understanding of the processes of socialisation and acculturation is vital for planning effective interventions with refugee children. Children's developing understanding of the world is mediated through a number of conduits: their own direct experience; that mediated through the family (accounts of parents); and that mediated through wider social structures, such as school, church or mosque (Ager and Young, 2001). When these channels are disrupted and lack coherence, it impairs children's capacity to assimilate new experiences in their under-standing, and may also question the basis of their previous experience.

Causes and precipitants of mental disorder in migrants

It is not surprising then to find that the experience of migration, with the nec-essary adaptation to a new life context, can be stressful. Elsewhere we have noted that although the cultural, historical, sociological, political, and eco-nomic context – *the content of context* – clearly varies greatly from one migrant situation to another, the *process of psychological adjustment* to new contexts may have some similarities (Gillespie, Peltzer & MacLachlan, 2000). Research sup-ports the idea that various broad factors influence the degree to which migrant stress may result in significant psychological disorder. Table 4.6 summarises the causes and precipitants of such disorder, once again as described by West-ermeyer (1989). Although some of the factors in Table 4.6 will affect most forms of migration, others will be particular to some types, and yet others can be found exerting deleterious affects in non-migrants too. Table 4.6 omits other factors that might be expected to cause mental distress or disorder in anybody

Table 4.6 Cases and precipitants of mental disorder in migrants.

Premigration factors	*Family factors*
Self-selection (drift hypothesis)	Absence of family/partial family
Biased migration	Family expectations
Forced migration	Marital conflict
National policy	Intergenerational conflict
Traumatic events	
Lack of preparation	*Psychological factors*
	Loss and grief
Cultural factors	Guilt and shame
Culture shock	Status inconsistency
Future shock	Maladaptive traditionality
Demodernisation shock	Life change events
Language and communication	Attitudes
Acculturation stresses	Expectations
Minority status	Homesickness
Social factors	*Biological factors*
Loss of social network	Acute travel effects
Social isolation	Organic brain damage
Role strain	Chronic illness
Marginality	Growing old
Unemployment	
Prejudice/bigotry	
Iatrogenic morbidity	

After Westermeyer (1989).

(e.g. certain genetic, biomedical, environmental or familial factors) and focuses on those that are particularly relevant to the experience of migration. Such migrations could include refugees, guest workers (*gastarbeiter*), permanent emigrants, students studying abroad, temporary expatriate workers. The unifying theme among them all is one of transition between cultures. Some of the factors reviewed below will be more relevant to some groups than to others.

Pre-migration

Self-selection, or the 'drift hypothesis', refers to the notion that migration may be particularly attractive to people who are predisposed to mental disorder. Following on from this is the idea of biased migration where a country actually facilitates the migration of its least desirable citizens (e.g. paupers, criminals and those with chronic mental disorders). Forced migration may occur to escape death, imprisonment or poverty, for example, and it seems to be the case that the more involuntary a migration is, the more likely it is to act as a precipitating factor in mental disorder. Migration as a national policy does not necessarily imply that it need be official government policy, e.g. in the 1970s and 1980s many Irish university graduates migrated each year because of difficulties in finding employment within Ireland, yet there were no attempts to cut back on the number of graduates that the state produced. Thus, migration may be seen as a default policy. Perhaps the other end of the spectrum is migration that results from traumatic events. This is commonly associated with the migration of political prisoners or refugees who may have witnessed distressing events or been tortured and may present with various stress-related reactions, including post-traumatic stress disorder (PTSD). The final pre-migration factor described by Westermeyer (1989) is lack of preparation. Desirable preparation may include language training, prior experience of separation from those left behind and a plan for acculturation.

Culture

A number of cultural factors may explicitly cause or precipitate mental disorder. 'Culture shock' has already been described. 'Future shock' refers to the rapid technological advancement and social changes that many societies are experiencing. These changes may be unsettling, disorienting and lack integration, especially when encountered through migration as opposed to 'accelerated modernisation', which may also present challenges to social relationships and personal well-being (as discussed earlier in this chapter). Demodernisation stress can occur when people fail to adapt to their new environment, e.g. immigrants from tropical areas who fail to adapt their dress to colder northern climates may experience frostbite, whereas those from northern climates who migrate to tropical areas may risk dehydration and heat stroke by failing to dress appropriately. Similarly moving from humid to arid areas (or vice versa) or from low to high latitudes each have various maladies associated with them. Perhaps more expectedly the term 'demodernisation stress' also describes the difficulties encountered when an individual moves from what he or she considers to be a 'more modern' (usually technologically sophisticated) to a 'less modern' environment. We have already reviewed the importance of language/communication including verbal and non-verbal communications. 'Acculturation stresses' refers to the conflicts in the long-term adjustment to a new system of living and has also been described else-where. Finally, minority status is often a new experience for many migrants who originate from places where 'their type' is in the majority. This new status may single the individual out as different and through prejudice of the major-ity, or fear within the minority, produce many concomitant stresses.

Social factors

A related but distinguishable category of causes and precipitating factors for mental disorder is social factors. Migration usually involves the loss of an indi-vidual's social network and this will obviously influence the amount of social support available to a person, which might enable him or her to cope more effectively with a stressful situation. Social isolation may therefore not only be stressful, but also act as a vulnerability factor. Such isolation may be height-ened unless immigrants move into areas where 'their type' are accepted (recall the earlier discussion of group density). Role strain may occur where people are attempting to fulfil roles (e.g. work roles) that their background, experi-ence or, more generally, their culture has not prepared them for, e.g. women from cultures that have traditionally put them in the role of homemaker may struggle to adapt to the role of factory worker. Also similar social roles in their country of origin and in their new country may involve quite different skills. The process of transition may also result in a person no longer feeling part of a group. This 'marginality' may become a dual marginality if an immigrant neither identifies with their own ethnic group nor identifies with that of the place into which they have moved (marginalisation).

Unemployment may be a major stressor because it can encompasses many other negative factors such as poverty, or lack of an occupational role, social network, or opportunities to maintain or enhance self-esteem. Prejudice and bigotry will inevitably lead to increased psychological burden on immigrants. It is likely to be at its worst in situations of high local unemployment, com-munities with little ethnic diversity and communities with a history of dom-ination by one ethnic group where unwritten rules about access of certain ethnic groups to particular areas, residences, jobs, etc. apply. The last example listed by Westermeyer (1989) under the social category is 'iatrogenic morbid-ity'. Iatrogenic refers to the induction of further (or a different type of) dis-tress or illness in a person as a result of a clinician's attempts to treat that person. Westermeyer argues that treating people from different cultures may result in failures to communicate different understandings surrounding their problems (i.e. diagnosis, treatment, expectations of each other), coupled with factors such as poor social support, and may result in worsening or additional problems for the person. The importance of such communication is discussed further in Chapter 6.

Family

Various factors relating more directly to the family may also cause or precip-itate mental disorder. Sharing the same past, the same migration and the same new environment can strengthen family relationships, whereas solo migra-tion, or migration of only some members of the family, reduces this poten-tially positive effect and may psychologically distance family members from each other. However, family expectations of, for example, a son excelling aca-demically at a university abroad, or of a daughter sending money back home, may place significant additional demands on the migrant. As well as this the (different) experiences of migratory transitions can place strains on close rela-tionships, as can being separated from a partner for months or years. Differ-ent acculturation experiences may also relate to age, with younger people finding it easier to adapt to the different lifestyle of a new culture than older people. Also many immigrants may leave behind a society where being older is associated with greater wisdom and being shown more respect, and enter into a society where elderly people are seen as 'spent'. Naturally such a change in status can be very distressing and fuel intergenerational conflicts.

Psychological

For those migrating permanently or for prolonged periods a sense of loss and grieving after what has been left behind, including a particular self-identity, are a common reaction. Homesickness, obsessively longing for the 'home', may be an aspect of this. Self-perception may also be an important issue for those with experiences of combat or civil unrest, where they may feel guilt or shame about their own behaviour. Status inconsistency (already discussed) and the difficulties of integrating a meaningful self-concept may produce sig-nificant stress for an individual. Sometimes people will continue to identify with the place from which they have migrated. This reluctance to re-define oneself, 'maladaptive traditionality', may prohibit opportunities to enjoy life in a new culture. Psychological research has highlighted how an accumula-tion of negative life change events (e.g. divorce, unemployment or the loss of a loved one) or, indeed, positive life change events (e.g. marriage, childbirth or promotion in work) can be detrimental to health, especially for those already with low self-esteem.

Clearly the experience of migration not only includes a massive array of life changes but also, as has been mentioned, can often reduce personal resources to deal with such changes. Westermeyer (1989) also notes some potentially troublesome attitudes and expectations among some migrants. In the case of victims of pre-migration horrors he suggests that they sometimes behave as though they are owed or entitled to something as a result of their unjust persecutions. They may also project their hostility towards their persecutors as rage against those who are now trying to alleviate their suffering. Such individuals may also have unrealistically idealised expectations of what their new country can offer them.

Biological

The acute travel effects of the migratory experience are often overlooked. Travel across time zones may produce fatigue, hypoxia in jet flights, dehydration, and a plethora of other experiences that can exacerbate existing problems and stressors. In certain types of migration, where people have experienced extreme deprivation or dangerous environments, malnutrition, famine, hyperthermia, hypothermia, untreated infections, war wounds, etc. these may have led to organic brain damage. Similarly unborn infants, exposed to such problems *in utero*, as well as infants and children, may also develop organic brain damage. Add to this the presence of certain dangerous diseases that may be endemic to areas that emigrants leave (e.g. malaria or measles) and it can be seen that organic disorders may also be an important factor in precipitating or causing mental disorder. Chronic physical illnesses may be more difficult to cope with and therefore worsen in unfamiliar environments, especially where these are associated with a reduction in social support. The relevance of old age to migration has already been mentioned in a number of contexts; it is, however, noteworthy that several North American research studies have found that elderly migrants have a higher rate of psychiatric hospitalisation than elderly native-born 'Americans'. The reasons for this are not clear but may well relate more to the psychosocial factors (described above) than to strictly biological ones (Westermeyer, 1989).

Other factors could surely be added to Westermeyer's list and some people would argue about the relative strength and prevalence of the factors presented here. However, there should be no attempt to neglect the diversity that exists within any group of refugees, students, sojourners, *gastarbeiter*, tourists or whoever, by developing a caricature of them. I see Westermeyer's list of factors as a useful checklist of issues that may be influencing how well people are adapting to their migration experience and how this may interact with their health, both mental and physical. As we have focused on mental aspects of migration, let us briefly consider how these may interact with physical well-being.

Cancer and the stress of immigration

From the end of 1989 to June 1992, 380,152 Jews from the former Soviet Union immigrated to Israel, increasing that country's population by almost 10%.

Adverse conditions in the Soviet Union, such as political instability, economic hardship, national conflicts and fear of increasing anti-Semitism, motivated these migrants, many of whom knew very little about Israel. In Israel they confronted severe housing shortages and high levels of unemployment along with the radically different culture of Israel. During this time, Baider and colleagues (1996) from Hadassah University in Jerusalem studied the adjustment and psychological distress of 116 of these immigrants who had cancer and compared them with 288 healthy immigrants, who had also come from the former Soviet Union.

They found that all immigrants, whether physically healthy or not, reported significant adjustment problems. Sixty per cent of the physically healthy group reported that their employment, economic and social conditions were *worse* in Israel than in Russia. Among the cancer patients this was even stronger, with almost 80% judging their social situation in Israel to be worse than it was in Russia. Both groups scored highly in terms of mental distress, with the mean score in both the male and female cancer patients exceeding the cut-off (on the Brief Symptom Inventory) for mental disorder 'caseness'. The average age of cancer patients was significantly higher than that of the physically healthy control group and this factor might also have contributed to their distress, in that they may have been less adaptable. In addition the majority (almost 90%) of the cancer patients had been diagnosed since arriving in Israel. Putting all of these factors together – recent serious diagnosis, being older, recently arriving in a new country, being out of work, economically worse off and possibly having less social support – we can appreciate that the health of these migrants was influenced by many more factors than having to adapt to a different culture. So it is with any cultural group entering into a different culture. They do not bring only their culture with them but also a plethora of demographic and psychosocial factors that may place them at risk and make their recovery more problematic.

The study by Baider and colleagues further illustrates the complexity of the health of immigrants in its findings about social support. It is well recognised that social support, especially support from the spouse, can be of great benefit to people attempting to cope with cancer. For the male patients in Braider et al.'s study, and for both the healthy male and healthy female immigrants, the perception of strong family support was associated with less distress. Not so for the female cancer patients, where there was no significant relationship between the level of perceived family support and psychological well-being. It may therefore be very important to note such a gender difference (also reported in other studies of adjustment to chronic disease) in designing interventions for such immigrant groups. While illustrating the complexity of individual differences within an immigrant group Baider et al.'s (1996, p. 1082) general conclusion seems justified:

> . . . cancer patients who have to cope with an additional stress (immigration in this study), should be regarded as highly vulnerable patients who, as a consequence, develop extreme psychological distress.

Refugees

Physical symptoms and distress may also be an aspect of the migration experience, even when these are not associated with pre-migration illness. I now review some interesting German research on this topic. With over one inhabitant in every 50 being a refugee, Germany has one of the highest proportions of refugees to nationals in the world. This includes recognised asylum seekers and their dependents, quota refugees accepted on account of international humanitarian actions, asylum seekers (i.e. applicants) and *de facto* refugees, i.e. people without right of asylum but who have not been expelled for humanitarian or political reasons. Clearly, this again illustrates that refugees are not a homogeneous group and that entitlement to 'refugee status', which may carry with it benefits of access to health and welfare services, does not accrue to every individual seeking refuge in a foreign country (see later).

Schwarzer, Jerusalem and Hahn (1994) from the Free University of Berlin investigated the effects of prolonged unemployment and lack of social support among 235 East German refugees. In fact, although most of their sample were indeed refugees, 62% of them having come to West Berlin before the opening of the Berlin Wall on 9 November 1989, the remaining 38% were technically legal migrants because they arrived after this date. These two groups were, however, treated together because there were no significant psychological differences between the two groups.

The outcome variable for the study was a 24-item self-report measure of physical symptoms including heart complaints, pains in the limbs, stomach complaints and exhaustion. Each item was scored on a five-point Likert-type scale. Measures of physical symptoms, social support and employment status were taken at three different times over the 2 years after their transition to West Berlin. Those who were always jobless over the 2-year period reported significantly more physical symptoms than those who were employed. In addition, those who received less social support (determined by a median split) reported significantly more physical symptoms than those who received more social support. However, the really interesting question was how these factors would interact. Figure 4.3, which documents these results, illustrates a significant interaction between employment status and social support. Those who experienced both unemployment and relatively low levels of social support reported the highest levels of physical symptoms at each of the three points of measurement. Those who remained jobless from time 1 to time 3, but who received high levels of social support, showed a dramatic improvement in reported physical symptoms over time. This effect appears to reflect the 'buffer' effect of social support, i.e. receiving a high level of social support buffers, or reduces, the detrimental effects that stress can have on health.

It is clearly desirable for refugees, migrants or anyone else entering a new society to have the opportunity for employment. Employment not only gives

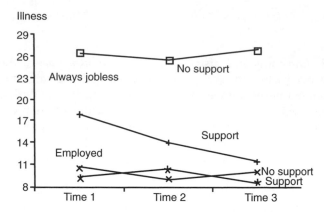

Figure 4.3 Employment, social support and physical symptoms among East German 'refugees' (reproduced from Schwarzer et al., 1994, with permission).

economic benefits but also provides psychological benefits through giving a sense of purpose and social benefits as a result of the social role(s) that go hand in hand with a job. In addition to this it also acts as a gateway to social support from colleagues. The unfortunate reality is that many immigrants find it very difficult to get a job in their new country, at least initially. Studies such as that by Schwarzer and colleagues (1994) illustrate how unemployed immigrants living in communities that afford them little social support are likely to experience more symptoms of physical illness. It is also quite possible that this increased level of illness will ultimately place greater demands on health services than would be the case if more social support were available.

On the basis of this line of argument it is therefore very important for health professionals actively to advocate the settlement of immigrants in environments that will afford them the maximum social support and therefore the maximum buffer against the development of certain physical symptoms. The health of people travelling across cultures is not simply determined by what they have left behind them or by what they bring with them, but by how they are received. Their reception into communities capable of providing meaningful social support may be the greatest help that we as clinicians can give them. It should not be assumed that such a community will necessarily be a clone of their culture of origin, because other research suggests that too strong an identification with the culture of origin may make the acculturative experience more stressful (see Dona & Berry, 1994). Nevertheless, the social context into which immigrants are expected to commune must be one that knows how to welcome, embrace and support its new members in ways that recognise their customs. The case study below describes the situation of a refugee family after leaving their home country. It conveys something of the circumstances that refugees may have left behind them before becoming permanent residents in another country.

Case study: running from fear

The following referral letter is based on my own case material.

The letter was addressed to a Senior Protection Officer, resident at a United Nations High Commissioner for Refugees (UNHCR) office, and recommends that UNHCR evacuates a family to elsewhere.

Mr S. Naik,
Senior Protection Officer,
UNHCR,

Dear Mr Naik,
At the request of an official of the Baptist Church in Bowali, I interviewed Mr and Mrs Zimba on the 10 June in order to assess their mental state.

Mr and Mrs Zimba and their five children have been refugees for some time. They experienced the trauma of imperative forced flight from their country of origin and several subsequent relocations. They have had difficulties integrating with local and refugee communities because of a continuing fear for their safety. They are concerned that certain factions from their country of origin are attempting to trace them with the purpose of killing them. The fact that close friends of theirs who were forced to leave the same country, recently died under suspicious circumstance appears to give some credence to their fears. The Zimbas, who might otherwise be expected to make a meaningful contribution to society, find themselves in a state of insecurity, bewilderment, disorientation and alienation.

In the case of Mrs Zimba this has recently driven her to attempt suicide. She has also expressed the idea of 'saving her children from the world'. At interview she presented with depressed affect and reported feelings of pessimism and helplessness. In addition I understand that she has been confused and disorientated in the past few weeks. Mr Zimba has been a constant source of support and strength to his wife throughout their exile. However, I feel that the pressures of this commitment are now beginning to affect his own judgement and that he is floundering, reporting both anxious and depressive experiences. In my estimation there is a real and frightening potential for self-destruction within the family. They continue to struggle with their perceived insecurity and an environment which offers little support and no realistic prospects of employment. There is very little professional support available to the Zimbas in the town of Bowali; the Zimbas do not speak the local language and there are significant cultural differences between this country and their country of origin.

I strongly recommend that the Zimba family be evacuated to a secure environment which can provide the level of professional support they require. Being fluent in English they have expressed a wish to be sent to an English-speaking country which has some experience in receiving

refugees. I would like to end on a positive note by saying that Mr and Mrs Zimba are clearly intelligent people with the ability to make a genuine contribution to a host society, rather than simply being 'accommodated' by one. I believe that in time a recipient country would benefit from accepting them.
Your sincerely,

Unfortunately in the case of the Zimbas, although they were evacuated to an English-speaking country, they had great difficulties in attaining any sort of employment. They found it impossible to gain employment at an equivalent level of professionalism as they were employed at in their own country. Such factors may have a profound effect on their health for as we have seen social support and employment may influence the psychological stress associated with pre-existing problems.

Migration and a loss of resources

In Chapter 2 we considered in some detail Berry's acculturation framework, and noted Lazarus and Folkman's (1984) cognitive model of stress, where an individual's appraisal of stressors in relation to their own ability to cope is seen as crucial. It may be argued that the former overworks the influence of cultural factors, whereas the latter overworks the influence of personal coping. This chapter ends by returning to the idea of stress and coping, and a recent application of it which takes into account the influence of migrants' official legal status. Hobfoll's (2001, p. 341) Conservation of Resources (COR) Theory of stress has as its central tenet the idea that: 'individuals strive to obtain, retain, protect and foster things that they value'. Resources are what one values. They vary from basic resources (food, housing, clothing) to more abstract ones (loyalty, positively challenging routine), the latter being more influenced by cultural differences. Psychological stress is seen to arise from the threat of loss, or actual loss, of resources, or where resource investment fails to produce the expected return. Two key principles of COR are that (1) 'resource loss is disproportionately more salient than resource gain' (p. 343), and (2) 'people must invest resources in order to protect against resource loss, recover from losses, and gain resources' (p. 349). In this theory resources are used to satisfy needs, pursue goals and meet demands. However, presumably some stressful things can be experienced – witnessing traumatic events – which although they could be construed as 'resource loss' are in reality more of a 'harm' than a 'loss' (see Lazarus & Folkman, 1984; Ryan, 2005).

Ryan (2005) used the COR model to explore the ideas of resource loss and gain, in the context of the migration process. He added the term 'cultural resources' to describe 'knowledge and beliefs that are learned within a particular cultural setting, and whose adaptation value is often intimately related to their being deployed in such a setting or in similar ones' (p. 33). Cleary these 'cultural resources' overlap with other 'psychological resources' and are patterned by the social norms and needs of the cultural context into which people are socialised. A consideration of migrants' resource pool during pre-migration, migration (flight) and post-migration phases may be illuminating. Ryan (2005, p. 43) argues that:

> Negative psychological outcomes are likely to arise when the host environment places constraints on, or depletes the migrant's existing resources, while offering few opportunities for resource gain. Psychological distress can be understood as the result of unmet needs, the loss or blocking of goals and exposure to an unmanageable level of demands.

Identifying methods to minimise resource loss and promote resource gain among migrants is therefore essential.

Ryan's (2005) own empirical work examined the experiences of forced migrants in Ireland – those who came to Ireland because they were involuntarily displaced from their home communities. His primary interest was the stress implications of either having legal status (refugees) or not having legal status (asylum seekers) – legal status being seen as a key resource. In a longitudinal study with a 12- to 24-month follow-up period, he followed up 70 of the original 162 participants, and showed that those who had obtained legal status in the intervening period were the ones who experienced a significant decrease in stress (including psychological and psychiatric symptoms). In addition to not having legal status, other distress risk factors included female gender, welfare dependency and separation from children, loneliness and the experience of discrimination. Protective factors included social support, the presence of a partner in Ireland and strong religiosity or spirituality (Ryan, 2005).

Conclusion

In this chapter we considered the complexities of charting depression across different cultures. Considering a particular disorder from different cultural perspectives can sharpen one's understanding and it can also question one's assumptions. It is when we see our own society as one of many cultures that we can operate most effectively as multicultural practitioners. This perspective is vital if we are to avoid making serious errors in the hazardous diagnosis of conditions such as personality disorder, where being exposed to the 'right ' kind of socialisation may be very important. Understanding how changing 'contemporary' social contexts, as well as different 'traditional' cultural practices, may contribute to mental health and suicide is very important. The social context of mental health is nowhere more clearly represented than in the plight of many minority immigrant groups who live at social, political and economic disadvantage. Yet these factors, and culture, do not divide our experience of the world into neat 'mental' and 'physical' boxes; rather they are each part of the same experience. In Chapter 5 I consider the physical aspect of culture and our experience of health.

Guidelines for professional practice

1. Research on cross-cultural mental health is very diverse and includes comparative, ethnic minority and transitional approaches among others. Although there is overlap between these areas of research they are undertaken with different questions in mind and in different contexts and settings. It may not therefore be legitimate to generalise results derived from one of these approaches to problems encountered in another approach.

2. Clinicians should avoid the temptation to assimilate an unfamiliar form of suffering into a familiar diagnostic system. An example of this may be seen in attempts to 'fit' a range of somatic symptoms (which occur in many and diverse cultures) into the diagnostic category of depression.

3. Clinicians should attempt to understand the meaning of a person's problem within that person's terms of reference. Such 'terms of reference' are likely to reflect not only cultural norms but also social, economic and political factors.

4. Cultural identity is a community resource that is relevant to healthcare. The individuals within a community may be healthier if their culture is in the majority or is at least a sizable minority. Clinicians should inform people of the possible negative health consequences of moving from communities where their cultural group is in a majority to communities where their cultural group is in the minority. Higher rates of psychological disturbance are generally associated with group minority status.

5. The use of western-based diagnostic systems may misclassify certain cultural behaviours as disorders. An example of this is the category of personality disorder, which describes socially inappropriate ways of behaving within most western cultures. Clinicians should seek to understand the intended function of unusual behaviours and explore the extent to which the observed behaviour might be functional within their client's culture.

6. Although a cultural perspective on suicide dates back to the nineteenth century, contemporary thinking emphasises primarily biological and cognitive factors. Of course these are very important, particularly with regard to the proximate causes of suicide. However, to understand why suicide rates vary so dramatically among age groups, genders and ethnic groups, we need to consider much broader cultural and social change factors. These factors are very relevant both at the social policy level and for planning community support and intervention.

7. The experience of transition may constitute a serious stressor in itself and/or may aggravate existing mental and physical health problems. A number of factors detailed in Table 4.6 may be related to the onset of a migration-related disorder.

8. Migration involves not only a change of cultural settings but also economic, political and social factors that may all impact on health. Clinicians should broaden their own frame of reference to include the many factors that impinge upon an individual's health. Although individual clinicians may

not be able to influence many of the broader issues directly, the clinician's acknowledgement of them can legitimise the distress experienced by their clients.

9. One of the issues becoming increasingly important in managing the acculturative stress of refugees is the response of people in the country into which they migrate. Recent research has shown that the legal status of refugees contributes significantly to their level of psychological distress. It is important for practitioners to recognise that legalistic and administrative aspects of a refugee's experience may interplay with the disorders with which they present.

CHAPTER 5

Culture and physical health

This chapter reviews the influence that cultural differences may have on physical health. It is once again worth emphasising that cultural differences do not occur in isolation. They can be associated with socioeconomic, environmental, dietary, behavioural and genetic variations. It is therefore often a matter of relating physical health to cultural variation through one of these routes, e.g. the relatively high incidence of sickle-cell anaemia among west African men can be attributed to genetic factors. Different 'dietary cultures' may also account for the high incidence of rickets in some immigrant groups. The effects of dietary variations are also evident in the well-known difficulties that Chinese people have in metabolising milk-based products, or which Europeans have in dealing with a genuine Vindaloo curry! However, before reviewing this literature I would like to argue for culture having a much broader impact on physical health than suggested above. There are two aspects to this argument: the first is that psychosocial processes influence physical health and the second that some cultural differences relate also to health (perhaps through the psychosocial processes that have been shown to be important). Following our review of these issues I consider to what extent cultural groups may differ in their health problems, whether cultures understand the physical body in different ways and how different cultures react to various diseases.

Psychosocial processes and physical health

Steptoe (1991) has described three ways in which psychological and social factors can be linked to physical disease states: psychophysiological hyperactivity, disease stability and progression and host vulnerability. The first of these, psychophysiological hyperactivity, refers to the effects that continuous stress can produce on the body. Many people react similarly to severe momentary stress with, for instance, palpitations, sweating, breathlessness and perhaps trembling. However, if an individual is continuously in a stressful environment this level of physiological responding cannot be sustained, so physiological arousal declines and there may be few visible signs of stress. Nevertheless the body is in quite a different physiological state from when it is relaxed. After prolonged stress and the attempts of body's systems to adapt to their increased physiological demands, the body becomes depleted of its ability to fight off infection and to supply its various organs with sufficient resources. Physiological damage may occur in any of the body's systems or organs. Individuals differ in the physiological problems that they develop in response to prolonged stress. It is almost as though we have a physiological 'Achilles' heel', a relative weakness in our physiological make-up that is therefore relatively more vulnerable to the effects of prolonged stress.

Psychosocial processes may also be linked to disease through their influence on disease stability and progression. In this case we are not talking of psychosocial causes of disease but of how psychosocial processes may influence existing disease, whatever its cause, e.g. a person may suffer from asthma, but exactly when he or she has an asthma attack or how severe the attack is can be influenced by psychosocial factors such as the degree of stress in their immediate environment.

A third way in which psychosocial factors are linked with disease is through their influence on host vulnerability. In this case the physiological effects of stress have no direct influence on disease. However, as described above, the prolonged effects of stress deplete the resources of the body. One aspect of this is that the body's immune system is suppressed so that its ability to fight off invasive pathogens is diminished. The body becomes more susceptible to infections. So, for instance, it has been found that people are more likely to develop a common cold when they are under stress. Although there are 'colds' out there all the time, usually we are able to fight them off. Thus stress does not give you the 'cold', but, should you encounter the cold virus, it makes you more vulnerable to it.

There is now a convincing literature to support the existence of the above pathways between psychosocial processes and physical disease, and these pathways incorporate a diverse range of factors (see Steptoe & Wardle, 1994). Wilkinson and Marmot (2003) recently summarised evidence regarding the link between psychosocial factors and health – *both mental and physical health*. The 10 that they highlight, and their accompanying summary statements, are quoted below:

1. *Social gradient*: 'Life expectancy is shorter and most diseases are more common further down the social ladder in each society.'
2. *Stress*: 'Stressful circumstances, making people feel worried, anxious and unable to cope, are damaging to health and may lead to premature death.'
3. *Early life*: 'A good start in life means supporting mothers and young children: the health impact of early development and education lasts a lifetime.'
4. *Social exclusion*: 'Life is short where its quality is poor. By causing hardship and resentment, poverty, social exclusion and discrimination costs lives.'
5. *Work*: 'Stress in the workplace increases the risk of disease. People who have more control over their work have better health.'

6. *Unemployment*: 'Job security increases health, well-being and job satisfaction. Higher rates of unemployment cause more illness and premature death.'
7. *Social support*: 'Friendships, good social relations and strong supportive networks improve health at home, at work and in the community.'
8. *Addiction*: 'Individuals turn to alcohol, drugs and tobacco and suffer from their use, but use is influenced by the wider social setting.'
9. *Food*: 'Because global market forces control the food supply, healthy food is a political issue.'
10. *Transport*: 'Healthy transport means less driving and more walking and cycling, backed up by better public transport.'

The social gradient effect – the further down the social ladder people are the worse is their health – is independent of levels of poverty, such that, even among middle-class office workers, the lower ranking staff suffer much more disease, as well as earlier death, than higher ranking staff.

Cultural differences and physical health

The summary statements above derive from a panel of distinguished international experts, whose purview is backed up by thousands of research papers on the topics. For our purposes it is clear that marginalised ethnic, minority or migrant groups fall victim to many of these: often being lower down the social gradient, experiencing greater stress, often with unstable early life situations, marked social exclusion and poorer access to work, and higher rates of unemployment, often accompanied by poor social support, and sometimes higher rates of consumption of addictive substances and less healthy food. In fact, about the only thing that may be in the favour of some minority groups is their greater reliance on their feet, as opposed to their car, to get about!

We have already reviewed in Chapter 4 how the stress associated with migration may result in the worsening of existing physical illness, such as cancer, or the development of new physical problems. We have also noted that minority cultural groups may exist in social and economic contexts that are stressful and threatening to their health and general well-being. These factors must be kept in mind when examining the more abstract concept of culture in relation to health and disease.

Dimensions of culture associated with disease

In Chapter 2 we reviewed some large-scale studies of how cultures differ along certain social dimensions, which had the virtue of being empirically identified (rather than simply being a product of theorising) and can be related to health in as much as they may relate to the social processes described above, e.g. it has been suggested that cultures that put an emphasis on collectivism have a prophylactic effect on disease because they promote harmony within small supportive groups. This would imply that levels of disease in collectivist cultures are lower than in individualist cultures (see Triandis et al., 1988).

Bond (1991) specifically addressed the relationship between different cultural values and physical health. First of all, Bond explored the extent to which people from different countries held certain values to be important. The variation among 23 countries was simplified statistically into two dimensions. The first of these dimensions has 'social integration' at one pole and 'cultural inwardness' at the other pole. Social integration refers to holding values of tolerance towards and harmony with others. This pole also emphasises patience, non-competitiveness, trustworthiness and persistence. Social integration thus reflects the coming together of people, perhaps from different cultures, in an environment that nurtures social relationships. The polar opposite of this is cultural inwardness, which includes values of respect for tradition, a sense of cultural superiority and the observation of rites and social rituals.

The second dimension identified by Bond had 'reputation' at one pole and 'morality' as its polar opposite. Here reputation is concerned with protecting your 'face' (in the sense of not losing face), reciprocation of favours and gifts, and the possession of wealth. Morality, on the other hand, is concerned with a sense of righteousness, keeping oneself 'disinterested and pure' and chastity in women. This second dimension could therefore be thought of as a dimension of 'appearing good'–'behaving good'. What is intriguing about Bond's study is that these dimensions, which initially appear rather abstract and hard to grasp, do indeed appear to have relevance to physical diseases.

It is well known that the level of economic development within a country influences the health of its citizens. However, the relationship between Bond's dimensions and disease held up even after the influence of gross national product (GNP), per capita, was controlled for. It therefore appears that variations in cultural values can account for at least some of the variation in disease prevalence across countries. Furthermore, although these two dimensions could predict the occurrence of a range of diseases in different countries, the dimensions were not themselves associated with life expectancy. In other words, their ability to predict the occurrence of disease is not confounded by variations in average life expectancy in different countries.

Let us look at some of these relationships in more detail. There was a statistically significant association between holding the values of 'social integration' and the increased incidence of cerebrovascular disease, ulcers of the stomach and duodenum, and neoplasms of the stomach, colon, rectum, rectosigmoid junction and anus. This array of ailments would suggest that strong endorsement of the values of social integration may, somehow, be particularly deleterious to the functioning of the digestive system. Endorsement of the values at the other end of this dimension, 'cultural inwardness', was not significantly related to any of the diseases studied. On the basis of these data it could therefore be argued that 'cultural inwardness' is a healthier outlook than 'social integration'. However, a careful consideration of these findings suggests a more complex situation.

We have already noted suggestions that collectivism could be a health-promoting attribute because it encourages harmony and social support between members of an 'in group' (e.g. the extended family, work colleagues or neighbours). It seems that individuals living in a collectivist society exhibit these positive behaviours only towards other members of their 'in group' and not towards other individuals in the society at large. This focuses the therapeutic impact of 'cultural inwardness' at the community level. It is at this level that 'cultural inwardness', through processes such as collectivism, may benefit the health of people. Communities that do not offer social support or foster harmony between their members will strip individuals of an important coping mechanism, and the resultant 'cultural isolation' may, somehow, cause a high incidence of cerebrovascular disease and diseases of the digestive system.

This is another argument for allowing different cultural groups to establish a genuine 'sense of community' wherever they are living, rather than support the 'melting pot' notion of different cultures finding a common denominator. Bond's research can thus be interpreted as supporting the integrity of cultural communities as a mechanism for promoting health. However, communities also function in a wider context. For communities to provide their potential benefits, the societies in which they live need to be tolerant towards them. In recent years there has been much debate on whether immigrants should locate in areas where their predecessors settled or whether they should 'integrate' with the nationals of the host country. It would seem that 'cultural inwardness' is the healthiest option in the short term, for the reasons outlined above. In the long term, when immigrants are genuinely accepted as a part of a local community, they may then accrue the same health benefits from such communities as they do from their own 'cultural community'. It would, however, also be important to investigate how the effect of group densities (Halpern, 1993; see Chapter 4) interacts with long- and short-term integration strategies.

Bond's (1991) second dimension, 'reputation–morality', was also related to physical health. The 'reputation' end of this dimension was significantly associated with acute myocardial infarction and other ischaemic heart disease. In addition, it was, as with the other dimension, associated with neoplasms of the colon, rectum, rectosigmoid junction and anus, as well as of the trachea, bronchi and lungs. The influence of the 'reputation' end of this dimension thus seems to be quite pervasive, influencing cardiac function and the digestive and respiratory systems. The opposite end of the dimension, 'morality', was significantly associated with only one disease, cirrhosis of the liver. Taking the two dimensions together, the strongest relationship was with neoplasms of the rectum, rectosigmoid junction and anus. However, among the diseases studied by Bond, neither of these dimensions was related to the occurrence of other diseases, such as chronic rheumatic disease, atherosclerosis, hypertension or neoplasms of the breast and cervix uteri.

Why statistically significant relationships exist between each dimension and some diseases, but not others, is not clear. It may be that some diseases are more influenced than others by the psychosocial processes on which cultures have an impact. It may also be that some diseases are influenced by psychosocial or cultural factors of which we are as yet unaware. Clearly much research is needed to clarify such links. From the point of view of our present argument, the point to be taken on board is that cultural variations in values are associated with the occurrence of some diseases, so cultural differences are indeed related to physical health.

Are some cultures healthier than others?

If cultural differences are related to health, this begs the question 'Are some cultures healthier than others?' The simple answer seems to be 'yes'. Of particular interest here are the Seventh Day Adventist studies. One of the factors that influence the lifestyle of Seventh Day Adventists is their belief that the human body is the 'temple' of the Holy Spirit. As such, the body is a sacred place to be treated with respect. You may recall from Chapter 1 that the word 'culture' derives from the ways in which people seek to 'cultivate' a positive relationship with their god(s). As different cultures encourage different ways of living, this is another way in which culture can influence physical health.

Seventh Day Adventists constitute a culture (or at least of particular 'religious culture') that has communities throughout the world. Ilola (1990, p. 287), reviewing studies on Seventh Day Adventists, states that 'numerous studies from different countries have shown that Seventh Day Adventists (SDAs) live longer and are healthier than their country-men'. The diet of Seventh Day Adventists, based on biblical principles, is around unrefined foods, grains, vegetable protein, fruits and vegetables. A survey of 40,000 Seventh Day Adventists in the USA found that half were vegetarian, 90% did not consume alcohol, 84% drank less than one cup of coffee a day and 99% did not smoke. Compared with the general population Seventh Day Adventists appear to have a lower incidence of lung cancer or breast cancer, in fact cancer of any sort. For those Seventh Day Adventists who do develop cancers, they have better survival rates. Similarly, Seventh Day Adventists have a lower incidence of circulatory diseases. Australian studies have found lower systolic and diastolic blood pressure, lower plasma cholesterol levels and higher lung ventilator capacity in Seventh Day Adventists, compared with the general population. Thus both risk factors and serious diseases appear to be less prevalent in Seventh Day Adventist communities than in the general population of their co-nationals.

Ilola also suggests that the degree of adherence to the Seventh Day Adventist lifestyle constitutes a dose–response relationship, in that less adherence is associated with greater health risk. The Seventh Day Adventist studies illustrate the importance of lifestyle for health. Every culture encourages a particular 'style' of living. When these styles are analysed in terms of the ingestion of foods and other substances, they produce powerful predictors of physical health. Indeed it is through 'consumption customs' that culture, quite literally, 'gets inside of you'.

More recently Willcox, Willcox and Suzuki (2001) studied the world's longest-lived population and claim that by following 'the Okinawa way', health and longevity can be improved dramatically. The Okinawa islands (of which there are 161) are a state (or prefecture) off Japan to its south (formally known as the Kingdom of Ryukyus). In Okinawa, the three leading causes of death in the west – coronary heart disease, stroke and cancer – occur with the lowest frequency of anywhere in the world. Through the Okinawa Centenarian Study, Willcox et al. gathered data over a 25-year period. They recorded over 400 centenarians in a population of just over 1.3 million – about 34/100,000, compared with a rate of about 5–10/100,000 in the USA.

This 'culture of health' is characterised by a combination of a low-calorie, plant-based diet high in unrefined carbohydrates; their stress-reducing psychospiritual outlook' related to Taoism and Confucianism; their life-long commitment to exercise through different aspects of their life (martial arts, traditional dance, gardening and walking); their socially supportive practices (e.g. deep respect for others, obligations to help others and expectations of reciprocity); and the integration of eastern and western healthcare practices. Although the authors are aware of the potential influence of genetic factors, they see lifestyle factors as much stronger causal agents and note that when people (particularly the younger generation) deviate from these (and adopt a more western lifestyle) they do not have the associated health benefits. The authors believe 'it's not the cards we're dealt, but how we play them' that is the greater influence on longevity, at least in the case of Okinawa.

Cultures and their health problems

It would be wrong to suggest that cultural variations, be it in terms of behaviour, nutrition or other factors, can account for diseases of all kinds. This is certainly not the case. Some diseases are caused by factors quite unrelated to sociocultural processes. Even here it is worth acknowledging, however, that the way in which such diseases are experienced, expressed and treated may well be influenced, to some extent at least, by cultural factors. Notwithstanding this important point, I would like to review some forms of physical suffering that are found more commonly in certain cultural groups. Black (1989) describes four types of disease categories that are especially relevant to different cultural groups: genetically determined diseases, acquired diseases, diseases that result from the use of indigenous medicines and practices, and diseases related to the poor socioeconomic conditions in which many immigrant groups find themselves (discussed earlier). In this section we consider some examples from the first three of these categories, giving particular emphasis to the first.

Genetically determined diseases

One hereditary blood disease, sickle-cell anaemia, is so called because the blood cells contain abnormal haemoglobin and, when the supply of oxygen is low, these cells, rather than being rounded, adopt the quarter moon shape of a sickle. They then carry less oxygen than the normal rounded blood cells, and also gather together in the bloodstream, preventing their passage along capillaries and causing infarction blockages. As a consequence the supply of oxygen to vital organs may be reduced or interrupted. This may result in progressive organ failure and brain damage.

Sickle-cell anaemia is caused by a recessive gene, and most people who have this gene are carriers but not sufferers. However, if two people with the recessive gene have a child, that child could experience sickle-cell anaemia. The sickle-cell gene has a high frequency of occurrence in a number of countries, especially western parts of Africa and southern India. Although its high rates of occurrence in the West Indies and the USA may be historically accounted for by the slave trade, it is also found in the indigenous population of the north coast of the Mediterranean, the Persian Gulf and Saudi Arabia. Thus, immigrants from any of these areas will have a 'higher than local average' chance of having or transmitting the disease. Sickle-cell anaemia is of course just one of many genetically determined blood diseases that occur with different frequencies across cultural groups. For those involved in diagnosing and treating such diseases knowledge of these cultural variations is vital.

Although sickle-cell anaemia may be genetically determined it is important to note that, although more common in black people, it appears to result not from 'race' but from geographical origin (Williams et al., 1994). In Africa, it is believed to have occurred for hundreds of years along the Nile, and to have an adaptive function – to increase resistance to malaria transmission from the mosquito *Anopheles* species (Giger & Davidhizar, 1999).

A second example of a genetically determined disease is lactase deficiency, which is caused by a recessive gene with high penetrance, i.e. although the gene responsible for lactase deficiency is recessive, it usually manages to penetrate into the phenotype and its effects are expressed. The symptoms of lactase deficiency become apparent when an individual consumes milk-based products. In older children (aged 6–7 years and above) and adults the consumption of milk results in abdominal distension, flatulence, abdominal pain or discomfort, and occasionally diarrhoea. Although not necessarily a serious condition it is nevertheless interesting: it is a product not of genetics alone, but of an interaction between environmental (actually ecocultural) factors and genetics. I first learnt about lactase deficiency through being told that Chinese people were unable to tolerate a high intake of milk-based products. The rather ethnocentric inference was that 'the rest of us' were. In fact, the great majority of the world's population is 'lactase deficient'.

At birth we are all endowed with intestinal lactase and this helps us to break down and metabolise our mother's milk. For most people, the amount of lactase produced in their intestine declines to relatively low levels by about the age of 6 or 7. It remains at this lower level from then on. However, for the majority of north, central and western Europeans, and their descendants, as well as some nomadic cultures that depend on the consumption of large amounts of milk from goats or camels, the level of intestinal lactase remains undiminished throughout life. This lactase retention appears to be the result of a dominant gene with high penetrance. Once again, because of the genetic basis of lactase intolerance, its incidence varies geographically. People of Chinese decent do indeed appear to have one of the highest levels of lactase intolerance. However, only a minority of these may become symptomatic after drinking, say, a glass of milk. Nevertheless it is important for clinicians to recognise the cultural distribution of this disease and to avoid confusing it with milk allergy.

As a final point on genetically determined conditions, it is important to acknowledge that sometimes these diseases are, in fact, a direct product of cultural practices, e.g. among Asian Moslems, marriages between first or second cousins are more common than in other cultures. This practice increases the likelihood of their children falling victim to recessive metabolic disorders and possibly of a child being born malformed. However, it is also very important to emphasise that, among such consanguineous marriages, the probability of such occurrences is still extremely low.

Acquired diseases

Nutritional rickets refers to faulty or inadequate bone growth and it has proved a particular problem among Asian immigrants to Britain. Black (1989) describes a number of factors contributing to rickets in Asian children: inadequate exposure to sunlight (possibly as a result of the Moslem custom of covering the arms and legs); strict vegetarian diet (especially for Hindus); use of cows' milk for infant feeding (having little vitamin D); maternal deficiency of vitamin D; and a poor uptake of vitamin preparations. The 'Stop Rickets' and 'Asian Mother and Baby' campaigns specifically targeted Asian communities in Britain. These initiatives aimed to create awareness of the role of vitamin D in maintaining good health, with programmes recognising that each cultural group had to be targeted in a manner that acknowledged differences in their dietary customs, religious beliefs and socioeconomic conditions. Once again this example of nutritional rickets in immigrant Asian communities illustrates direct links between cultural customs and physical disease. However, these campaigns have also been criticised for problematising the culture of immigrants rather than recognising socioeconomic aspects of rickets as a disease of poverty (see also Chapter 8).

Traditional healing and iatrogenic diseases

Culturally 'traditional' treatments, similar to many 'modern' treatments developed in industrialised societies, sometimes produce side effects. For some treatments the unwanted effects are as predictable as the wanted, or desired, effects. This brief discussion does not therefore suggest that traditional treatments are somehow more primitive because they can produce unhealthy responses in their recipients. Anyone who doubts this need only consult the *British National Formulary* (the BNF, or 'pharmacological bible') to be aware of the huge range, sometimes fatal, of unwanted effects produced by modern medicines. Clinicians should, however, be aware of some of the more common iatrogenic problems that can result from traditional treatments or practices.

In some Asian communities there is a practice of placing black make-up (surma) around the eyes and inside the eyelids in order to prevent infections and for cosmetic effect. This 'make-up' can be made from a variety of substances, one of which is lead sulphide. Over time, with repeated use, dangerous levels of lead may be absorbed through the eyelids. The use of non-lead-based substances for this eye make-up is, however quite safe.

'Coin rubbing' is a traditional practice common among Vietnamese people, but this can produce lesions on the skin. In some unfortunate cases these marks have been misinterpreted as indications of physical child abuse. Some people of Chinese origin believe that pinching or squeezing either side of the trachea will alleviate persistent coughing. This procedure can produce considerable bruising, which might also be misinterpreted.

For another example, recall the 'female circumcision' or 'genital mutilation' described in Chapter 1. This is still practised by many peoples throughout the world, including immigrants to more industrialised societies. It can, however, without doubt produce suffering. Beyond the immediate distress that may be experienced, girls can subsequently develop serious medical conditions and find sexual intercourse painful.

Nevertheless it is important to recognise each of the above practices in their cultural context. This does not necessarily mean accepting them. Instead the clinician will be more successful in changing undesirable practices if he or she can understand them to the extent of being able to offer suggestions for their safe replacement, while still retaining some aspect of their cultural function.

Cultural understandings of the human body

It can be difficult to understand the function of a healing practice without also being aware of the rationale upon which the practice rests. Different understandings of how the human body works should, and do, lead logically to different ways of 'fixing it'. It is therefore useful briefly to consider some of the different cultural metaphors for understanding the workings of the human body. Perhaps the most widely held view is that which refers to the notion of balance and imbalance in the body. According to this concept the various systems within a healthy body are seen as being in harmony. Imbalance, causing illness, can result from physical, psychological, nutritional, environmental or spiritual influences that tip this balance.

The humoral theory is an example of a balance metaphor. This theory was developed into a systematic account of disease by Hippocrates and subsequently elaborated upon by Galen in the second century BC, spreading throughout the Roman and Arab world. Whether the presence of this theory elsewhere (e.g. throughout Latin America) derives from the same source, or can be accounted for by indigenous beliefs, is unclear. Hippocrates saw the body as being made up of four liquids or humours: blood, phlegm, yellow bile and black bile. Too much, or too little, of one of these humours would put the body 'out of balance', resulting in disease. It is also interesting to note that Hippocrates understood these humours to be linked to behaviour. His term 'melancholia' (an excess of black bile) is still in use in today's 'modern' medicine to describe behaviour of depressive affect. His other terms are also in common parlance: sanguine (meaning animated, hopeful or florid, resulting from too much blood), phlegmatic (meaning lethargic or placid, resulting from too much phlegm) and choleric (meaning bad tempered resulting from too much yellow bile). Excesses of these humours were treated by bleeding, purging, vomiting and starvation; deficits were made up through the ingestion of special medicines. Of course, these ideas continue to influence popular thinking in industrialised countries, especially with regard to maintaining an 'optimal' or balanced weight. The person with bulimia, who vomits or purges in order to retain 'a balance', is a distressing example of this.

In Latin America a common theory of disease relates to the balance between 'hot' and 'cold'. However, this categorisation does not refer to temperature as such, but rather to the 'power' intrinsic to different substances. Illness is treated by ingesting substances that counteract an imbalance. Some illnesses are 'hot', others 'cold'. Somebody who is suffering from a 'hot' condition, e.g. menstruating, would be given only 'cold' food. Another example of the concept of balance is the Chinese notion of the 'yin' and 'yang' forces. Yin has the attributes of darkness, moistness and femininity, whereas yang is characterised as being bright, hot, dry and masculine. Different organs of the body possess yin and yang in different proportion, e.g. the heart and lungs have an excess of yin, whereas the stomach and gallbladder have an excess of yang. Illness results from inappropriate combinations of yin and yang at different points of the body's interconnected energy system. One well-known way of treating such an imbalance is through acupuncture.

There are, of course, also other philosophical systems emanating from different cultures that give other accounts for how our well-being is mediated. However, once again, there is a danger of oversimplifying the relationship between culture and health. Health systems, especially those found in the western world, reflect many understandings of health. To appreciate that western healthcare does not have an absolute and definitive approach to understanding illness and well-being, let us briefly consider the work of Rogers (1991).

Rogers described seven metaphorical accounts, found in contemporary western societies, of how diseases interact with bodily function (Table 5.1). These metaphors are embraced by different subcultures to varying extents. Whatever metaphor is embraced will have consequences for understanding the cause and treatment of a disease, e.g. the 'body as machine' metaphor welcomes biomedical interventions because they represent the way to 'fix' what is 'broken'. On the other hand, the 'inequality of access' metaphor calls for

Table 5.1 A summary of Rogers' (1991) metaphors for health and illness.

Metaphor	Themes related to poor physical health
Cultural critique	Inequality, exploitation, disadvantage; modern medicine as an institution of hegemonic power often ineffective in caring or curing, possibly feminism
Willpower	Illness as a challenge; power of positive thinking will aid recovery; individual in control rather than social factors, medicine as assistance to own efforts
Health promotion	Can be avoided or delayed; due to inappropriate lifestyle, lack of equilibrium, environmental concerns, commercial exploitation, poor eduction
Body as machine	Pharmaceuticals critical in 'fixing' dysfunctions; medical excellence through technological expertise; personal responsibility for body maintenance
Inequality of access	Injustices between rich and poor; impact of capitalism; health a fundamental human right, modern medicine effective but inequitably distributed because of differences in income, class, education
Body under seige	Struggling in a hostile world; germs exploiting emotional distress; not a 'challenge'; conversion of stress into illness; self-denigration, needing help
Robust individualism	Stress and pollution of modern life; health a valued investment; self-determination; personal responsibility; consumer selection of expert opinions; healthcare in the market place

socioeconomic intervention that will distribute resources more evenly. The 'God's power' metaphor calls for the restoration of a spiritual balance through a deity that has the power to cure or kill. It is quite common for people to endorse more than one of these metaphors. Professional disputes often arise when metaphors clash and clinicians are intolerant of alternative explanations. Endorsing one metaphor over another usually has resource implications, e.g. the 'health-promotion' metaphor may call for resources to be channelled into creating healthy lifestyles, whereas the 'body under siege' metaphor encourages the development of resources for coping with problems as they arise. This might include the manufacture of vitamins or antidepressants, or the provision of relaxation exercises and rehabilitative services.

In many ways the health professions are health subcultures, each endorsing certain metaphors over others, and therefore understanding the relationship between health and disease in different ways. Within each professional subculture, as within each social group or culture, there is great variation. However, seeing different health professions as different 'cultures', which work through different 'communities', may help us to understand the interprofessional rivalry that can be a feature of multidisciplinary work. This organisational interpretation of the link between cultures, communities and health, although intriguing, is at a tangent to the purpose of this chapter. I therefore return to consider how social and cultural factors may be implicated in disease.

The colour–hypertension relationship

It is well established that dark-skinned people have significantly higher rates of hypertension than light-skinned people (e.g. Krieger & Sidney, 1996). Some people consider the relationship between 'black' skin and hypertension to be indicative of a common genetic link. For some, the finding that, among 'black' people, the darker their skin the greater the prevalence of hypertension, further reinforces this assumption. However, challenging this is the possibility that the relationship between skin colour and hypertension is entirely caused by social and psychological factors. There is now very good evidence for the link between stressful experiences and the development of hypertension (e.g. Uchino & Garvey, 1997). Could it be that black people experience more stressful prejudice than white people, and that 'black' people with darker skins experience more stressful prejudice than black people with lighter skins? If so, perhaps the colour–hypertension relationship is accounted for by differences in stress, rather than differences in skin themselves.

Klonoff and Landrine (2003) used the 'Schedule of Racist Events' (SRE) to explore exposure to stressful situations arising through racial discrimination, in a sample of 300 black men and women in the USA; (a study examining the darkness–hypertension link in a predominantly black culture, say in an African country, where we might expect loss colour prejudice, could provide illuminating data). The SRE measures both the frequency of such events and how stressful they are experienced as being. Participants also rated their skin colour along a five-point scale ('very light skinned', 'light skinned', 'medium skinned', 'dark skinned', 'very dark skinned'). Splitting the sample into two groups who experienced either relatively high or low levels of racial discrimination, they found that 65% of the group that reported high levels of racial discrimination also rated themselves as 'dark skinned', whereas only 8.5% of the group who rated themselves as 'light skinned' fell into the high discrimination group. These results therefore support the possibility that hypertension is more prevalent in dark-skinned black men because they experience more stress-related discrimination.

There was also an interesting gender difference in the results: 75% of the light-skinned groups were women, who therefore tended to be in the low discrimination group. The likelihood that black women's self-rated skin colour actually was lighter than that of the men's self-rated skin colour is supported by other studies that have found the same result when skin colour has been measured objectively (e.g. Krieger, Sidney & Coakley, 1998). It seems that not only do black women have greater concerns about skin colour than black men, but they also use more skin-bleaching creams (Russel, Wilson & Hall, 1992). For those who doubt the extent to which darker black skin may be seen as less socially desirable and associated with greater racial discrimination, it is worth reflecting on the motivation of some black women to diminish their darker appearance – their attempt to construct a different bodily appearance in order to be seen as more socially acceptable.

Constructions and reactions

When people from different cultures suffer with the same disease they will naturally use different terms to describe it, because their languages are different. However, even when the same language is used, in the same country, confusion can still arise. Ilola (1990) describes a young physician, trained in a metropolitan centre, but undertaking an internship in rural Tennessee, USA. There he encountered 'sick-as-hell anaemia', 'very close veins' and 'smiling mighty Jesus' (spinal meningitis)! In this section we look at how cultures understand the same illness in different ways. In essence, human suffering is explained by different cultures in different ways. The form of explanation may reflect the projection of a culture's values into the experience of suffering. In the following sections we review cultural perspectives on pain, deafness, cancer and obesity. Although there is a large literature on cultural aspects of many physical conditions, I have chosen these for specific reasons.

Pain is a problem common to most physical conditions that cause suffering. It is often the 'signal' that something is wrong and so, as a 'medium' of communication, it is important to understand pain in a cultural context. I review research on deafness, taking it to be one example of a physical disability. Deafness was specifically chosen because many people would assume that its cause is so 'obvious' that it cannot be influenced by cultural factors. The third condition, cancer is a commonly feared disease with much mythology arising from it. Finally, obesity is considered due to its rapid rise and pervasive influence on health, particularly in 'westernised' countries. Many of the themes noted in relation to these conditions are relevant across many physical health problems. HIV/AIDS is considered in some detail in Chapter 9.

Pain

Here again we encounter the warning to refrain from simplistic stereotyping of cultural groups, this time with regard to people's experience of pain:

> . . . everyone has a cultural heritage which is part and parcel of an individual's health practices. The practical answer is not to learn in detail the infinite varieties of culture but to be aware of these varieties and how they might affect one's health practices. I am totally opposed to training anyone in the details of a particular ethnic group, for this will ultimately squeeze people into unreal categories, and 'typecast' their culture just as we have rigidified diagnoses. What I favour is making practitioners

sensitive to the patient's heritage, their own heritage, and to what happens when different heritages come together.

Zola (1983, p. 227)

Over the last 50 years there have been a good number of investigations into the interplay between culture and pain experience. However, differences in methodology have made the results hard to integrate, although generally it is believed that culture does influence pain experiences and/or pain behaviour. To delineate more clearly the relationships between culture and pain, Lipton and Marbach (1994) studied consecutive referrals to a facial pain clinic in New York. They randomly selected 50 patients from each of five prominent groups in the hospital's catchment area (Black, Irish, Italian, Jewish and Puerto Rican). Note that these categories reflect potentially overlapping criteria of colour, religion and geography, regarding culture (presumably black Italian Jews were screened out of the study!).

The pain patients completed a comprehensive questionnaire concerning the physical experience of pain, its cognitive and emotional aspects, how it inter- feres with daily functioning, and the patient's health-seeking behaviour. Regardless of ethnicity these patients gave equivalent responses for two-thirds of the items on the questionnaire. They did not, for instance, differ in the degree to which they experienced their pain as 'stabbing or sharp' or in the extent to which they worried about their pain. Each group gave equal importance to seeing pain as a warning that something was wrong and described themselves as being able to 'take pain' equally well. Most patients from each group claimed that they never cried or moaned about their face pain, whereas an equivalent number of patients from each group claimed that they would not worry about having an operation as long as it cured their facial pain. Thus differences in culture did not extend to influencing these pain patients on most items.

Nevertheless, of equal interest are those items on which there were cultural differences. We have already noted that cultural groups live in a variety of socioeconomic conditions and that these conditions can influence health. Lipton and Marbach (1994) therefore investigated a range of factors, which they believed were not intrinsic attributes of different cultural groups, but which might differ between different groups and so make it appear that cul- tural differences existed, when in fact they did not. The results of this inves- tigation are fascinating in themselves. Table 5.2 shows the results. Patients attending the clinic from each cultural group differed significantly in their average age, the ratio males:females, their income and education, the pro- portion who identified themselves as 'American' and the proportion who were third generation, or more, born in the USA.

The cultural groups did differ not only on social and demographic vari- ables, but also significantly on psychologically more immediate measures, including social assimilation, medical acculturation, psychological distress and symptom history. The term 'social assimilation' describes the extent to which a minority culture group member has integrated into the dominant

Independent variable	Ethnic group										F ratio
	Black		Irish		Italian		Jewish		Puerto Rican		
	X	SD	X	SD	X	SD	X	SD	X	SD	
Sociodemographic											
Age (in years)	47.2	18.4	36.2	15.6	33.7	13.3	42.2	17.2	36.4	11.4	6.42†
Sex (percentage male)	25.0	43.7	0	0	9.1	29.0	18.9	39.5	37.5	48.9	7.71†
Position (percentage youngest and middle)	60.0	49.5	71.4	45.7	54.5	50.3	66.0	47.8	68.7	46.8	0.99†
Income (percentage greater than US $18,000)	30.0	46.3	73.3	44.7	71.4	45.6	50.9	50.5	31.2	46.8	9.79†
Education (years completed)	11.0	4.1	13.1	2.6	12.8	2.2	13.5	2.6	11.2	2.2	8.29†
Generation American (percentage third or more)	85.0	36.1	73.3	44.7	45.4	50.2	41.5	49.7	6.2	24.4	26.27†
Ethnic identification (percentage 'American')	55.0	50.2	26.7	44.7	45.4	50.3	71.7	45.5	12.5	33.4	13.49†
Social assimilation (score on index) (higher score indicates greater degree of acculturation)											
Ethnic exclusivity	1.10	0.54	1.73	0.45	1.64	0.57	1.31	0.58	1.25	0.56	12.15†
Friendship solidarity	2.60	1.44	3.00	0.85	2.48	0.97	2.64	1.09	1.53	1.32	10.44†
Family tradition	1.44	1.18	1.85	1.11	2.15	0.97	1.84	0.99	1.33	1.20	4.25†
Medical acculturation (score on index) (higher score indicates greater degree of acculturation)											
Scepticism	0.70	0.91	1.33	0.71	1.09	0.91	0.88	0.89	1.19	0.81	4.32†
Dependency	1.00	0.78	1.33	0.80	1.27	0.62	1.26	0.68	0.94	0.66	3.17†
Health knowledge	5.90	3.14	5.87	2.47	5.73	2.51	6.72	2.98	4.37	2.83	4.62†
Level of psychological distress (score on index)	4.35	4.71	3.13	4.11	5.52	4.27	5.72	3.82	6.73	4.22	5.19†
Symptom and treatment history											
Duration (percentage chronic)	35.0	48.2	60.0	49.5	72.7	45.0	69.8	46.3	75.0	43.7	6.23†
Other pain (percentage none)	35.0	48.2	73.3	44.7	55.0	50.3	34.5	48.0	43.7	50.1	5.65†
Change in location of pain (percentage no change)	45.0	50.2	41.7	50.0	41.2	49.9	56.2	50.1	56.2	50.1	1.04†
Pain severity	70.0	31.5	61.7	31.8	62.5	31.2	63.7	29.7	54.7	29.9	1.57
Number doctors previously consulted (percentage seeing three or more)	25.0	43.7	66.7	47.6	59.1	49.7	56.6	50.0	25.0	43.7	8.99†
Number different treatments previously received (percentage two or more)	20.0	40.4	53.3	50.4	50.0	50.5	32.1	47.1	0	0	13.47†
Diagnosis (percentage TMJS)	50.0	50.5	73.3	44.7	68.2	47.0	66.0	47.8	81.2	39.4	3.12*

*Significant, $p < 0.05$; †significant, $p < 0.01$.
Reproduced from Lipton and Marbach (1984). (With kind permission from Elsevier Science Ltd.)
TMJS, temporomandibular joint syndrome.

culture, e.g. by having close or intimate relationships outside their cultural group. The degree of ethnocentricity, friendship solidarity within one's own group and strength of family traditions each differed significantly across the five cultural groups. 'Medical acculturation' refers to the exchange of cultural health norms for the biomedical norms of the 'mainstream' American culture. The extent of biomedical health knowledge, scepticism about it and the adoption of a dependency role when sick all differed across cultural groups. Puerto Rican patients reported the highest levels of psychological distress and Irish patients the lowest levels. There were also significant differences across the five ethnic groups in the reported chronicity of pain, the occurrence of other pain, the number of medical doctors previously consulted, the number of different treatments sought and even the diagnosis given. In contrast to the previously noted difference between Puerto Rican and Irish patients' psychological symptoms, they were both more likely to be given a diagnosis of temporomandibular joint syndrome (TMJS) than were Black patients.

These variables therefore represent a broad spectrum of life experiences and all varied across the five cultural groups studied by Lipton and Marbach (1994). It is little wonder that the provision of multicultural health services is so complex, because there are many aspects of health that could be influenced by the above differences, e.g. with regard to the pain clinic patients, these 'confounding variables' accounted for apparent cultural differences in reported fear of cancer, ability to enjoy oneself, belief that 'I probably deserve this pain', attending a medical doctor once pain is experienced and willingness to take medication to alleviate suffering. It is therefore not only the cultural differences between groups themselves that influence health, but also differences between them arising from the different contexts in which they exist.

What, then, of the 'pure' cultural differences in pain? Culture did account for differences in the extent to which pain was experienced as 'a dull ache' or 'very severe, almost unbearable'. There were also significant differences in the extent to which patients wondered about what they had done to have the pain, in their feeling that they might 'lose control', about the benefit of complaining and the importance of trying to hide pain. The likelihood of becoming emotional when describing the pain and the desire to have other people around when experiencing the pain also differed. Finally, whether the pain affected appetite, the ability to work and the likelihood of having been to many medical doctors were also influenced by cultural group membership.

The most compelling finding to come out of Lipton and Marbach's (1994) research is not, however, about the similarities or differences across cultural groups in their experience of pain or their pain behaviour; instead it is that each cultural group appeared to have different 'triggers' for their pain experience. Different factors appear to be associated with pain in each cultural group. In the case of Black patients, the greater their degree of dependency (during sickness) on 'lay' social/cultural group members, the greater was their emotional and expressive response to pain, and the greater was their disturbance in daily functioning. For Irish patients, longstanding close relationships ('friendship solidarity') with other ethnic Irish individuals was related to greater reporting of disruption in daily functioning and a non-emotionally expressive response to their pain. Italian patients' response to pain was best predicted by the length of time that they had the pain. Chronic pain (for at least six months) was associated with an emotional and expressive response, as well as a disruption in performing physical activities. The level of reported psychological distress was most important for explaining the pain of Jewish patients, because a high level of distress was strongly associated with an emotionally expressive pain response and with interference in daily functioning. Finally, for Puerto Rican patients, high psychological distress, strong 'friendship solidarity', dependency on other Puerto Rican individuals when sick and suffering chronic pain were all associated with an emotionally expressive pain response and significant disruption in daily activities attributable to pain.

Overall, this research suggests that although cultural groups may report similar responses to pain, different factors influence their responses. Different cultures present different settings and conditions for the expression of pain. Nevertheless, we should not expect all Irish, or all Italian or all Black individuals to be equally influenced by intracultural factors. Lipton and Marbach's research does, however, help us to understand how, within different cultural groups, individuals are influenced by particular psychosocial processes. A very practical clinical example of this would be that not all cultures are equally willing to use 'pain-killing' medication. Poliakoff (1993) suggests that many Chinese people fear that such medication may give them a feeling of being out of control. In addition to this, some Chinese people also have a belief that pain-killers cause sweating and that this loss of body fluid will induce weakness.

People of particular faiths may accept pain as their due, e.g. Hindus who believe that they are facing death may wish to do so 'clear headed' rather than sedated. Negative feelings, such as pain, may be attributed to wrongs that they have committed in the past. Thus, the reluctance of some patients to accept analgesics may have no relationship to the severity of their pain experience, but instead be to do with the extent to which psychosocial factors particular to their own culture impact upon them as individuals. This level of analysis moves us beyond the stereotypical 'one culture–one type of person'; perspective to a 'one culture–several salient psychosocial processes that individuals will encounter' perspective. This is a much more sensitive and realistic level of analysis. It recognises the dynamic between the individual and his or her social context, which the will of the individual and the 'grain' of his or her cultural setting, each contribute to the person's behaviour. Although it is more sensitive to the realism of clinical practice, we must also acknowledge that it allows for less specificity and predictability.

We cannot say with certainty that, because Simon is Jewish and experiencing facial pain, and because he reports a high level of psychological distress, he will necessarily also report significant disruption in performing his usual activities. We can, however, say that this would usually be the case for a member of the Jewish culture in the USA. The fact that he may not adhere to this relationship may be very significant, not only in understanding him as a person, but also in providing an effective intervention to help him. As a final thought, it is important to acknowledge that much remains unknown about pain and we may not expect great clarity from cultural perspectives on pain when more conventional perspectives produce results that are both paradoxical and incomplete (MacLachlan, 2004).

Cancer

We have already discussed cancer in connection with folk taxonomies, the stress of migration, etc. but, given the pervasiveness of this disease, it deserves some consideration in its own right. This is particularly so as Meyerowitz et al. (1999) have argued that the vast majority of research on cancer, particularly in the USA, is entirely on White people. They wanted to explore the possible link between ethnicity and cancer-related outcomes, with regard to people's response to cancer and its treatment. They were concerned to consider both years of survival after cancer and the quality of life post-cancer. Using the National Institutes of Health's (age-adjusted) statistics on 'Racial/Ethnic patterns of Cancer in the US 1988–1992', they report the following breakdown for the incidence of prostate cancer per 100,000 people:

- Black (180.6)
- Non-Hispanic white (137.9)
- White Hispanic (92.8)
- Japanese (88.0), Hawaiian (57.2)
- Native American (52.5)
- Chinese (46.0).

Clearly there are massive differences for prostate cancer. More generally, across all cancers they highlighted some important trends:

- Latino (or Hispanic) individuals have a low incidence of cancers except for *cervical cancer* (where they have the highest rate).
- Asian individuals have low incidence of cancers except *stomach* cancer.
- Native Hawaiian individuals have relatively very high rates of cancer.
- Native American individuals have relatively very low rates of cancer.
- Five-year survival rates are highest among Japanese individuals.

It therefore seems that the relationship between ethnicity and cancer may differ in terms of the *anatomical site* of the disease, its *treatment* and its *prognosis*. Meyerowitz et al. (1999) developed a framework to take account of the effects of ethnicity in terms of cancer outcomes, *after* a diagnosis of cancer (the framework does not refer to the causes of cancer). Within their framework 'ethnicity' incorporates aspects of minority status, culture and identity. Minority status is seen to be associated with poorer socioeconomic status and poorer access to health services, which in turn affects adherence behaviours

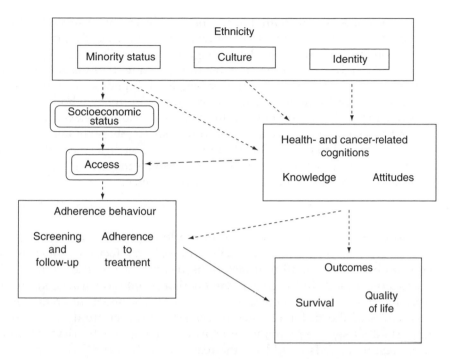

Figure 5.1   Possible culturally relevant mediational framework for cancer outcomes following cancer onset. (Adapted from Meyerowitz et al., 1998.)

such as attending screening, sticking to the treatment and being effectively followed up. Thus factors such as the cost of screening, transport and lack of alternative childcare are minority-related barriers. Cancer and identity are seen to relate to the way in which people think about cancer and their health in general (health- and cancer-related cognitions). The resultant knowledge of cancer and attitudes towards it, in combination with adherence behaviours, influence both survival time and the quality of life during that time (Figure 5.1).

To illustrate the role of knowledge and attitudes, for example, Chavez et al. (1995) reported that physicians working in the USA (as a group) ranked family history as the highest risk factor for breast cancer, whereas Mexican immigrants to the USA ranked it twelfth, with the following included in those ranking higher: injuries to the breast, never breast-feeding, excessive fondling, taking drugs or smoking, and using birth control pills. A more detailed insight into an individual's cultured construction of cancer is given by Donna King, aged 35, who described her feelings about breast cancer being a white woman's disease. Here she recalls her initial diagnosis two years earlier:

When I was first diagnosed I never knew any other Black women with this disease. You hear all this about the war on cancer, then the war on breast cancer, but I never saw any Black women with breast cancer,

I never saw any of us with it. And I never saw any of us surviving breast cancer either. I saw tons of White women, though, on TV just as happy and smiling that they had been diagnosed early. They all kept talking about the fight to win the war. I just did not know that Black women get breast cancer. I had pain with my cancer, but I did not know it was breast cancer. I went to the library to find out more. In this one book they said breast cancer lumps are not painful. I know I should have checked it out, but I had so much on my mind. I did not have a job, no money, no insurance. I wanted to believe. I had so much going on and since I did not see any of us living with breast cancer and with all that going on. I'd just as soon not know I was going to die of breast cancer.

Moore and Spiege (2000. p. 116)

This quotation clearly illustrates how cultural understandings of physical illness are not only associated with intracultural factors (issues within a culture) but also intercultural factors (issues between cultures). It also illustrates a point made in Chapter 1, namely that people construct cohesive identities by differentiating themselves from those who seem different. Although awareness of the different rates of cancers across cultural groups may be important for service planning and surmounting access barriers, a good deal more research needs to address the reasons for the variation in cancer onset between cultural groups.

We already know that lay perceptions of the *causes of* cancer can be strongly influenced by culture, e.g. Kohli and Dalal's (1998) study in Allahabad, India, of Hindu women receiving radiotherapy for cervical cancer found that they mostly attributed their illness to metaphysical beliefs – fate, God's will, karma. Belief that God's will had caused their cancer was associated with a lack of perceived controllability over their illness; however, it was also associated with stronger feelings of recovery from cancer. Thus although an attribution of 'beyond my control' may be considered undesirable in cultures where people are encouraged to 'take control over' their illness, in other cultures the same attribution may be seen in a more positive light. As Kohli and Dalal (1998, p. 125) state:

Metaphysical beliefs help individuals in comprehending even apparently senseless events. . . . These beliefs render life meaningful.

and as such strongly direct their health-related behaviours – they guide their own health psychologies:

While medical causes may lie at the core of explanatory models in the West, in Indian settings metaphysical beliefs are prominant.

The theme of cultural transition – both across time and between places – has already been discussed. In the classic migration model, as it relates to physical health, the health profiles of migrants come to assume the same characteristics as those of their 'host' country. However, as Abbotts, Harding and Cruickshank (2004) note, this well-established model – particularly with regard to cancer among Japanese individuals migrating to the USA – is, in fact, too simplistic, e.g. Irish individuals in Britain have over a 20% increased all-cause mortality rate, relative to the UK average. Furthermore this increased mortality rate has persisted not only into the second generation (parents born in Ireland), but also into the third generation (grandparents born in Ireland, but parents born in the UK). This is despite intergenerational improvements in socioeconomic position: Abbotts et al. (2004, p. 301) suggest that this may be at least partially attributed to smoking and 'reflects a lag in lifestyle modification between generations in spite of upward social mobility', which would usually be associated with reduced mortality. Close study of intergeneration changes in health-related behaviours presents a sort of 'natural experiment' from which we can gleam a better understanding of the relationship between culture and health, and more research in this area is also clearly needed.

Deafness

Hearing loss is one of the most common health problems in industrialised societies. People suffering from loss of hearing are often stigmatised, e.g. problems in communication are often attributed to the person with a hearing loss being rude, uninterested or stupid. One of the major causes of hearing loss appears to be working in a noisy environment. Migrant workers are often over-represented in noisy industries such as manufacturing or construction. Even when companies do provide ear protection and information leaflets on the importance of avoiding loud noises, employees often continue to expose themselves to potentially harmful levels of noise. Migrants may be at a particular disadvantage if they are not proficient in the language of the health promotion literature provided by the company. However, a more pervasive problem may be that migrant workers have different 'explanatory models' for deafness.

Westbrook, Legge and Pennay (1994) at the University of Sydney have conducted a series of studies on disability within a multicultural society. They have looked at the causal attributions for midlife deafness among the Anglo, Chinese, German, Greek, Italian and Arabian communities. The participants in the study were 665 community health practitioners who were members of each of the above cultural groups, and included medical practitioners, nurses, dentists, physiotherapists, occupational therapists, speech and language therapists, and social welfare and community health workers. These practitioners completed a questionnaire that gave 18 different potential causes for hearing loss in a 35-year-old man. The practitioners rated each cause in terms of how they believed members of their own cultural community would explain hearing loss. They did not give their own personal ratings. Table 5.3 summarises the results of the study.

Table 5.3 Causal attributions for deafness.

Attribution	Community attribution score[a] (rank in brackets)						f[b]	p
	Anglo	German	Italian	Greek	Chinese	Arabic		
Ageing	(1) 3.06	(2) 2.68[c]	(1) 2.83	(2) 2.75[c]	(1) 2.75[c]	(2) 2.61[c]	3.15	<0.01
Industrial noise	(2) 2.99	(1) 2.71[a]	(2) 2.69	(1) 2.82[c]	(5) 2.42[c]	(4) 2.45[c]	9.21	<0.0001
Heredity	(3) 2.74	(5) 2.38[c]	(6½) 2.26[c]	(7) 2.28[c]	(6) 2.34[c]	(10) 2.10[c]	10.33	<0.0001
Loud music	(4) 2.70	(4) 2.50	(6½) 2.26[c]	(5) 2.31[c]	(7) 2.32[c]	(13) 1.87[c]	8.99	<0.0001
Chance, could happen to anyone	(5) 2.55	(3) 2.57	(3) 2.50	(3) 2.53	(3½) 2.43	(6½) 2.25	1.54	>0.05
Past injuries	(6) 2.41	(6½) 2.23	(5) 2.38	(8) 2.27	(3½) 2.43	(5) 2.42	1.30	<0.01
Infectious germs	(7) 2.10	(6½) 2.23	(8) 2.13	(6) 2.29	(2) 2.52[‡]	(3) 2.57[‡]	5.61	<0.0001
Person's temperament (doesn't bother listening)	(8½) 1.87	(11) 1.78	(11½) 1.85	(11) 1.95	(15) 1.70	(15) 1.72	1.47	>0.05
Stress and tension	(8½) 1.87	(8) 2.16[c]	(10) 1.86	(9) 2.13[c]	(12½) 1.74	(11) 1.97	3.83	<0.01
Person in poor health, 'run down'	(10) 1.82	(9) 1.94	(13) 1.78	(13) 1.92	(8) 2.24[‡]	(12) 1.94	5.60	<0.0001
Drugs	(11) 1.81	(10) 1.81	(9) 2.00	(13) 1.92	(11) 1.75	(16) 1.67	2.07	>0.05
Poor medical care	(12) 1.73	(12) 1.64	(11½) 1.85	(10) 1.96[c]	(9) 2.04[‡]	(9) 2.15[c]	5.44	<0.001
God's will	(13) 1.52	(14) 1.49	(4) 2.43[c]	(4) 2.46[c]	(10) 1.81[c]	(1) 3.09[c]	50.16	<0.0001
Upsetting or disturbing event	(14) 1.49	(13) 1.54	(14) 1.75[c]	(15) 1.81[c]	(12½) 1.74[‡]	(6½) 2.25[c]	10.48	<0.0001
Poor diet	(15) 1.39	(15) 1.45	(17) 1.43	(17) 1.43	(16) 1.69[‡]	(18) 1.45	3.39	<0.01
Karma	(16) 1.13	(16) 1.24	(18) 1.25	(18) 1.32[c]	(14) 1.72[‡]	(17) 1.63[c]	15.62	<0.0001
Person's bad actions, sins	(17) 1.09	(18) 1.09	(16) 1.53[c]	(16) 1.58[c]	(17) 1.65[‡]	(14) 1.77[c]	19.04	<0.0001
Evil influences, e.g. evil eye curse	(18) 1.07	(17) 1.10	(15) 1.64[c]	(13) 1.92	(18) 1.58	(8) 2.24[c]	41.13	<0.0001

[a] Scores ranged from 4 (almost always explanation) to 1 (rarely).
[b] Degrees of freedom (d.f.) ranged from 5/654 to 5/585.
[c] *t* contrast between Anglo and other cultural groups' scores yielded $p < 0.01$.
Reproduced from Westbrook *et al.* (1994). (With permission; © 1994 Harwood Academic Publishers.)

Two audiologists independently rated the likelihood of each of the attributions in Table 5.3 being the most probable cause of hearing loss. They each agreed that industrial noise, followed by drugs and past injuries, would 'often' be cited as the cause of the patient's hearing loss, and that infection, heredity, loud music and poor medical care could 'sometimes' be the cause. As can be seen from Table 5.3 none of the ratings from any ethnic group agreed with the ratings of these two specialists. Analysis of variance showed that there was a significant difference across the six ethnic groups for every one of the 18 possible attributions. 'God's will' was the cause over which there was greatest disagreement. It was predicted that the Arabic community would give this top ranking, the Greek and Italian communities would rank it fourth, and the Chinese, Anglo and German communities would rank it 10th, 13th and 14th, respectively. It was predicted that the 'ageing' explanation would be rated either the first or second most likely cause by all the cultures.

Another way of looking at these data is by considering whether the top-rated attributions were endorsed by the audiologists. Across the six cultures the top eight attributions included the following explanations, not endorsed by the audiologists: chance (all cultures), God's will (Italian, Greek and Arabic), stress and tension (German and Anglo), person's temperament (Anglo), poor health (Chinese), upsetting event and evil eye (Arabic). It is clear that each culture would have a distinct profile for the probable causes of hearing loss, and that they would all differ from the specialists' opinion. This sort of research is especially useful to the community clinician because it emphasises how she or he may need to act as a go between for members of minority cultural groups and clinicians in the 'mainstream' centralised health services. This research also points to a problem with health promotion, because, if the 'official' line on what causes deafness is different from that which you have been brought up to believe, adopting health-promoting behaviour may also involve a rejection of your own cultural values. This issue is dealt with in more detail in Chapter 8. We now turn to consider the confusing context of rapidly changing cultural values and practices and their implications for one dramatically increasing health problem – obesity.

Obesity

Let us return to the idea of cultural evolution, i.e. ideas within a culture changing over time, and apply it to one of the most demonstrable aspects of our physical health, body mass and its relationship to contemporary culture (or consumer culture). Of North American citizens 61% are so overweight that they will experience health-related problems, whereas 20% meet the criteria for morbid obesity and qualify for gastroplasty, a radical surgical technique that prevents food being digested (Critser, 2003). The percentage who are under 19 and overweight or obese has doubled in the last 30 years. Of course it is changed social norms about consumption that have fuelled this feeding frenzy: a serving of McDonald's 'french fries' rose from 200 calories, in 1960, to 320 calories in the late 1970s to the contemporary 610 calories. As I have noted elsewhere (MacLachlan, 2004) people have come to see 'big' as the norm, at least in the USA, banishing notions of gluttony and shame. Astride galloping globalisation and the broader adoption of western consumption norms, obesity has now been identified by the WHO as a major health concern.

Like so many other disorders, obesity is socially, culturally and economically 'patterned'. Its greatest effects, at least in the USA, are felt among 'the poor, the underserved, and the underrepresented' (Critser, 2003, p. 109), e.g. 33% of black people, 26% of Hispanic individuals and 19% of white people with an annual household income of less than US$10,000 are obese in the USA. For those same groups in the US$50,000 plus bracket, the respective figures are 23% (black), 22% (Hispanic) and 16% (white). In trying to partition the causative factors Critser (2003, pp. 110–11) states:

> The point is not that culture or race does not matter. They do. The point is that class almost always comes first in the equation: class confounded by culture, income inhibited by race or gender, buying power impinged on by ethnicity or immigration status.

Bogin and Loucky (1997) have described the contemporary clash of culture and metabolism, the seeds of which were planted by European conquerors hundreds of years ago. They argue that cultural exploitation of the Guatemalan Maya, with the resultant poverty, produced an environmentally adaptive metabolic proclivity to retain fat in their context of scarcity. However, when they migrate into a culture of abundance, such as that in the USA, this proclivity predisposes them to obesity. It is not thus a 'regular' immutable genetic inheritance that causes the high rates of obesity in the Guatemalan Maya who migrate to the USA, but rather an adaptive metabolism inherited from generations of poverty that just cannot 'turn off' a survival mechanism that has worked over many generations. It is in this sense, Bogin and Louckey argue, that metabolically the original traumas of conquest are played out daily on the streets of Los Angeles.

Weight and body composition are a reflection of daily consumption, whereas height reflects health and nutritional history. Thus increases in body weight precede increases in height when people from impoverished regions migrate to regions of abundance (Bogin & Louckey, 1997). This lineage shows just how complex is the pattern of health woven through the physical, the psychological and the cultural. Metabolic changes that adaptively arise as a result of cultural and economic exploitation can subsequently and dramatically disadvantage their 'carriers' – witness clinical obesity among Mexican–American children: for 5–11 year olds it is 27.4% for girls and 23% for boys. The rate peaks in the fourth grade for girls at 32.4% and in the fifth grade for boys at a staggering 43.4% (see Suminski et al., 1999).

In the culture of abundance, it is, perversely, those who are best at restraining who present the iconic bodies of leanness and thinness. The body has become the canvas of intrasexual competition as well as cultural change. It seems that the extreme forms sought by both men and women are not necessarily those that are seen as attractive to potential partners, but more those seen as 'hard to achieve' within one's own sex (MacLachlan, 2004). Once the more explicit concern of women, men too are now increasingly body conscious and dissatisfied with bodies that once would have been quite acceptable. 'Reverse anorexia nervosa' is concerned with an excessive focus on fat-free muscularity and may involve the abuse of anabolic steroids (Anderson, 2002).

Male mannequins now possess larger genital bulges (!) and more defined muscular build than previously and, mimicking the changes in female cultural sexual iconic imagery, over the last 25 years the average *Playgirl* centrefold has lost 12 pounds of fat and gained approximately 27 pounds of muscle (Leit, Pope & Gray, 2001).

Corson and Andersen (2002, p. 194) suggest that 'males want to be heavier but see themselves as lighter, and females want to be lighter but see themselves as 10–15 pounds heavier than they really are'. Although females may want to lose weight, males want to lose body fat while maintaining lean muscle mass. It has been argued that the relative empowerment of woman in most western societies has had a consequential disorienting effect on men and that, because of their threatened masculinity, they are seeking increasingly to define themselves through what distinguishes them most from woman – their bodies (Olivardia, 2002).

Elsewhere I have noted how psychological, social and cultural concerns can express themselves through ailments of the body, and how the mind–body distinction so prevalent in western thinking is not apparent in other cultural views. In Chapter 6, while considering more 'physical' aspects of treatment, I place especial emphasis on the therapeutic and healing relationships that may be common across different types of health practitioners. In many cases we implicitly expect healing relationships to have physical as well as psychological effects.

Guidelines for professional practice

1. Clinicians should be aware that the relationship between psychosocial stress and health is complex and often indirect. Psychosocial factors can influence health through at least three pathways: producing physiological hyperactivity, exacerbating existing disease and reducing the body's immunocompetence. Stressful psychosocial experiences should therefore be addressed in any treatment plan, even when the clinician does not see them as directly related to the presenting complaint. At the very least such experiences may reduce the beneficial potential of treatment interventions.
2. Cultural differences, the experience of migration or the experience of being a member of a minority group can produce psychosocial stressors

that have been shown to influence physical health. Such experiences should therefore be considered risk factors in themselves. Thus, even when these experiences are shrugged off as easily dealt with, further investigation may find that they have been problematic but difficult to articulate or that it has been difficult to find a suitable person in whom to confide.

3. Even rather abstract cultural values, such as social integration and cultural inwardness, appear to be related to health. Although the mechanism for such links is unclear, these relationships may be important for health planning and policy making. It is therefore important not to discount research findings simply because they do not indicate how to work with individuals. Such findings may be of great importance to public health planners.

4. Cultural inwardness may be a health-promoting attitude that community clinicians can utilise as a resource. Clinicians may therefore build on this by investigating how their interventions can incorporate cultural values and practices. Beyond this, clinicians should resist being seen as representatives of 'modernity' with concomitant biotechnological skills and aligned to moves away from tradition.

5. Some cultural groups, such as the Seventh Day Adventists, appear to have a healthier lifestyle than other cultural groups. Clinicians must remain open to the possibility of finding healthier ways of living than those prescribed by their own culture or profession. Clinicians should make a case for healthier living by referring to evidence-based research studies and avoiding evaluative comparisons about what is the 'right' way to live.

6. Different cultural groups experience different diseases to varying extents. This arises through diseases that are genetically determined, acquired, iatrogenic or related to socioeconomic conditions, in addition to those that are influenced by other cultural factors. Acknowledgement that some diseases have genetic causes more strongly associated with certain physical features (such as skin colour) than others need not be seen as problematising culture.

7. Cultures vary in the way in which they understand human body functioning. A balance metaphor appears to be the most common way of viewing the internal working of the body. This metaphor need not be inconsistent with the way in which health professionals work with their clients. Practitioners should try to translate their own thinking into the metaphors used by the cultures with which they are working.

8. Explanations for disease vary not only across cultures but with the health professions found within one culture. Many disagreements between health professionals can be understood better if they are seen in and analysed through a cultural perspective. Here the challenge is to be able meaningfully to communicate with and understand the position of other people.

9. The topic of pain has attracted much cross-cultural research that has led clinicians to develop somewhat stereotypical ideas about how different

cultural groups experience pain. Recent research suggests that different cultural groups report similar responses to pain, but that different factors influence these responses. Clinicians should not assume that a lower level of pain complaint or declining the offer of pain-killers is associated with a lower level of experienced pain. Patients should be given the choice to cope with their pain in ways consistent with their cultural beliefs, even if these are inconsistent with those of the clinician.

10. Community clinicians must develop a role for themselves where they can negotiate for healthy behaviour between the models of illness offered by their own profession and the community that they seek to serve. Neighbouring communities may have quite different ideas about the cause and necessary preventive action for a particular disease.

11. Obesity has become a major modern epidemic with rates rocketing within the last decade. Although obesity rates do very across cultural groups these differences are also conflated with income and gender.

12. The growing emphasis on ideal bodies in the contemporary 'success' society effectively further disadvantages those who live on the margins of that society, and stigmatises them for failing to achieve their standards. In the age of abundance, restraint is king.

13. The colour–hypertension relationship describes the significantly higher incidence of hypertension reported in black American compared with white American individuals. Furthermore, among darker-skinner black American individuals the incidence is higher again. Although some people may intuit that this suggests a genetic link between skin colour and hypertension, recent research suggests that a skin colour discrimination–stress–hypertension causal route may also be involved to some extent.

CHAPTER 6

Culture and treatment

The topic of 'treatment', taking into account the many health professions whom might benefit from this book, is so broad that this discussion needs to be tightly circumscribed. However, it is also going to need to be rather general in order to have some relevance across different professions. We cannot therefore specify how Hungarian counsellors should treat the phobia of a Nigerian client, how Scottish dentists should evacuate the cavities of Pakistani children, or how Malaysian physiotherapists ought to remedy the complaints of Australian athletes! Instead we will consider what is involved in a therapeutic encounter. This will mean trying to develop a way of thinking about and approaching intervention that goes beyond making the patient or client the *object* of treatment. Instead we must acknowledge the patient or client as the *subject* of concern, giving credence to their subjective experience and personal construction of their problems. This sort of analysis of treatment is something that may have great value across the scope of clinical encounters.

Case study: finding help

Peter was interested in unorthodox ideas about ecology and animal communication. Aged 45 he was lean, handsome and fit and worked as a biologist. He collapsed suddenly at work and awoke three days later to be told that he had cancer of the brain. Orthodox treatment with chemotherapy began almost immediately; meanwhile Peter began to research the condition himself. While under treatment from his doctors in Paris, he came across, on the internet, a Canadian doctor who offered an unorthodox treatment that Peter felt offered a reasonable chance of success. Despite being quite ill, Peter flew to Canada, undertook the complementary treatment, and met other sufferers with his condition. Impressed by his experience in Canada, where he began to fell much better, he set about starting up a self-help group.

Peter's complementary treatment was 'holistic', incorporating changes in diet, lifestyle and how he looked at the world. It seemed to fit his own views on life very well. Continuing both orthodox and complementary treatment simultaneously, Peter came increasingly to dislike the orthodox treatment: he lost his hair, constantly felt tired and found the other side effects of chemotherapy quite debilitating. He also found some of the doctors and nurses to be arrogant and patronising; they were dismissive of his interest in complementary medicine. Peter was quite shocked at how lacking in inquisitiveness they were, accepting the orthodoxies of medicine so unquestionably, even though they seemed to accept that many cancers were incurable. He began to feel that they all thought that he would soon die.

Complementary therapy offered such a contrast. Rather than feeling sick and depressed after sessions, he felt elated. He was, however, sceptical about the efficacy of some of the 'mixtures' that he had to take. Nevertheless after these consultations he felt calmer and as though there was something that he could do to help himself.

Peter's relapse was sudden. He died only 3 weeks after he started to feel distinctly unwell again, despite having brain surgery during this period.

(Adapted from Furnham and Vincent (2001) with permission.)

Peter's story is clearly a sad one but one from which we should learn. As Furnham and Vincent (2001) point out, Peter was an intelligent, educated person who participated in complementary therapy while continuing with orthodox treatment. This alternative to orthodox medicine was evidently offering Peter something *additional*, something he was not getting through orthodox treatment. Perhaps the practitioners were less patronising than the orthodox 'health professionals'? At the very least complementary therapy had the effect of empowering, rather than of sickening, Peter. Although ultimately neither approach cured him, perhaps it would be fair to say that one was of more help to him that the other.

I wanted to use Peter's story to introduce this chapter because it does not relate a miraculous cure; it relates something that all health practitioners should aspire to: the need to understand how people understand their illness, what sort of help *they need* and what effect treatment has on them – *as people*, rather than as biological systems. Ultimately therapy should be about giving people a degree of faith in their ability to overcome illness, and a degree of dignity in their response to it. Just how these aims can be achieved is one of the themes running through this chapter.

Practitioner–client communication

The way in which people relate to each other reflects social norms and roles. When is the last time you were a patient? You become a 'patient' when you consult a doctor (or some other clinician), regardless of whether or not there is something wrong with you. When you leave the doctor's consulting room and go to buy a newspaper in the shop next door, you are no longer a 'patient', regardless of whether you continue to adopt, or have just had validated, a 'sick role'. In most cultures there is a well-worn path to becoming legitimately sick. The gatekeepers along the Western biomedical pathway are convention-ally general medical practitioners. GPs decide whether or not the complaints presented to them are legitimate forms of sickness. If a doctor says that there is nothing wrong with you, while you maintain that you are indeed sick, you may experience some degree of marginalisation. Radley (1994, p. 88) has described the patient's dilemma thus: 'how to present one's symptoms in a way that does justice to one's feelings, without prejudicing one's status as a responsible person i.e. without being seen to be "making a fuss"'. Clearly knowledge of social norms and rules is central to being able to present as a convincing patient. It should therefore be of no surprise that communication between practitioners and clients from different cultural backgrounds can be highly problematic and indeed prohibit effective healthcare.

Before considering some of the complexities of cross-cultural practi-tioner–client communication, first I review some of the difficulties and limi-tations of such communication between individuals of the same culture. The vast majority of research on this theme has concerned the communication between medical practitioners and the patients who attend them. It is now well established that patients often fail to act on the advice given to them by a doctor. Often this is because patients do not understand what the doctor is trying to communicate to them, or they fail to remember what it was that they understood the doctor to say during the consultation. Consequently patients fail to comply with the doctor's advice and this may well lessen their chances of recovery, or slow their speed of recovery. About a third to a half of patients either fail to take their medicine as prescribed or fail to follow medical advice. Thus patients' compliance with, or adherence to, doctors' suggestions con-tinues to be an important area of research. The best informed and most skilful of clinicians is effective only to the extent that he or she can influence the behaviour of their patients in the desired direction (e.g. taking medication, avoiding certain foods, attending specialists). If the clinicians' communication with patients does not afford them this degree of influence, the potential benefit of their knowledge will not be felt in practice.

Radley's (1994) review of the importance of the healing relationship high-lights the neglected area of the influence of faith in healing. We may talk of faith in the practitioner, and faith in the treatment, or the 'placebo effect'. It is amazing how quickly people (including myself!) recover from a headache after taking a tablet for it. Long before any chemical action can have done its work the headache is out of mind. Of course, trials of new drugs try to take this effect into account by using a control procedure that may involve some people receiving a tablet that, despite being inert, looks and tastes the same as the active drug. More sophisticated trials employ placebos that not only look and taste like the active agent, but also produce some of the unwanted (side) effects of the drug being tested. This sophisticated technology of exper-imental control has evolved because of the well-accepted notion of the placebo effect: the mere act of engaging in pro-health behaviour (e.g. taking a drug) can improve health. If you believe that you are doing something to make your-self better, then this will – to some extent – make you feel better. The often quoted phrase 'we should use the new drugs while they still have the power to heal' nicely encapsulates the role of faith in medicine(s). The placebo effect works not just on patients, but on their clinicians too.

The role of faith in practitioners is no less important than it is in medicines. The actions of a clinician can be seen as having a placebo effect. The doctor who looks at your throat and tells you that it will get better soon is encouraging you to avoid sick role behaviours and to engage in healthful behaviours. The doctor's reassurance may make you feel better. Similarly the doctor's involvement in prescribing some treatment may give you greater faith in the treatment. However, without faith in your doctor, treatment or no treatment, you may continue to be ill.

Surely I am not the only clinician to avoid certain treatments until my clients have had a chance to establish some faith in me! For example, if I am working with a person with agoraphobia, in which I think hyperventilation is influential, I would very rarely ask the person to hyperventilate in my first session with them. Now I can justify this in all sorts of ways and in truth one of them is to allow the person an opportunity to build trust and confidence in my ability to take care of them during a hyperventilation provocation test. Likewise, I would never use hypnosis with someone during our first session.

There are ways of short cutting the faith-building process. One is to present yourself as a person in whom others can have faith for particular treatments. A doctor may wear a white coat or a stethoscope, 'advertising' his or her status as a trustworthy person and someone with special knowledge (or powers). Someone who advertises as a specialist in hypnosis may use the technique right away. Such 'advertising' is essentially similar to the placebo that looks like the active agent but may not be. Most practitioners, at least in the clinical specialties, believe that it is the techniques that they use, rather than their persona or appearance, that are the active agents. Although not disregarding their own behaviour or appearance, they see these as assisting the active agent in the treatment, of which they are but a conduit. However, clinicians may also have faith invested in them by their patients and sometimes this faith may exceed the clinician's ability to deal with the patient's ailment. This presents us with a rather tantalising notion, that of the 'placebo practitioner'.

What exactly would a placebo practitioner be? It would be somebody who looks like and perhaps acts like a competent practitioner but who does not have access to truly therapeutic tools (e.g. effective medicines, techniques or procedures). The theme of placebos and faith is highly relevant to health practices across different cultures. Within one culture the idea of the placebo practitioner is at the root of much professional rivalry. Alternative, or complementary, practitioners are often castigated as presenting themselves as having therapeutic knowledge but in fact being inert. Furthermore within conventional health services the jibe that some specialists may look good but are not very effective is not unheard of. When we consider practitioners from a different culture the situation becomes even more complex. We may well accept that people from their own culture have some faith in them but we dismiss the efficacy of their methods, e.g. we may not believe that the amalgam of various herbs presented by an Indian traditional healer has any intrinsic value in alleviating an illness, but we may acknowledge that the way in which it is prescribed does have a therapeutic effect. Figures 6.1 and 6.2 outline some of these relationships.

Figure 6.1 portrays a matrix of faith in clinicians and their treatments in a monocultural context. In this hypothetical situation there is only one sort of clinician and one sort of treatment. The patient or client either does or does not have faith in the treatment, and either has or does not have faith in the clinician. This analysis at the micro-level of the individual indicates that the double-placebo condition of faith in both the clinician and the treatment renders the best chance for the recipient of their joint efforts, e.g. I go to my GP, whose professional competence I greatly respect, and she prescribes me a drug, which I understand has been highly effective in treating my sort of problem. In contrast to this, the scenario in quadrant 4 might go something like this: I go to my GP whom I have previously found to be rather rude, lacking in sympathy and unable to prescribe effective treatment. He tells me to take a drug that I have taken before and found not only to be ineffective but also to have unpleasant 'side' effects. The other two quadrants describe the situation where, although one does not like the individual doctor, one still believes that the treatment prescribed will be effective (quadrant 2). Finally we have the situation where, although we feel that the doctor is a lovely fellow, we also believe that there is no effective medicine for the ailment. In these two cases the placebo effects of faith may still be present but perhaps modified.

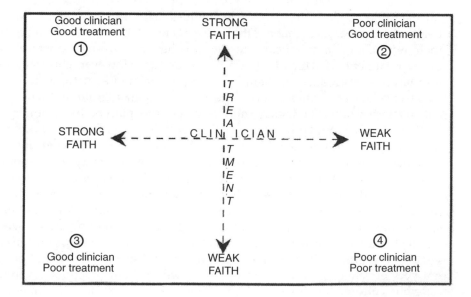

Figure 6.1   Faith matrix for clinicians and treatments in a hypothetical monocultural context.

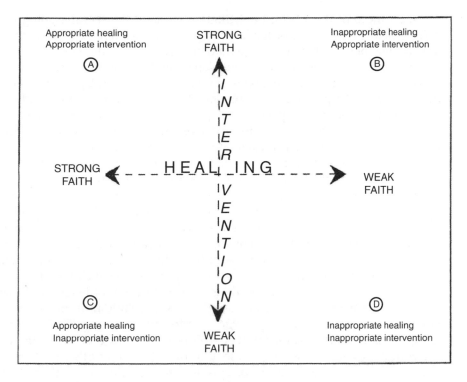

Figure 6.2   Faith matrix for healing and intervention in a hypothetical multicultural context.

Figure 6.1 makes the assumption that the general therapeutic approach of the clinician (or healer) and the general mode of treatment (or intervention) are acceptable to the client or patient. Thus, the patient accepts that the condition should be treated, e.g. by a Western medical practitioner (healer) using pharmacological methods (intervention). Clearly this simplistic assumption does not hold even for people of the same cultural background who may differ in their opinions as to the most appropriate sort of person and means of intervention for a particular problem. The cross-cultural perspective extends this complexity into numerous different understandings about health and illness, how they are caused, who should treat them and in what way.

Figure 6.2 provides a generic matrix for understanding this broader, or macro-level, interaction between faith in the healer and faith in the intervention. At this level, quadrant A represents the situation where the sort of intervention for which the person is looking (say, a spell of protection) is the same as the intervention being offered by the healer, and the healer appears to be able to produce an effective intervention of this sort (their spell of protection will indeed afford protection to the recipient). Thus, both the mode of intervention and the healer to carry out the intervention are seen as appropriate. In quadrant D of Figure 6.2 neither of these conditions exists.

An example of this might be a Chinese student in Australia going to the college medical practitioner for relief of pain. The student feels that the most appropriate help for his problem would be given by a healer familiar with traditional Chinese ideas of energy imbalances and the most appropriate treatment would be acupuncture. The Australian doctor naturally enough sees the problem from the perspective of his own training and prescribes medication to lessen the patient's experience of pain. Unfortunately he dismisses the student's ideas as unscientific and primitive and is experienced by the student as being rude. The student consequently lacks faith in the healer and the intervention. It is worth reflecting on this for a moment. It has been argued that having faith in both the intervention method and the healer can engage a double-placebo effect, such that the patient is helped to get better, partly as a result of this faith. A lack of faith in both the healer and the method of intervention may not only remove this positive placebo effect but may actually produce a negative effect – it may worsen the health of the individual. Such negative consequences may well result from the situation described in quadrant 4 of Figure 6.1, but it is likely to be even greater when an individual experiences a mismatch between their own philosophy of health and that of a healer whom they consult. For immigrants or ethnic minorities this may enhance feelings of alienation, marginalisation and isolation. This undermining of their psychological state may well result in a further deterioration in the condition with which they present, or the addition of other problems.

Quadrant B of Figure 6.2 could represent the situation of a GP conducting acupuncture where the patient feels that this is the right sort of intervention, but lacks faith in the GP's knowledge of the technique and the ability to carry it out. Such instances may be particularly frustrating for practitioners who attempt to be more eclectic in their practice by also offering 'alternative' therapies. Paradoxically, in the present example, the GP may be ineffective with a Chinese patient who has faith in the technique but lacks faith in the healer, while being effective with an Australian patient, who lacks faith in the techniques but has faith in the healer. This case is the scenario represented by quadrant C in Figure 6.2.

The interaction of faith has been examined at the micro-level of individual clinicians and treatment and at the macro-level of different types of healer and intervention. In reality both these levels interplay when a person seeks help from a healer and the healer suggests a particular intervention. Figure 6.3 subsumes the previous two figures, representing them on three dimensions. There are 16 different combinations possible through this matrix, e.g. A1 represents a match between the sort of healer and sort of intervention that a person is seeking and that which is offered, as well as a belief in the ability of the individual healer encountered and in the particular treatment recommended.

D3 describes the situation where somebody goes to a healer (e.g. a GP) whom they do not see as having the necessary skills to alleviate their problem (e.g. feeling anxious because someone has put a spell on them, or because they have been made unemployed) and also where the sort of intervention

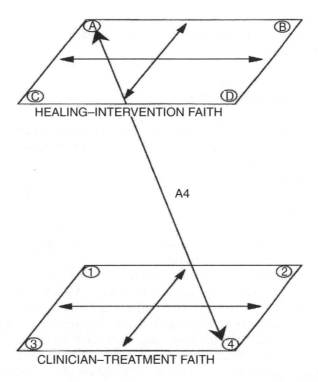

HEALING–INTERVENTION FAITH

A4

CLINICIAN–TREATMENT FAITH

Figure 6.3   Faith matrices illustrating a possible interaction between the micro-level of clinicians and treatments and the macro-level of healers and interventions.

(e.g. medication) being offered is not seen as an appropriate method of helping. Nevertheless they see the clinician as a very nice person who is truly trying to help, but the diazepam prescribed as being of no help. Such complexities may produce confusion and conflict both within the patient and within the clinician, but also *between the two of them*. Their frustration with a mismatch between their two paradigms may spill over into an uneasy relationship between them.

Clearly some of the permutations in Figure 6.3 are more likely than others. Some of them may occur very rarely, if at all. The frequency with which they do occur is open to empirical investigation. If we take seriously the positive influence that belief in a treatment and belief in a healer may have, it is important to analyse where client–clinician interactions lie within this two-dimensional grid. It is likely that a person's coordinates on this grid have a significant impact on recovery from an illness or a distressing experience. The grid is intended to emphasise the dual effects that faith in healers and faith in interventions can have on the recovery of a client or patient. It is also intended to help the clinician to think through where they are in relation to the people whom they are trying to help. The 'faith grid' may be especially useful in understanding the therapeutic process between people from different cultures, or subcultures. We now consider one particular way in which culture influences the interaction between clinicians and clients of the same culture.

Diagnostic disclosure

The idea that 'treatment begins with assessment' is central to many health professions. However, what then becomes of the assessment? A particularly sensitive part of assessment is the decision about whether the clinician's opinion should be shared with the patient. Although such diagnostic disclosure is common in some cultures there is by no means a universal understanding, either among clinicians or among patients or their families, about to what extent diagnostic information should be disclosed. As expectations about diagnostic disclosure vary across cultures, the practitioner should be aware of how such differences can operate.

Of course within any one culture there will be great variation in the extent to which patients actively seek information about their condition and in the extent to which clinicians feel that it is appropriate and/or helpful for patients to know their condition, especially if they have a poor prognosis. However, psychological research has suggested that certain people do benefit from knowing their prognosis, even if it is poor. It has also been shown that *some* surgical patients, who receive information about their condition, treatment and rehabilitation before surgery, make a better recovery than those given less information (Anderson, 1987). However, much of this research has been undertaken in North America and no doubt, to some extent, reflects cultural norms such as openness, democracy, individualism, etc.

Seen from another point of view, say a Japanese perspective, North American diagnostic disclosure may be experienced as mechanical, direct, blunt, thoughtless and irresponsible. Japanese attitudes towards diagnostic disclosure can be quite different from North American attitudes and naturally these reflect different aspects of life that are valued in each society. An especially notable difference is in clinicians' attitudes towards the disclosure of a diagnosis of mental disorder. It appears that in Japan there is a particularly strong stigma attached to the diagnostic label of schizophrenia, and that Japanese clinicians often substitute a less stigmatising diagnosis in their discussions with such patients and their families. It may be argued that, historically, this has its roots in a context of authoritarian clinicians dealing with uneducated patients who were expected to comply with instructions, any serious challenging of an expert's opinion being seen as an arrogant assault on their authority. However, in offering a less severe diagnosis to a person with mental disorder, the clinician may also be seen as assuming a paternalistic and protective role. McDonald-Scott, Machizawa and Satoh (1992) from the Japanese National Institute of Mental Health describe this practice as 'benevolent diagnostic deception'. They have investigated this 'deception' by comparing the diagnostic practices of North American and Japanese psychiatrists.

The psychiatrists, all of whom were affiliated with medical schools, were presented with six case vignettes and for each case they indicated if they would tell the patient their diagnosis. The case vignettes represented a variety of clinical conditions. Over 90% of both North American and Japanese psychiatrists said that they would inform patients of a diagnosis of affective or anxiety disorder. However, where the psychiatrist believed the patient to have schizophrenia, only 70% of North American and less than 30% of Japanese psychiatrists would disclose the diagnosis to the patient. In general Japanese psychiatrists preferred to give a vague alternative diagnosis such as neurasthenia. This relatively greater reluctance of Japanese psychiatrists to disclose the schizophrenic diagnostic label persisted even in the case where a patient presented with a 5-year history of continuous psychopathology and specifically asked if he had schizophrenia or psychosis. This illustrates how powerfully cultural values can influence clinical practice. Clinicians are themselves the vehicles of culture and respond to the broader context in which they are consulted. We might therefore also find that patients' expectations of diagnostic disclosure vary across cultures.

A further aspect of the study by McDonald-Scott et al. (1992) was that the psychiatrists were asked to indicate whether they would inform the patient's family of the diagnosis. The majority of both Japanese and North American psychiatrists indicated that they would disclose a diagnosis of schizophrenia to the patient's family. However, this statistical similarity belies an important cultural difference. North American psychiatrists would disclose the diagnosis to family members only with the patient's permission, whereas Japanese psychiatrists would do so without informing the patient of the diagnosis or seeking permission to tell family members. Once again this difference may be explained in terms of cultural values. The critical relationship for the North American psychiatrist is between the clinician and the patient, the patient's autonomy being highly valued and the family seen as a distinct, somewhat distant and ethically separate entity. In contrast, for the Japanese psychiatrist the burden of care for the patient is likely to fall on the family. Furthermore, other family members may be seriously jeopardised by a diagnosis of schizophrenia within the family, with its attendant social stigma. Here the psychiatrist has a wider social responsibility that can be fulfilled without informing the patient of the condition. Thus, what is seen as 'benevolent diagnostic disclosure' in one culture may be classified as malpractice in another. Likewise, adhering to the confidentiality of the clinician–patient relationship in one culture may be regarded as gross social irresponsibility in another.

Psychotherapy as myth and ritual

Frank and Frank (1991) have argued that 'psychotherapy's practitioners are almost as varied as its recipients' (p. 19) and that 'extensive research efforts have produced little conclusive knowledge about the relative efficacy of its different forms' (p. 19). Furthermore, they state 'features common to all types of psychotherapy contribute as much, if not more, to the effectiveness of those therapies than do the characteristics that differentiate them' (p. 20). They conceive people being drawn to psychotherapy because of their persistent failures to cope, resulting from 'maladaptive assumptive systems' (or, how they understand they world), and consequently producing demoralisation – *then people seek therapy*.

So what are the shared characteristics of psychotherapy? They may include: an emotionally charged, confiding relationship with a helpful person (or group); a healing setting; or a rationale, conceptual scheme or myth that provides a plausible explanation for the patient's symptoms along with a prescribed ritual or procedure for resolving them. The ritual or procedure should require the active participation of both patient and therapist and that mutual belief of it being the means of restoring the patient's health (Frank & Frank, 1991).

Frank and Frank consider that myth and ritual have various important functions in psychotherapeutic relationships. These include: combating the patient's sense of alienation and strengthening the therapeutic relationship; inspiring and strengthening the patient's expectation of help; providing new learning experiences; arousing emotions; enhancing the patient's sense of mastery or self-efficacy; and providing opportunities for practice. The point of the perspective offered by Frank and Frank, in their famous book *Persuasion and Healing*, is not to undermine psychotherapy but to acknowledge that it is a culturally constructed system of healing which, in fact, has much in common with other systems of healing, not in its content, but in the processes – enacted through myth and ritual – that it adopts. All healing is made up of myths and rituals, and it is these elements that often mobilise the 'recipient's' expectations, hopes and commitment. Although science seeks to distinguish the 'active' agents in treatment from more 'common' factors across interventions, or from straight out-and-out placebo effects, the appropriateness of this is increasingly being questioned.

Hubble, Duncan and Miller (1999), in their review of 'what works in psychotherapy', state 'we found that the effectiveness of therapies resides not in the many variables that ostensibly distinguish one approach from another. Instead, it is principally found in the factors that all therapies share in common' (p. xxii). These factors are the so-called 'common' factors. Importantly Hubble et al. are at pains to point out – unlike some previous critics – that psychotherapy works! They stress that different components of the psychotherapeutic process contribute to different extents to positive outcomes: extra therapeutic change (or what happens outside the consulting room); the therapeutic relationship (the common factors); expectancy or placebo effects; and specific techniques (e.g. empty chair, thought record sheets, dream analysis). Crucially they also stress that different sorts of psychotherapy work equally well for the vast majority of problems. Needless to say, these are not arguments that mainstream psychology is comfortable with; however, they are relevant to a broad range of health professions and interventions.

More recently Paterson and Dieppe (2005) argue that it is not meaningful to split complex interventions into the 'characteristic' (particular) and 'incidental' (more general in the sense of occurring because of the mode of intervention rather than the intrinsic aspect of the treatment). They argue that elements classed as incidental in drug trails may in fact be integral to non-pharmacological treatments. Taking the example of acupuncture and Chinese medicine they note that the simple additive model of randomised control trials (RCTs) is too simplistic and that therapeutic effects interact on multiple levels. They state:

> . . . treatment factors characteristic of acupuncture include, in addition to needling, the diagnostic process and aspects of talking and listening. Within the treatment sessions these characteristic factors are distinctive *but not dividable from incidental elements*, such as empathy and focused attention
>
> Paterson and Dieppe (2005, p. 1204, italics added)

They concluded that it is the underlying theory of a therapeutic intervention that should determine which elements are 'active' and which may be considered as a 'placebo', rather than a simple biomedical common denominator of therapeutics. It is clear that in many healing processes the healing agents, and the beliefs that surround them, may be distinct, but not necessarily divisible.

Service utilisation

Before proceeding with an assumption that communication about health occurs only once a patient gets to the consulting room, I briefly consider how culture may influence what gets into the clinic. One aspect of this is to consider to what extent available services actually get used. Sue (1994) has stressed the importance of understanding the role of 'shame' and of protecting (saving) 'face' in the underutilisation of health services by Asian groups in North America. Related to our previous discussion on diagnostic disclosure, *Haji* among Japanese, *Mentz* among Chinese, *Chaemyun* among Koreans and *Hiya* among Philippinos are terms used to convey concern over shame or loss of face. The individuals with problems such as juvenile delinquency, AIDS or depression may be seen as bringing disgrace on their whole family. Although people from many cultures may be reluctant to publicly engage health services – and by doing so to publicly admit they have problems – Sue argues that this tendency is especially pronounced among Asians. Such cultural differences in services utilisation have serious consequences for attempts to provide health across cultures, on an equitable basis.

Behaviours associated with shame or stigma are likely to be denied or under-represented to the clinicians, perhaps leading to the mistaken conclusion that certain problems are less common in particular cultures. Thus, the demand for services may not be equivalent to the need for services. The concept of the 'clinical iceberg', where only a small proportion of clinical problems are ever presented to clinicians, is well accepted. If we assumed that all cultural groups have roughly equivalent service needs, this second point would essentially mean that some 'icebergs' were more buoyant than others, and that perhaps there is an element of selective buoyancy. Thus Asians, or any other cultural group, may have service needs that are not met because their culture 'discourages' recognition of particular problems. Even when appropriate services do exist, their uptake may be delayed, or used only as a last resort, with the result that the time-line of a disorder may appear different from one culture to another.

Where the distressed person is not the person who decides to seek professional help cultural factors may also skew the presentation of problems, e.g. the high achievement orientation of many immigrant Asian families has been noted in North America, Europe, Australia and Africa. Where the admission of a problem may influence a child's opportunities for success, parents can be reluctant to seek appropriate help through formal channels. Thus there are many reasons why the expression and presentation of symptoms to a practitioner may be influenced by the status of a person's problem within their own culture. Likewise the estimation of service needs, as opposed to service demand or service utilisation, within any one culture may require great cultural sensitivity on behalf of service providers, and so cultural variations in help-seeking behaviour need to be taken into account.

As indicated at the beginning of this chapter 'treatment' must not be thought of only as something that occurs between a clinician and a client or patient. Treatment has to be conceived of as being much broader than this. After his review of the literature on mental health among Asians, Sue (1994) targets three levels of intervention. At the level of individual therapists he recommends the education and training of therapists around the challenge of how psychotherapeutic issues can be integrated with a client's cultural background. At the level of Asian families and communities he advocates the promotion of positive health messages concerning how stigmatised problems can be successfully treated. For administrators and policy makers, at the third level, Sue recommends the recruitment of more Asian therapists, more funding of research on cultural factors that may determine health, and the creation and financing of truly integrated training and treatment programmes.

These points are similar to those made by many others in trying to advance interventions for different cultural groups. One key aspect in such suggestions is the cardinal importance of working through the medium of the client's cultural assumptions. However, cultures change. '"Culture" cannot be thought of as a bag of memories and survival techniques which individuals carry about with them and of which they have forgotten to divest themselves. Rather it is a dynamic re-creation by each generation, a complex and shifting set of accommodations, identifications, explicit resistances and reworkings' (Littlewood, 1992a, p. 8). All cultures are in a process of change, even those that are replicating their present state. Transition is a part of every 'stable' culture. It is the means through which a social group reproduces a likeness of itself as a social group.

Cultural aspects of psychological treatments

Psychotherapies are products of their culture. Many cultures assume that their own culture is the closest interpretation of reality. Most cultures, defining the world in their own way, are understandably self-centred, or ethnocentric, the inhabitants of one culture often seeing the behaviour of members of another culture as being a variation (reinterpretation) of themes within their own culture. In essence, each culture assumes some degree of universalism: that other peoples are like themselves in some important respects. Clearly many cultures also assume that there are some important differences and if these are seen in a negative light then they can be the source of racism. Many Western societies put great value on objectivity and the scientific method. One tenet of the scientific method is that we should study universal laws. In the west there is therefore a (perhaps unconscious) drive to show that different phenomena throughout the world behave according to certain basic universal principles. Thus Western science believes that it should be able to discover these universal laws. If it can do so, it will be showing that, whatever goes on in the world and wherever it happens, these things can be accounted for by rules and principles that reflect the Western way of seeing the world.

There need be nothing sinister in this sort of endeavour. There does not need to be any conspiracy, or any explicit attempt to colonise the minds of other cultures. Yet there is a real sense in which attempts to apply a psychological treatment, developed in one culture, to the inhabitants of another culture may be imposing a theory of mind on people who have their own minds and their own theories. Psychologists or others, who work through psychological treatments, therefore run the risk of unwittingly becoming missionaries of the mind where they are the agents of a sort of Western psychological colonialism. When psychotherapies developed in the West are practised on members of a cultural group that is relatively disempowered (e.g. immigrants or people in low income countries), they may deny the validity and dignity of another human being's experience of the world; they may subjugate another person's distress to a foreign language where it cannot be heard, understood or alleviated. This is surely a most damning instance of cross-cultural psychology.

A counter-instance of cross-cultural psychology in this therapeutic domain is where one culture is not necessarily disempowered relative to another, and there is an exchange of ideas between the two. An example of this might be the adoption of Zen Buddhism in some western psychotherapeutic models, the use of Indian yoga exercises in western stress management training or the practice of Chinese acupuncture in western pain clinics. These are no lesser examples of one culture influencing another. The millions of people who make up the hundreds of different western cultures are no less subject to the possibility of hegemony (both from within and outside the west) than are those from South American, African or Asian cultures. The important difference is, however, that where a power imbalance exists there is a danger of one culture's way of seeing the world being (often deliberately) imposed on another.

Check in to a hotel in 'down-town' Harare, 'grab' a shower, 'flake out' on the bed and 'flick on' the TV. If this is your modus operandi you may not experience the next step: feeling like wallpaper, with CNN coming at you from around the world, i.e. the USA world! The west is in your bedroom. It is probably in your TV, your clothes and, before long, your thinking. This is where we are at. Modern technology and power imbalances can colonise minds in peacetime, probably more effectively than they ever could in times of war. Usually, in war there is a concerted effort at 'counter-propaganda'. Yet in peacetime where clear dependency relationships exist (again, for instance, between host nationals and immigrants, or between the more and less industrialised countries) the mobilisation of cultural forces necessary for resisting such influences may be lacking. Some practitioners who work with culturally disempowered groups are well aware of these problems, yet it is often in those most unaware of these problems that the greatest opportunities for change lie. Perhaps you are one of them?

Psychoanalysis is one of the icons of western psychotherapy. Its originator, Sigmund Freud, was a Jewish German. Many of the early psychoanalysts in Britain were of Jewish origin (having fled the Nazis in the 1930s). Yet at that time Britain was also quite anti-Semitic. However, rather than psychoanalysis being developed as a Germanic–Jewish therapy (which might have happened without the Second World War), it was identified with 'science', by postulating that certain intrapsychic processes were common to all people. This particular group of immigrants to Britain was unusual in that they were upper middle class and able to influence the health beliefs of another culture. Their influence was at the significant level of the intellectual British bourgeoisie who were willing to part with their money for this new Germanic–Jewish therapy. The therapy did not explicitly tackle issues of culture but instead focused on the inner life of the individual, safe from the sociopolitical context in which analyst and analysand lived. Yet it is within the middle class, with its white, cerebral and western subcultures, that psychoanalysis has largely restricted itself. Indeed, even today popular psychoanalytic folklore has it that to benefit from this treatment you must be smart, rich and white. If this is so, it would clearly be a 'culture-bound' treatment. I do not believe that it is, and indeed Freud's recognition of transference and counter-transference provides a mechanism for exploring all that analyst and analysand bring to the therapeutic encounter. The fact that their 'all' reflects not only intrapsychic processes but also cultural factors may be an aspect of psychoanalysis that has not been sufficiently developed.

Modifying psychotherapy across cultures

Many subsequent psychological therapies have followed psychoanalysis in their emphasis on individualism and autonomy. So, for instance, the maximisation of the client's potential and the successful negotiation of dependency relationships are keystones in many therapies. One line of research has explored how psychological treatments could be modified in order to take account of their application in non-Western cultures.

Varma (1988) has emphasised the close interrelationships of culture, personality and psychotherapy, and therefore the importance of adapting western models of psychotherapy if they are to be used in non-Western contexts. Varma's survey of Indian psychiatrists suggested a number of ways in which this could be done in the Indian context. It was recommended that the therapist should be more active in his or her role, making more directive suggestions and giving reassurance, and putting less emphasis on psychodynamic interpretations. Therapy should be brief, crisis oriented, supportive and flexible. It should also be eclectic (drawing on a range of techniques from different 'schools') and tuned to the cultural and social conditions, including recognition of and blending with religious beliefs. Finally, it was also suggested that the same level of professional training (as is usual in the West) would not be necessary to carry out this function in India.

Ilechukwa (1989), practising psychotherapy in Nigeria, notes a number of points that prohibit the benefits of a Western, especially psychodynamic, style of therapy. Perhaps at the most basic level individual therapy ignores the greater sense of collectivism, or group awareness, that prevails in Nigeria in comparison to the USA or Europe. At the level of presentation Nigerians rarely present with feelings, but with somatic symptoms. The focus is on their physical experience rather than their mental experience. Concerning mode of intervention, the usefulness of the individual approach may be limited; instead Ilechukwa sees the use of ritualistic therapies, which may help to reintegrate the individual into the group, as being more appropriate. It is also suggested that within the context of psychodynamic therapy many Nigerians find free association and passivity very threatening. Instead, a more directive approach is advocated where the therapist tells the client or patient what to do. This, it is argued, falls in with the cultural expectation of being given advice. The practitioner is regarded as *mzee*, a 'powerful stranger'.

Jilek and Jilek-Aall (1984) reviewed several factors that they recommended should be taken into account in psychotherapy with North American Indians. These included the fact that North American Indians generally do not partition 'illness' into the mental and physical dichotomy so often used in western healthcare. Furthermore, North American Indians are generally more comfortable with attributing incomprehensible events to supernatural forces than westerners, who usually prefer to attribute things beyond their knowledge to knowledge that is waiting – just around the corner – for them to discover. This western knowledge is, of course, to be unearthed by scientific endeavour. Although westerners cannot explain it now, they have sufficient *faith* in their methods to know that, at some point, an explanation in terms of what they currently understand will emerge. Is there not a sense of the supernatural about this? For North American Indians extrapsychic conflicts (i.e. social conflicts outside of the self) are seen as more important than intrapsychic ones (e.g. where parts of the self are in opposition). The focus is again on the social arena, social obligations, social status and social living. Here children are seen as universally desired and an absolute necessity for happiness.

Although various authors have emphasised the importance of taking the cultural background of clients into account in therapeutic relationships, others have sought to develop therapy that places culture in the foreground. This is a difficult task and to illustrate this point I consider the 'culture-centred' approach to psychological therapy.

Culture-centred intervention

Pedersen and Ivey (1993) have described the 'culture-centred' approach to counselling. Their emphasis is on how the assumptions and values that characterise a particular culture shape and direct the behaviour of individuals within that culture. This they have contrasted with several other approaches to counselling, e.g. a person-centred approach assumes that individuals are autonomous within their culture and that they have the power to act and think independently of their cultural context. A problem-centred approach sets its sights on solving externalised problems, often neglecting to appreciate the social and cultural function that a 'problem' may be serving for the owner of that problem. Behaviour-centred approaches attempt to manipulate behaviour without consideration for its cognitive or cultural representation. Situation-centred approaches may focus on the context of behaviour (including its cultural context) without taking into account the individual's own interpretation of the situation.

Pedersen and Ivey (1993) have attempted to develop a way of acquiring counselling skills that will make counsellors effective across many different cultures. Thus, rather than identifying the requisite skills to work in a particular culture, they attempted to identify skills to work with all cultures. An initial stage of their training programme is to release the practitioner from his or her own 'cultural encapsulation'. This term, originally used by Wrenn (1962), refers to a practitioner's inclination to use stereotypes of the world in order to make it more manageable and to assume that his or her own (culture's) aspirations for an individual are also those of the client. The first stage of Pedersen and Ivey's training programme therefore concentrates on making the practitioner aware of their own cultural assumptions. The second stage presents a conceptual framework, called the 'cultural grid', for distinguishing between personal and cultural aspects of interpersonal and intrapersonal relationships. This grid allows consideration of the variables that influence the values, expectations and behaviours of individuals.

The third stage of the model uses the concept of four 'synthetic cultures'. These synthetic cultures are based on Hofstede's (1980) four dimensions of culture (previously described in Chapter 2). The cultures, described as alpha, beta, gamma and delta, refer to Hofstede's dimensions of small to large power distance, collectivism–individualism, femininity–masculinity and strong–weak uncertainty avoidance. Practitioners are taught appropriate counselling skills for clients from each of these cultures. The practical value of this approach is that it illustrates how, for example, different questioning or reflecting skills may be required for individuals from 'alpha' and 'gamma' cultures. It is an interesting and mechanically intricate attempt to provide practitioners with a means of thinking through different cultures. Although Pedersen and Ivey argue (1993) for the various advantages of this approach, it is quite problematic.

The four dimensions described by Hofstede were derived from research initiated over 20 years ago, in an industrial not a therapeutic context, with one multinational company and on a data-set designed for a different purpose. This is not to detract from the usefulness of Hofstede's analyses, but, rather, to recognise their limitations. Can, for instance, 200 employees of IBM in Finland really be taken as a representative sample of the values of Finnish people? Is it possible to generalise from the views of people 30 years ago to the views of people from the same geographical areas today? In addition to these points there has for some time been concern with Hofstede's interpretation of some of the dimensions, especially the masculine–feminine dimension. This dimension, in particular, would have great significance in the therapeutic domain.

However, the major problem with the synthetic cultures approach is that the cultures are synthetic! They do not exist. They are caricatures, stereotypes based on psychological research that was conducted for quite a different purpose. In attempting to use abstractions for training there is a danger that counsellors will be skilled only in an abstract sense and not in the real sense of working with people from real world cultures. Here the counsellor may struggle to place the individual, or the culture, somewhere along the abstract dimensions with which they have been trained to deal. In doing so they may be distracted from the particular meaning of the presenting problem, for the particular person with whom they are working. The limitations of Hofstede's empirical dimensions for counselling work with individuals have also been noted elsewhere (e.g. Lago & Thompson, 1996).

Ten considerations when working psychotherapeutically across cultures

La Roche and Maxi (2003) discuss three distinct perspectives of understanding cultural differences in psychotherapy: universalism, particularism and transcendist perspectives. Universalism is concerned with common factors (e.g. warmth) as facilitators of successful therapy, and as such de-emphasises the necessity to address cultural differences. Particularism emphasises how difficult it is for individuals from different cultural backgrounds to understand each other; it sees cultural differences as generally insurmountable barriers between therapists and patients. Transcendism, on the other hand, sees discussion of cultural differences as an important skill for clinicians to develop, and as a key part of understanding the different perspectives that therapist and patient bring to therapy, whatever their cultural backgrounds.

Within this transcendent perspectives, which we have been reviewing here in other ways, La Roche and Maxie (2003) identify 10 considerations in addressing cultural differences in psychotherapy. These are also relevant to therapeutic/healing relationships outside the psychotherapeutic context and including more general healthcare settings. We briefly consider these ten factors below:

1. Cultural differences are *subjective*, and so one needs to explore the meanings that people ascribe to cultural differences. Cultural differences are *complex* in the sense that they include multiple interacting variables (re gender, sexual orientation, socioeconomic status, age, etc.), and they are also *dynamic* in the sense that meanings change and differences once important may no longer be so. Essentially, *culture cannot be presumed*, it has to be understood from the individual's own perspective. This echoes earlier discussions.
2. The most salient cultural differences should be addressed first.
3. Similarities should be addressed as a prelude to discussion of cultural differences.
4. The patient's levels of distress and presenting problem will often determine when and if cultural differences are discussed in psychotherapy. Those who are less stable and more acutely distressed are less likely to benefit from such discussions.
5. Cultural differences should be addressed as assets that can help in the therapeutic process, rather than being constructed as deficits.
6. The patient's cultural history and "racial identity" development are important factors in assessing how best to conceptualise presenting problems and facilitate therapeutic goals. In other worlds, cultural identity and acculturation affect understandings of what are 'appropriate' conceptualisations.
7. The meanings and saliency of cultural differences are influenced by ongoing issues within the psychotherapeutic relationship. What is meant here is that, if an issue such as gender identity was 'difficult' for a therapist and patient to discuss in any case, different cultural readings of gender roles may compound this difficulty and lead to avoidance of such discussions.
8. The psychotherapeutic relationship is embedded within a broader cultural context that affects the therapeutic relationship, e.g. public discussion of discrimination, refugees, AIDS or whatever may promote or inhibit their discussion in the therapeutic context.
9. The therapist's cultural competence will have an impact on the way that differences are addressed.
10. Dialogues about cultural differences can have an effect on the patient's cultural context, e.g. a culture that promotes materialism, competition and

heterosexuality may be challenged by a patient (and indeed the therapist) reflecting on alternative values, such as spiritualism, collectivism and homosexuality, in such a way that it actually initiates change in society.

How and when to address cultural differences will vary across healing contexts but the above themes are likely to be salient to most. The extent to which such considerations are explicitly addressed may influence the time that patients stay in therapy, their adherence to prescribed treatments, their likelihood to attend follow-up etc. What is needed here, as with so much of healthcare in a cultural context, is a stronger evidence base to inform our research, teaching and practice. However, such an evidence base does not need to come from large-scale studies alone; it can also come from understanding of individuals' particular experiences.

In any analysis of culture we must always remain aware that culture works through individual people. Yet culture also provides the social medium through which individuals work through life. Individuals and their culture(s) reciprocally influence each other. Even in the case of individuals who completely reject their cultural heritage, or who feel themselves to be between various cultural heritages, their attitudes can still be described relative to certain cultural values. We therefore return to an issue discussed in Chapter 1, i.e. the importance of keeping the individual foreground and the culture background in perspective, for every person. As both individuals and cultures are in a process of continual change, this seems to be a tall order indeed. I now set out an alternative attempt at unravelling this matrix, one that recognises that our worlds do not necessarily fit neatly into other people's categories, that we may not ourselves be aware of all the cultural and idiosyncratic assumptions that propel us, and one that uses as its primary data the immediacy of personal experience.

Analysing critical incidents as a therapeutic technique

We wish to find out what an individual considers important in his or her life. If we can unravel the goals and rules by which people live their lives we can get closer to understanding what will make them happy and sad, hopeful and pessimistic, angry and timid. Personality theory and psychology in general have attempted to come up with universally applicable explanations of why people are as they are (see Chapter 2). The search continues for grand theories that might explain the behaviour of not just one individual but of millions of people. In the technique described here the focus is idiographic and qualitative. We are concerned with how individuals experience life in their own terms, and not particularly concerned to compare this experience with that of others, to say whether it is more or less, better or worse, happier or sadder. The therapeutic use of critical incidents, which I am suggesting here, has its roots in occupational (or industrial) psychology and to put it into some kind of context let us briefly consider this.

The technique of critical incidents analysis was first described by Flanagan (1954) as a means of answering the question: 'What sort of skills are necessary to carry out a particular work role?' However, rather than the 'experts' in industrial psychology being asked this question, the question was directed at the 'on-the-job experts', those actually doing the job being studied. Now, simply asking somebody what skills are necessary to do the job is a deceptively easy question. In fact we often may not know exactly what skills we use, perhaps because we have become over-familiar with our work role. Flanagan therefore asked the same question in a different way. First he asked workers to define the objectives of their job, not as stated by their boss or in the company manual, but in their own terms. Second, he asked them to describe incidents that were critical to them achieving the objectives that they had described. The incidents could be critical in the positive sense of helping them to achieve their objectives, or negative in the sense of prohibiting them from achieving their objectives. Having thus identified a balance of positive and negative critical incidents, the workers were asked to reflect on the skills that they used (or failed to use) during these incidents which were relevant to them achieving their work objectives. In this way a catalogue of skills relevant to the job was built up.

Recently this approach has been used to identify job skills, not in the context of industry, but for people working with traumatised refugees. I therefore review some examples from my own research to illustrate the critical incident technique in a domain more clearly relevant to health and welfare work across cultures (MacLachlan & McAuliffe, 2003). During the height of the Mozambican war over one million Mozambican refugees poured into neighbouring Malawi. Many of these people had been traumatised through their war experiences. Relief work has usually (and understandably) targeted the immediate physical health needs of refugees. However, a sole focus on physical health neglects the fact that such efforts may be inhibited in their effectiveness by the mental state of traumatised refugees. Their trauma is, of itself, deserving of therapeutic intervention. In collaboration with the Finnish Refugee Council we investigated the job experiences of 15 counsellors who were themselves also refugees. Table 6.1 shows the objectives identified by those counsellors who were working with traumatised children.

The following is an example of a critical incident given by a counsellor who was working with a young boy:

> It was time to play football and a certain boy could not play with the others. Every time I tried to make this boy participate, he would complain of pain from a tiny wound on his left leg. On this day I chatted with the boy for a long time behind a fence, and learnt that the child's father was killed in Mozambique. I was also told that peers mock and segregate the boy saying that he is a fool. He stays with his mother and has no father. I also gathered that peers refuse to play with him. I felt sorry and

Table 6.1 Objectives of counsellers of Mozambican refugee children.

Statement of objective	Frequency
1. To play a variety of games with refugee children so that they can forget their war experience	5
2. To encourage group sharing of personal war experiences	3
3. To change the depressive feelings and thoughts of refugee children affected by war by inducing their participation in activities	3
4. To give advice to refugee children through telling them meaningful stories	3
5. To involve refugee children, without their parents, in singing, dancing, and other cultural activities	2
6. To create a sense of security	1

Reproduced from Kanyangale and MacLachlan (1995). (With permission.)

assured the child that he was free to play without being mocked, like any other child in the programme. Currently, the boy leads others in singing and dancing and he is good at riddles. The boy consults me for advice whenever he is provoked.

Kanyangale and MacLachlan (1995)

The counselling skills identified from this incident included the ability to create an environment of security/trust (from giving the child an opportunity to play without the fear of disapproval), the ability to probe (from having investigated the boy's home life and uncovering the fear of disapproval), and the ability to communicate a sense of being understood and cared for (from comforting the boy, showing interest and giving reassurance). In addition to these attributes identified by the counsellor himself, we also noted the counsellor's awareness of defence mechanisms (from the counsellor's recognition of the boy's projection of his fears on to the pain from the tiny wound) as an important attribute. The attributes identified from incidents such as these may then be synthesised into related themes.

Table 6.2 shows the complete list of skills identified in this way from 15 refugee counsellors. As can be seen, the technique of critical incident analysis provides rich qualitative information based on the acknowledgement of expertise that lives within the individual who is actually doing the job. This technique may therefore have the potential of uncovering some of the clinical skills, which particularly effective cross-cultural practitioners use, as well as highlighting the circumstances that many of us find particularly difficult to deal with. As the technique is so practically focused in terms of applied clinical skills, and because it acknowledges and utilises the skills of people actually doing clinical work, it could act as an important adjunct to training in therapeutic skills. However, the technique may also be able to make a more direct contribution to the clinician's approach to treatment across cultures.

As the critical incident technique describes authentic or real scenarios, its value has been recognised for training in cross-cultural awareness. Brislin

Table 6.2   Job-related attributes identified by refugee counsellors.

Attributes	Frequencies		
	Positive	Negative	Total
Interview process			
Create a sense of security and trust	4	6	10
Communicate a sense of being understood and cared for	1	8	9
Sympathy	4	5	9
Tolerance	4	7	11
Patience	3	4	7
Sensitivity to individual's needs	1	2	3
Non-judgemental	1	3	4
Prompt verbal communication	7	3	10
Facilitate open discussion	3	3	6
Probing	4	5	9
Analytical skills			
Interpret emotional reactions to be reasonable and normal	5	3	8
Challenge assumptions	2	1	3
Awareness of defence mechanisms[a]	2	3	5
Identify reinforcers of maladaptive behaviour	4	5	9
Sensitivity to emotional readiness to confront painful experiences[a]	1	3	4
Observe abnormal behavioural patterns	7	6	11
Awareness of step-by-step progression towards goal achievement[a]	1	2	3
Awareness of non-verbal behaviour	1	1	2
Self in relation to others			
Perception of self and others[a]	3	1	4
Being flexible in problem solving	1	4	5
Awareness of the influence of power relationships on communication[a]	1	1	2
Sensitivity to the communicative function of physical contact[a]	3	4	7

[a] Indentified by interviewer.
Reproduced from Kanyangale and MacLachlan (1995). (With permission.)

et al.'s (1986) cultural assimilator presents a series of critical incidents drawn from a range of different cultural settings. The trainee must choose the most culturally appropriate response from several alternative possibilities. Explanations are provided for each choice. By realising the rationale for their correct responses as well as the reasons for their errors, trainees are helped to assimilate a degree of sensitivity to issues of culture, especially communication across cultures. In addition to cross-cultural training, critical incidents have also been used to enhance clinical skills in various settings.

The original technique of critical incidents analysis sought to identify appropriate skills, or behaviours, from people 'on the job'. Critical incidents were defined as those incidents that specifically related to a person's job objectives. As such the objectives of the job defined the sort of incidents to be discussed, whether they were examples of the use of appropriate skills or of skills lacking.

In living, we are already doing a job. Every day we experience incidents that are critical to our mental and physical well-being. We find ourselves pleased with the outcome of some important events and disappointed with the outcome of others. Can we not, therefore, determine what our objectives must be?

If we can determine a person's objectives for living we are some way towards understanding how culture, family relationships, personal aspirations, etc. interact within any one of us. Thus, by examining what a person's critical incidents are, we can work backwards to unearthing their objectives. Sometimes we will do things for reasons that are perfectly clear to us, yet at other times our own behaviour can be a bit of a mystery. Conflicts between cultural identities for members of immigrant groups may be traced, for example, to conflicts in their objectives of living, where one objective is to retain traditional values, whereas another objective is to be accepted into the host society. These and other factors form important elements in the following case study, which explicates the technique that I have described as 'critical therapy'.

Case study: a cross-cultural example of critical therapy

Shagufta is a 16-year-old girl whose family came to England from Pakistan, 3 years after she was born. The family has returned to Pakistan twice since, on holidays, where Shagufta has enjoyed meeting with her extended family and taking part in family celebrations. In England she is an excellent pupil at the local comprehensive school and is popular both with other Asian girls and among the (majority) white English pupils. For the past 6 months Shagufta has been caught in a 'bulimic cycle' where she binges on sweet foods, vomits what she has eaten, feels great guilt over having done this and then sometime later binges, vomits and feels guilty again. Shagufta's mother had recently read an article called 'Eating disorders: The modern western plague'. After discovering her daughter in the middle of vomiting one night and being suspicious of her secret eating, Shagufta's mother brought her to their general practitioner who referred her to a clinical psychologist for treatment of bulimia nervosa. She has now seen the psychologist twice.

Shagufta has continued her bingeing behaviour. Last night at 2am after having binged on biscuits and bread for 2 hours she was making herself sick, vomiting into the toilet bowl, when she heard somebody coming along the corridor. She speedily cleaned up the vomit around the bowl and flushed the toilet. Her mother knocked on the door and Shagufta came out of the toilet reassuring her mother that everything was all right and that she had not been vomiting. While in the toilet her mother discovered a patch of vomit that Shagufta had missed. She went to Shagufta's bedroom and there ensued a huge argument. Shagufta described the incident as a clearly negative incident, identifying the following important aspects:

1. 'I had an argument with my mother.'
2. 'I lied to my mother.'
3. 'I gave in to a desire to binge.'
4. 'I felt so guilty and lonely before the binge.'
5. 'My mother said that she had never heard of anything like this before in Pakistan and that I am shaming my family.'
6. 'My mother said I was acting like a silly little English girl.'

To understand how these critical aspects of the incident are related to Shagufta's broader objectives we must ask: 'Why are they important?' Sometimes the relevant objective will be quite transparent, e.g. the first two points, in this case, related to a belief that Shagufta should respect her mother. The third point concerns the belief that one should use self-control, behave with some propriety and not over-indulge oneself. The fifth point, concerning how this had never happened to anyone else in the family, was about the expectation that Shagufta should make her parents proud, especially as she showed such promise at school. Shagufta was not sure why the final point should be so annoying to her, but she felt that it was important. Nor could she identify it with any major objective in her life.

In an attempt to clarify this, the technique of laddering was used:

Question: 'What would it mean if you were acting like a silly little English girl?'
Shagufta: 'It would mean that I was being foolish in an English way.'
Question: 'What does it mean to be foolish in an English way?'
Shagufta: 'It means I am not behaving as I should?'
Question: 'How should you behave?'
Shagufta: 'I should try to be sensible. . . . I should not try to be English!'
Question: 'What does it mean if you should be sensible and not English?'
Shagufta: 'It means I should be Pakistani.'
Question: 'Is this one of your objectives in life?'
Shagufta: 'I really don't know . . . but it's one of my mother's objectives for me.'

Thus the fifth and sixth points identified by Shagufta relate to her ambivalence about an objective that she feels her mother expects of her. Incidentally, the same scenario can also be used to find something positive: the problem was discussed, Shagufta is not being secretive at present, etc.

Clearly no two people will interpret an incident in the same way. The practitioner must be guided through the interpretation by the client. The practitioner's skill is in providing a framework to identify objectives and, where necessary, asking appropriate questions to clarify them.

The critical incident to be analysed in the form described in this case study need not be one of emotional outburst, it could be a stomach pain, a worry or any incident that makes the person feel uncomfortable. The strength of the critical incident process becomes apparent in its reflectivity, i.e. identifying the objectives relating to the incident may not simply give the practitioner a better idea of the cultural context and personal values of their client; it may also allow the client to reflect on the meaning of the problem. In short, it may be therapeutic in itself. However, at the very least, in the cross-cultural context, it should clarify the beliefs, values and expectations that clients have and how these relate to particular problem areas in their lives. But no therapeutic technique can be effective if it fails to take account of the much broader social and cultural context in which it is being sought and offered. The work of the Nafsiyat Centre has been distinctive in confronting and integrating this perspective in its clinical work.

Intercultural therapy

The Nafsiyat Intercultural Therapy Centre was established in London in 1983 to provide a specialist psychotherapy service to minority cultural groups. The centre provides a clinical service, training courses for health personnel and consultation to clinicians in related fields, and undertakes research into the efficacy of therapy. Kareem, the founder and clinical director of Nafsiyat, describes the objective of intercultural therapy as being 'to create a form of therapeutic relationship between the therapist and patient where both can explore each other's transference and assumptions. This process attempts to dilute the power relationship that inevitably exists between the "help giver" and the "help receiver"' (1992, p. 16). Before unpacking this description, it is important to appreciate that Kareem's approach to therapy, unlike many contemporary alternatives, acknowledges that individuals' distress results not necessarily from within themselves but from much broader economic and sociopolitical influences that colour the context in which they experience the world. Therapy therefore becomes a means for understanding the various factors – social, political, economic, psychological and cultural – that may contribute to the creation of distress experienced by members of ethnic minorities. Thus, prejudice, racism, sexism, poverty, social disadvantage and the internalisation of these experiences are confronted as tools of social injustice, which may fully account for the distress with which a person presents. Hopefully intercultural therapy also becomes an occasion for empowerment and self-affirmation of minority cultural groups and individuals.

Intercultural therapy is based on a psychodynamic model. I have already noted that any therapy is a product of certain cultural assumptions. However, it has also been argued that this need not prohibit the application of certain therapeutic techniques outside their culture of origin. One psychodynamic therapeutic technique that was noted earlier and which may have wide relevance is the interpretation of transference and counter-transference, which is an important element of intercultural therapy. Transference refers to the idea that in any encounter between two people there is also an encounter between two histories. These histories may be consciously or unconsciously presented.

A simple example would be where a client in therapy was behaving towards the therapist, and other authority figures, as though he were his father. The client is transferring the feelings that he has about his father into his relationship with his therapist. In turn his therapist also has a personal history. Again he may be consciously aware of certain ways in which his past experiences influence his current relationships, but he may also be unaware of other ways in which his past experiences are influencing the way in which he relates to his client. The therapist may also transfer his feelings, perhaps about his son, on to the client who relates to him in a paternal role. This describes the counter-transference. In this example the therapeutic encounter is explicitly between the therapist and his client, yet implicitly it may be between the client's father and the therapist's son. Psychotherapists therefore may 'work through' and make interpretations about 'the transference'.

Personal histories are not just about what has happened to an individual. They are also about the way in which an individual has come to understand the world and his or her place in it. Personal histories reflect culture, heritage and social history. Building on our simplified example, if the client is black and his father worked on a colonial-run British tobacco farm in Africa, and the therapist is white and his father was in the British colonial service, what histories do they each bring to this encounter? How do their histories interplay? What assumptions does each make about the other? And so on. It would be very surprising if an encounter between a 'help-seeking' member of a disempowered cultural minority and a 'help-giving' member of the white, middle-class intellectual elite did not have some resonance (perhaps literal but more usually symbolic) with their cultural histories. How such factors interact with other aspects of their transference and how these should be worked through is beyond the focus of this book. But it is to this hinterland of culture and health that intercultural therapy addresses itself.

Littlewood (1992), another proponent of intercultural therapy, emphasises that there can be no 10-point prescription for the clinician working across cultures (see La Roche and Maxie, 2003, discussed earlier). He also states that intercultural therapy should not be allowed to become a specialised psychotherapy targeted only at one culturally defined section of a society. Instead it is simply therapy that acknowledges and confronts the broader sociocultural context in which we all operate, whether as members of a powerful majority or of a repressed minority. In this sense we are all potentially 'part of the solution' because we are all an element in the matrix of the problem. For the therapist of white European descent Littlewood (1992, p. 41) powerfully encapsulates the dilemma thus:

'The obvious "liberal" approach is one which simply seeks to offer the European therapeutic model to others on the basis that this is the best we have and that common justice invites us to extend its application. Unless the very problem for which we extend it is ourselves?'

For example, if black people present with distress (psychological or physical problems) that results from their negative experience of white dominance over blacks, offering them 'white' therapies is problematic. It may be seen as denying the legitimate expression of oppression, by transforming its consequences (distress) into a form of pathology treatable by 'white' medicine. In short, it adds insult (of superior white intervention) to injury (of oppression of black people). This is without doubt an extreme sociopolitical interpretation, but not one without value. It is unfortunate because it pits one culture against another, which is neither necessary nor desirable. An interesting alternative approach to therapy for relatively disempowered groups has been to embellish the value of their cultural perspective. Reclaiming one's culture may be incorporated as a key element in reclaiming a healthy self-identity. Let us examine how this can work in settings as diverse as Canada, Australia and Scotland.

Culture as treatment

Alcoholism and drug abuse are a major problem among many indigenous minorities, in both rural and urban settings. Brady (1995), of the Australian Institute of Aboriginal and Torres Strait Islander Studies, has reviewed the high incidence of alcoholism among First Nation North Americans (American and Canadian 'Indians') and Australian Aborigines, and the recent emphasis on the use of 'culture' as a mode of treatment by these groups. These treatment programmes, which attempt to reassert a positive native identity through the practice of traditional customs and valuing traditional beliefs, expound the philosophy that *culture is treatment*.

Why has 'culture' become 'treatment'? A good part of the reason for this probably lies in the contemporary indigenous understanding of the cause of drug and alcohol abuse, which attributes these to social deprivation and the erosion of cultural integrity (acculturation) through colonialisation. The individual alcoholic is seen as a social expression of the experience of cultural repression. Re-connecting individual aborigines with their cultural heritage not only provides a medium for intervention but also regenerates traditional values that are increasingly being portrayed as counters to drug abuse. The Nechi Institute in Alberta is one of the leading indigenous drug abuse treatment centres in Canada. The treatment policy of the centre incorporates various indigenous practices with a disease-based model and an adaptation of the 12 steps used by Alcoholics Anonymous. One of the traditional cultural elements that may form part of the Nechi treatment programme is the sweat lodge. The use of sweat lodges is the most common feature of native alcohol treatment programmes in North America.

The sweat house is a sort of ritualised sauna that takes place in a small rounded structure made by placing blankets or canvas over a frame of willow saplings. Inside, a central pit of hot stones is splashed with water in order to produce steam. Participants, usually wearing shorts, sit around the stones in total darkness for several sessions of up to 30 minutes each. Various ritual practices may take place within the sweat house and tobacco may be used. Although sweat houses are traditionally used by many indigenous North American groups, it is not common to all of them and its actual purpose and associated rituals may differ from one region to another. Nevertheless it is not attributed to any one tribal or linguistic group and has in recent times been seen as a central part of a broadly based First Nations resurgence. The sweat house, through the powerful physical and mental experiences that it produces, therefore allows an individual to embrace a sense of cultural re-awakening.

Brady (1995) suggests four ways in which sweat houses, while being used as a treatment for alcoholism, are also an important mechanism for the revival and development of a positive cultural identity. First, the sweat house is a symbol of Indianness. For those who have lost touch with many aspects of their traditional culture (e.g. language or religion) the sweat house offers an instant and dramatic way of immersing oneself in Indianness. The second suggestion, relating specifically to alcoholism, is that the 'overwhelming physical sensation of undergoing a sweat is of detoxification and cleansing' (Brady, 1995, p. 1492). It therefore is consonant with the idea of physical, psychological and spiritual purification, a fresh start. Third, the drama of the occasion and the fortitude required to proceed with it provide a clear rite of passage and demarcation of an individual's commitment to a new way. The final suggestion refers to the sweat leaders. In the treatment programmes these individuals are often ex-drinkers who now serve as positive role models. The sweat house helps them to maintain their own sobriety. The sweat lodge is an intervention both for the individual and for the community. It signifies an alternative to modern Indian life, one that empowers traditional aspects of culture. It endows historical culture with goodness, wellness and value.

Australian aboriginal treatment of alcoholism

A particularly intriguing aspect of the resurgence in First Nations traditional healing methods for alcohol addiction is their adoption by another indigenous group who are geographically distant and culturally distinct, the Aboriginal peoples of Australia. They are also a people who have suffered dispossession of their land, historically poor 'race relations' and woefully inadequate access to health services. Brady describes how a central part of some alcohol addiction programmes among Aboriginal peoples have stressed the spiritual relationship with the land. Regaining a meaningful relationship with 'Mother Earth', with the 'Aboriginal Mother', is seen as an important pathway out of alcoholism. Many Aboriginal religious practices and beliefs are linked to features of the landscape, created by their ancestors during the 'Dreaming'. Once again, 'culture' is being presented as 'treatment'.

Addictions are, however, seen as a 'non-traditional' problem among Australian Aborigines and therefore to lie beyond the knowledge of Aboriginal traditional healers. This is one major drawback in seeing 'culture', historically, as traditions and customs from the past. In Aboriginal traditional healing there is no tradition of the group as a therapeutic medium; instead a healer and client meet on a one-to-one basis in relative privacy. Based on certain commonalities in their historical experiences and their contemporary marginalisation, Australian Aborigines have recently innovatively incorporated First Nations North American customs into their treatment programmes for alcoholism. Canadian Indian consultants have been employed to advise on and take part in the development of treatment programmes in Australia. There have been numerous exchanges between the Aboriginal peoples of North America and Australia concerned with incorporating traditional methods into the treatment of addictions. In some centres, North American traditions never previously seen in Australia have been incorporated into treatment programmes. This includes the Medicine Wheel (as a symbol of wholeness and strength), beginning each day by the burning of sweet grasses (as a ceremony of prayer and welcome), and the institution of ritual morning hugs and handshakes. Indeed, according to Brady, a Canadian Indian visiting Western Australia was recently asked to build a sweat lodge.

Although we may well have concerns (also expressed by some Australian Aborigines) about the appropriateness of grafting traditional First Nations customs on to contemporary Australian Aboriginal treatments for addiction, Brady (1995) makes the much more positive observation that a major synthesis between these two healing traditions is now taking place. Aboriginal treatments for addiction also adhere to the 12 steps (disease model) of Alcoholics Anonymous and incorporate methods for getting people back 'in touch' with 'Mother Earth'. However, it is also recognised that certain aspects of Aboriginal culture, such as a reluctance to confront (interfere with) people who are having personal problems, deriding ('pulling down') those who seek to escape from a (drinking) group norm, perhaps to 'better' themselves in some way, or not using groups as a medium of help, should not be seen as immutable customs.

This Australian situation provokes important questions about health and cultural healing:

- 'Are the First Nations of North America partially proselytising Aboriginal Australians?'
- 'Is the exchange little more than a form of psychological colonialism?'
- 'Does this synthesis reflect a recognition of the function of "culture" as a medium for self-affirmation?'

- 'Is there anything wrong with benefiting from the customs of another culture?'

And perhaps finally:

- 'Why is it so important to retain our own cultural heritage if any one will do?'

In an attempt to address some of these issues I briefly consider a longitudinal study of a 4-year-long Tibetan Buddhist retreat conducted in Dumfriesshire, Scotland, from 1989 to 1993. This retreat may be seen as another example of 'culture as treatment'.

The Samye Ling retreat: an alternative culture

Buddhism is a religious way of life that is based on the 'awakening' of Siddharta Guatama, later known as Buddha. He was a rich and pampered prince who, lacking fulfilment, decided to turn his back on his privileges and to become homeless. He achieved enlightenment through meditation. Although the contemporary practice of Buddhism varies according to different interpretations, some concepts may be identified as central. The law of *karma*, or cause and effect, ties people to a cycle powered by the results of their good and evil acts. Through *reincarnation* one must live with the consequence of previous lives. The 'Four Noble Truths' of Buddhism describe: how suffering is the effect of past karma; how misplaced values, particularly those of material wealth, are self-limiting; and how suffering can be overcome and that there is a path to achieve this. This path, known as the 'Noble Eightfold Path', identifies 'right' knowledge, attitude, speech, action, occupation, effort, mindfulness and composure as its basic elements. By following this path the goal of *nirvana*, a transformed mode of human consciousness, may be reached. Tibetan Buddhism is one particular interpretation of these ideas.

Buddhist ideas have recently become popular in Europe and North America where they represent not only a culturally foreign religion but also a way of life, a way of being, that is quite foreign. Various reasons may account for this popularity. Buddhism may be seen as more tolerant than, for example, Christianity, the order of natural justice – reaping what you sow – may also be appealing, and many of the high moral standards of Buddhism are certainly praiseworthy.

The Kagya Samye-Ling Tibetan Centre in Scotland was the site for a 4-year retreat undertaken by 46 people from all over the world, including each of the five continents. Artists, journalists, engineers, teachers, lawyers, receptionists, nurses, unemployed individuals and a prisoner on parole were among them. This was the largest Tibetan Buddhist retreat ever undertaken outside Tibet. As we have described (McAuliffe & MacLachlan, 1994) the retreat involved a number of discrete stages. The first year was dominated by prayers (incorporating chanting and visualisation) to remove obstacles to the retreat, promote long life, 'purify negativity' and develop generosity and a devotion to the 'enlightened beings'. To assist in the transition from the busy world to the relative tranquillity of retreat, the first year also involved vigorous physical exercise to use up energy and settle the mind. The second year of retreat involved 'shrine (*samatta*) meditation'. Using techniques such as focusing on the breathing helped to 'still the mind' and to prepare the retreatant for a six-month period of 'intensive practice', again requiring much chanting and visualisation. This period also required retreatants to minimise their activities in order that the mind would have as few distractions as possible. To this end, talking and writing were prohibited for the 6 months. In the third year of the retreat there was much less chanting, and physical exercise was introduced for 1 hour each day until the end of the retreat. The third year continued with the more complex prayer and meditative practices used during the 'intensive period', these being seen as the heart of the retreat. In the fourth year simpler practices were used (with less chanting) to help the retreatant 'wind down'.

Certain aspects of the retreat no doubt seem quite foreign, e.g. the fact that the retreatants were housed only with members of their own sex and essentially stayed within their retreat houses for the whole four years suggests the uniqueness of this form of voluntary 'withdrawal' – and more so given that some of the retreatants were married with children, and that in some cases both partners went into retreat. Also, for a six-month period retreatants abstained from washing. Such 'bizarre' aspects of the retreat's culture surprise or even shock some people. Yet within the ethos of the retreat they make perfect sense. Are there really any cultures in which people knowingly engage in senseless activity? Yet from outside a culture we may not be able to make sense of certain activities (see Chapter 3). Perhaps the most significant question is 'Was the retreat's culture of benefit to its participants?'

Participation in our research was voluntary and, although most participants initially agreed to take part, by the end of the four years only nine people had completed all of our yearly assessments. Many were concerned that our activities might be a distraction from the ethos of the retreat, particularly during the 'intensive period'. We used a range of different quantitative and qualitative techniques to investigate retreatant's experiences. Over the first six months of the retreat (based on data from 29 retreatants) we found a significant decrease in their sleep disturbance and in their ratings of the severity of personal problems. Despite the substantial transition in their daily lives – which we had expected would be quite stressful – we did not find any significant increase in their reporting of perceived stress or psychological disorder. Three and a half years later there were further significant reductions in the reported severity of personal problems and no increase in perceived stress or psychological disorder, both of which, on average, fell well within the 'normal' range.

Despite this lack of stress 'symptoms', many retreatants did initially describe difficulties with adapting to the retreat. Following this many indicated a process of becoming increasingly aware of their own limitations, subsequently growing in self-confidence, and then being anxious about the finishing of the retreat. This process of deconstruction and then reconstruction has similarities to some forms of psychotherapy. Wray (1986, p. 165) has described Buddhism as:

> the cultivation of increasingly ethical conduct, of a concentrated, tranquil but vibrantly energetic and joyful state of mind, and of the subsequent Transcendental Wisdom and compassion arising like a flower on a healthy plant.

Clearly Buddhism offers a unique perspective on life and how to confront life's problems. In the case of the Samye-Ling retreat, people from all over the world were immersed in the culture of Tibetan Buddhism. To the vast majority of retreatants this culture was very different from the one in which they were reared and socialised. Indeed, for some, this may have been the very attraction of Tibetan Buddhism. However, it also transpired that some cultural aspects of the retreat (e.g. having to learn and read scripts in Tibetan) were problematic, and indeed distressing at times for some people. Inasmuch as the retreat and the religion may be seen as a means of improving people's state of mind and body it too can be seen to be a case of 'culture as treatment'. However, the increasing interest in the relationship between religious belief and well-being deserves some further consideration.

Religion and health

Freud (1927/1989) rather dismissed religion as merely neurosis exhibited at the cultural level and, paradoxically, there followed very little interest in the psychological study of religion, with that which was undertaken usually emanating from quite biased perspectives, either for, or against, it. A recent heightened awareness of religion has perhaps been one of the consequences of the 9/11 attacks in 2001. The image of those two planes crashing into the World Trade Centre embodied a level of religious/political fanaticism that most of us had not contemplated. Yet, writing in 1994, Iannaccone, had reported that 'strict churches' in the USA had been growing in strength and membership more rapidly than their mainstream counterparts. Pargament (2002) suggests that more extreme religious beliefs create:

> an unambiguous sense of right and wrong, clear rules for living, closeness with like-minded believers, a distinctive identity, and, most important, the faith that their lives are *sanctioned* and supported by God. (p. 172, italics added)

Although the dark side of more fundamentalist religious interpretations is their association with prejudice, narrow-mindedness and bigotry towards 'out groups', their brighter side is the greater degree of optimism, religious and spiritual well-being, and marital happiness, that is reported by at least some of these groups (Pargament, 2002; see also Chapter 1 and the discussion of the psychological function of cultural world views).

Although fundamentalism obviously expresses the extremes, some themes run through the spectrum of religious beliefs. One of these is the degree of intolerance towards other religions. Although some forms of some religions are more tolerant than others, most religions maintain that they are, in fact, on the truest path towards God, enlightenment, or whatever. In fact, this is necessarily so because religion, at its best, is not a private matter; it is a public matter, in the sense that it binds people together, creates a collective identity and helps them live in harmony. To do this, however, religious beliefs and the moral values that go in tandem need to be shared. Without a shared 'language' communication becomes fraught with difficulties and individual identity becomes threatened (Berger, 1967). This line of argument about why religious intolerance is inevitable also echoes our earlier discussion (in Chapter 1) of why culture exists. As Baumeister (2002, p. 166) states 'Pluralism and tolerance represent a major defeat for any religion because they force it to the margins of life.'

Whatever the mechanisms of maintaining religious belief – whether or not these are extremist – the question that has excited much recent debate is 'Is religion good for your health?' It is fair to say that much research does support this association, e.g. George, Ellison and Larson (2002) conclude that there is increasing evidence that religious involvement is associated with both better physical and better mental health, and longer survival. They also suggest that various psychosocial mechanisms may account for this: positive health practices adopted by more religious people; the greater social support available to them through a larger social network; better psychosocial resources, such as self-esteem and self-efficacy; and the presence of belief structures that create a sense of coherence (or make the world seem meaningful, predictable and manageable).

The motivation of much psychological research is to disaggregate 'packages' of behaviour to find the source of the 'main effects' and 'interactions'. Thus specific beliefs, rituals, piousness, faith, spirituality, confession, atonement, prayer, miracles and virtuous striving could all be isolated, but in doing so we may fail to capture any benefit that arises as an emergent property (something greater than the individual parts) of the system. Furthermore, the sort of instrumental evaluation of religion that I have discussed is not necessarily acceptable to those with strong spiritual beliefs who may well feel that the path to God does not have to be 'good for you', if it is the right path.

Research on religion and health is fraught with difficulties in terms of defining each of these constructs and then operationalising them, i.e. how you measure them (see Shreve-Neiger & Edelstein, 2004). Although religion is often an indivisible component of culture our interest in it here is to illuminate the role of belief and faith in therapy, e.g. Phillips, Ruth and Wagner (1993) explored the belief in Chinese astrology that the year of a person's birth influences that person's fate. They compared over 28,000 adult Chinese Americans with over 400,000 white American controls. When people with a belief in Chinese astrology got a disease that was in some way associated with the phase of their birth year, they were more likely to respond with feelings of helplessness or hopelessness or stoicism. Furthermore, those with stronger faith in Chinese astrology were more likely to die significantly earlier from their disease than those in the comparison group. Clearly, faith can work *for* you as well as *against* you, as illustrated in Figures 6.1–6.3). If the role of faith and religion in health are current 'hot topics', then another, perhaps from the other end of the spectrum, is the role of biological factors, and it is to this that we now turn to complete this chapter on culture and treatment.

Race-based therapeutics

With the advent of patented drug combinations targeted at specific physical ailments, Bloche (2004) poses the question: 'Are we moving into a new era of race-based therapeutics?' Previous research has found that African–Americans have a higher incidence of congestive heart failure than other cultural groups in the USA. Taylor and her colleagues (2004) in the African–American Heart Failure Trial (A-HeFT), noted that a certain combination of drugs (isosorbide dinitrate and hydralazine), given in addition to standard therapy for heart failure, seemed – in retrospective analysis – to have been particularly effective in patients who identified themselves as being 'black'. Taylor et al. (2004, p. 2049) speculated that this may be because people 'who see themselves as black may have, on average, a less active renin–angiotensin system and a lower bioavailability of nitric oxide than those self-identified as 'white'. They therefore set out to undertake a prospective study of the efficacy of isosorbide dinitrate and hydralazine in a sample of 1,050 black people who had heart failure with dilated ventricles (New York Heart Failure Association class III and IV), approximately half of whom were treated with a placebo.

The study was terminated before completion as a result of the significantly higher death rate in the placebo group (who were still being treated with standard therapy) where 10.2%, compared with 6.2% of the treatment group, had died after an average of 10 months on the treatment regimen. These results, which were highly statistically significant, indicate an impressive reduction in mortality from a very common disease, and must therefore be welcomed. The cultural – or racial – conclusions that may be drawn from these results, and indeed the motivation for undertaking the research, do, however, need further scrutiny.

In 1996 a biotechnology firm obtained the intellectual property rights to a fixed-dose combination of isosorbide dinitrate and hydralazine, and then sought approval for its use from the US Food and Drug Administration (FDA) to market this as a new drug. However, they were declined, presumably on the grounds of unproven efficacy. In 1999, having run retrospective analysis on how the drug combination performed among patients from previous trials who 'self-identified' as black, NitroMed obtained the intellectual property rights to the fixed-dose combination and sought FDA approval to market the formulation as a therapy for heart failure in black people only. Bloche (2004) reports that the FDA indicated that a successful clinical trail of the fixed-dose combination in black people would most likely result in them giving their approval. That commitment, according to Bloche, gave rise to A-HeFT.

NitroMed have not only the combination patent noted above, but also a patent on its use in black people – 'the first ever granted to a pre-existing drug for a new, race-specific, use' (Bloche, 2004, p. 2036). The effect of these patents is that they prevent any other drug manufacturer producing a less expensive but equivalent 'generic' drug for another 16 years. Bloche (2004, p. 2036) therefore argues that 'the emergence of the combination treatment as a race-specific drug was driven in large measure by regulatory and market incentives', because the treatment for all patients (regardless of colour) would not have allowed NitroMed to extend its intellectual property rights' protection on the combination.

Bloche (2004) notes that this research does not of course offer evidence of the distinctive therapeutic efficacy of combined isosorbide dinitrate and hydralazine in black compared with other colours of people, because only those 'self-identified' as black took part in the study. Nevertheless, he does acknowledge that the combination may well have differential effects correlated with 'race' (colour), and that black people may be more susceptible than white people to heart failure because of their relatively poor production of nitric oxide in their coronary and peripheral vasculature. Furthermore, he also concedes that other drugs are likely to have 'race-linked' differential effects.

There is of course an argument that we need to exploit these biological differences to the best therapeutic ends, and that here 'race' is used only as a 'placeholder', or marker, for underlying genetic, but as yet undiscovered, differences that result in differential responsiveness to some drugs. Proponents of this view generally acknowledge that skin colour (and other physical features that define 'race') is a poor proxy for genetic variation that might influence the expression of disease. They would see 'race-based therapeutics' as an interim step on the road to personalised pharmacotherapy. However, as Bloche notes, markets and regulatory agendas are possibly more influential in setting research agendas than is the quest for scientific knowledge, or the desire to alleviate human suffering.

There is also a moral issue here in that NitroMed's patents can now effectively 'hike' the price of the combination to one colour of patient, but not to others. What, one may wonder, is now NitroMed's incentive to explore the underlying (possibly genetic) mechanisms, having just publicly 'floated' the company and raised US$66 million, following the above drug trial results. Such research would, if successful, surely only shrink the number of people for whom the combination is indicated, because not all black people will have the underlying genetic predisposition that it hypothetically treats, and NitroMed do not hold the combination patent for non-black people? As a final thought, recall the discussion of the colour–hypertension relationship in Chapter 5: it was suggested that another cardiovascular disease – hypertension – that also has higher prevalence in black people may have more to do with higher rates of stress experienced through racial discrimination, than with a biological predisposition. It would indeed be a sad social commentary on the role of 'race-based therapeutics', if the *ultimate* source of NitroMed's good fortune was not a less active renin–angiotensin system as such, but a 'more active experience of prejudice related stress' among black people. Now, there's a thought: any offers for an anti-prejudice drug?

It is, however, important to acknowledge that pharmacological differences in reactivity have been known of for some time, particularly in the mental health area. As Gaw (2001, p. 137) states there are 'significant differences in the metabolism of psychotropic drugs among various cultural/ethnic populations; these differences affect the treatment of psychiatric disorders', e.g. the percentage of those categorised as poor metabolisers of psychotropic medication varies. For the antidepressant amitriptyline it is 2–6% for white compared with 20% for Asian Americans. For the antipsychotic risperidone it is 5–10% for white and 1–2% for Asian Americans. Lithium, a mood stabiliser, is reported to have a half-life in hours of 14.1 for Asian, 15.9 for white and 20.9 for African–Americans. Thus, in psychopharmacology, levels for therapeutic doses may well vary between different cultural groups (Gaw, 2001). These biological differences are not issues that we should run away from for fear of their connotations of 'race'. They deserve our careful and principled consideration and to be protected from the dangers of inappropriately zealous commercialisation. We need to establish the best way of alleviated people's suffering regardless of their differences, but not necessarily without regard to those differences. This applies as much to biological as it does to socioeconomic and political contexts.

Conclusion

Emerging from studies of 'culture as treatment' is the idea that the attributes of a culture – a context, language, rituals, symbols, etc. – can offer people a vehicle for confronting their problems. Culture as treatment may offer a means of countering a sense of cultural anomie, i.e. in countering the aimlessness that a person may experience through the rejection of the norms of his or her original cultural group. In such cases, 'culture as treatment' offers the individual another 'system of living'. Treatments are ritualised in different ways in different cultures. Whether we experience healing through sweat lodges, 'Mother Earth', psychoanalysis or key-hole surgery may not matter, but what does matter is that the healing is presented in a context that gives our experiences meaning. A strong belief in any particular meaning, be it biomedical science or spirit possession, is likely to heighten our faith in its treatments and practitioners. A pluralistic belief in different modes of intervention may allow us more ways of getting better. However, it is not simply a matter of adopting a laissez-faire attitude of 'whatever works for you', or of imposing a system of healing to which you are passionately dedicated. Instead, healing across cultures must start from the individual's conception of the world, and working through the model the clinician must strive to find mechanisms appropriate to the client's context, while keeping faith with his or her own powers of healing. Sometimes this will involve introducing new elements into the way in which individuals live their lives and understand their world. The utopian aim of the clinician working across cultures is to build healthy communities and allow them to reproduce themselves in ways that represent an adaptation to their current context. This is how 'culture' strives to survive, renewed each and every day.

Guidelines for professional practice

1. In most cultures there is a well-worn path to becoming sick. People from a different culture may not be conversant with the 'right way' to be sick. However, such a role will be facilitated by establishing good communication between patient and clinician. Clinicians should allow for more time, and perhaps more visits by the patient, before making a formal diagnosis.

2. Clinicians may well find that the practitioner placebo effect is less strong with patients from a foreign culture than with those from their own culture. Judgements about who is an effective clinician are subjective (initially anyway) and usually based on faith in the clinician rather than objective data about clinical success. Clinicians should therefore be prepared for patients from a different culture to be more sceptical of their healing powers.

3. The idea of faith in clinicians and faith in treatments can be broadened further to include faith in different healers in general and faith in different types of intervention. This broader level of analysis may help clinicians appreciate how they can be liked as individuals but dismissed as therapeutic agents, or many other combinations of reactions to them as individuals and as healers. These faith grids may help clinicians to think through the interactions between themselves and their patients.

4. People from different cultures will have varying expectations about the information that clinicians will/should share with their patients. Benevolent diagnostic deception may seem unethical to some, whereas others will view the sharing of a stigmatised diagnosis as gross social irresponsibility. As clinical work is increasingly multicultural, in the sense of working with colleagues from different backgrounds, the manner in which cultural values influence clinical decision-making must be considered. Likewise, the patient's expectation of what will/ought to be disclosed should also be taken into account.

5. In attempting to plan for necessary treatment services, service utilisation may be misleading. Some cultural groups may avoid presenting particular complaints because of the shame associated with certain problems. In such cases the role of a cultural representative may be very important in service planning.

6. Treatments are products of cultures. A particular form of psychotherapy, for instance, may strongly reflect particular cultural values. Psychotherapy may also problematise legitimate distress, which arises out of the oppression of individuals of a particular culture. Therefore, sometimes clinicians can adopt a stance to a client that makes them more a part of the problem than a part of the solution. In offering treatment clinicians should think through what their role implies for the client's complaint.

7. Clinicians should not be hesitant about adopting approaches to treatment that emanate from another culture. However, where a power imbalance exists between cultures there is a danger of one perspective being imposed on people who have another perspective.

8. The concept of transference offers a powerful tool for understanding how the interaction between a client and clinician from different cultural backgrounds may mirror important themes concerning how these two cultures have related to each other in the past. Clinicians, of all types, should therefore make themselves familiar with the concept of transference.

9. The 'culture-centred' approach to counselling encourages clinicians to think through abstract and hypothetical cultures, derived from the results of Hofstede's international IBM studies. This approach places culture in the foreground and risks minimising consideration of the extent to which an individual conforms or discounts the values of his or her own culture.

10. The analysis of critical incidents may be used as an adjunct or as a more central part of a treatment intervention. The advantage of this technique is that it allows one to examine what is critical to a person and in doing so to derive at least some of the goals and values in his or her life. Such an understanding should enhance the clinician's ability to intervene in a manner that is sensitive to the client's values.

11. Intercultural therapy provides a medium for therapist and client to explore the influence of many contextual factors, including social, political, psychological, cultural and economic factors, on the distress that may be experienced by members of minority cultural groups. Although many clinicians will feel poorly equipped to deal with such issues, awareness that these broadly based contextual factors may contribute to mental and physical ill-health is crucial.

12. Rather than clinicians operating across cultures, it may be useful for them to consider the potential benefits of operating *through* cultures. Culture may be seen as treatment in itself. Culture can offer a system of living from which marginalised groups have been displaced with the consequence that self-identify and self-esteem have been damaged. The benefits of 'culture as treatment' need not, however, be prohibited to one's own culture. Involvement with different cultures or different religious groups, which offer alternative ways of living, may also benefit some people.

13. Recently, there has been an increasing interest in the role that religious belief and practice may play in health, both physical and mental. Although definitions and the operationalisation of both religion and health have made this a complex area to explore, most reviews find some

support of the relationship. At the level of practice it is important for practitioners to be aware of any beliefs that motivate people to adopt, or
indeed avoid, health-related behaviour. Clinicians should therefore be
interested in elucidating the religious beliefs of the people with whom
they work, to the extent that they influence their health behaviour and
regardless of the clinicians' own religious beliefs.

14. The possibility of 'race-based therapeutics' raises the spectre of being able
more effectively to target and treat diseases that are particular to, or more
prevalent among, a particular group of people. Of course, any treatment
that enhances health is to be welcomed. However, it is important to consider to what extent commercial interests may promote new 'innovative'
colour-targeted therapies, and how such interests may not only affect
the cost of such therapy, but also obscure the motivation to address
ultimate (and possibly social) as opposed to *proximate* (biological) causes
of diseases.

CHAPTER 7

Culturally sensitive health services

> For practising health professionals, it is timely to take pluralism or diversity into account, to re-examine the important role culture plays in how people view and make decisions about their health. We all need periodically to re-examine our own cultural and professional biases, and to be cognisant of the current diversity in the communities we serve.
>
> Mensah (1993, p. 39)

This chapter is concerned with enhancing the cultural sensitivity of health services. It goes beyond the individuals who constitute the service to consider the systems and policies that health services must develop in order to be sensitive to the diverse needs of multicultural communities. We begin by recognising that people's health may be served through various sectors, including the popular, folk and professional sectors. Each person seeking healthcare brings with them their own ideas, or explanatory models, of why they are suffering. Often these models will include a pluralism of ideas that do not necessarily accord with the models of those from whom they seek help. The central concept of any culturally sensitive health service should be 'tolerance of pluralism'. Only through such tolerance can a health service perform its many social and therapeutic functions. I consider what barriers exist to the provision of culturally sensitive health services, and how professional training must address multicultural skills; then I review the sort of policy initiatives that can help to create culturally sensitive health services.

Case study: a clinical challenge of pluralism

Although the ethos of cultivating pluralism in our health services can stimulate a warm glow of good will, it can also present significant challenges to practitioners and researchers. The following case study, reproduced from MacLachlan (2001), illustrates how incorporating pluralism into clinical practice has its difficulties; how, in fact, it may complicate and possibly even compromise the practice of healthcare.

In 1978, Mary, who lived in Central Malawi was brought to a Sing'anga (traditional healer) because of her strange behaviour, including wandering aimlessly, entering other people's houses and attempting to undress herself in public. The Sing'anga treated the woman for *vimbuza* (being troubled by spirits) and the treatment is likely to have included making some sort of offering to appease the spirits and being part of a ritualistic dance/ceremony that possibly included others of her family or social network. This intervention seems to have worked in that she did not seek further help for 15 years.

In 1993, she presented at a psychiatric hospital, run by African nurses and clinical officers (a grade 'in between' nurses and doctors), along a western-oriented biomedical model. Here she was prescribed anti-psychotic medication for the same sort of behaviour that she had presented with in 1978. Again she went through a period of being symptom free, this time for five years. Then in 1998 she presented to a small rural psychiatric facility, with voices telling her not to eat or talk, and directing her actions. This admission coincided with a change in her medication. This was necessary because her local dispensary had run out of her prescribed drug.

Various staff were involved in her assessment at this stage, but the diagnosis arrived at differed between European expatriate and local African staff. The local staff, who had been trained through a western biomedical model, diagnosed the woman as psychotic and wanted to prescribe chlorpromazine (an antipsychotic drug). Expatriate staff, however, felt that much of her behaviour was explicable in terms of cultural norms, but that she was depressed, and wanted to prescribe imipramine (a non-psychotic antidepressant). It would seem that both expatriate and Malawian staff were trying to be pluralistic in the sense that they were taking into account cultural beliefs beyond their own. Ultimately a diplomatic 'compromise' diagnosis was made: psychosis with depressive features! The woman was prescribed chlorpromazine and imipramine! Thus, although the clinicians illustrated a degree of pluralism in the explanatory models involved, their choices of treatment clearly 'privileged' (Shweder, 1991) a biomedical model. Although different approaches to health and illness may exist alongside each other, they are rarely integrated; each treatment context seeks its own (partial) solutions to problems presented in a broader pluralistic environment.

Transcultural, cross-cultural or multicultural care?

The way in which we care for people is influenced by the cultural and social systems in which we live. However, our modern urban communities often present a plethora of cultural and social systems. This makes the task of providing appropriate healthcare extremely complex and challenging. In essence we need a way of conceptualising what it is that we want to achieve. Can the UN initiative of 'Health for All' ever be achieved across many different cultures? Can cultural diversity be retained while providing for equal standards of healthcare to be achieved? Mensah (1993) describes three perspectives on healthcare in the context of cultural variations.

Transcultural care

This care is concerned with a comparison between cultures in terms of their caring behaviour, health and illness values, their beliefs and patterns of behaviour. The focus of this approach is on the care-giver, who has to develop expertise in understanding the groups with which he or she is working in order to deliver care effectively. Thus the clinician is taught to recognise and understand the values, beliefs and practices of different cultures, and in so doing is enabled to deliver care in a culturally sensitive and appropriate manner. In a sense this perspective seeks to make an anthropologist out of the clinician.

Cross-cultural care

A second perspective is that of cross-cultural caring. The implicit assumption here is that the giver of care and the receiver of care are from different cultural backgrounds. Key issues in this approach are how well the cross-cultural bridge can be established in order to allow, for instance, a white English obstetrician to care for an Indian woman. Also of concern in this approach would be the extent to which different cultures within a community health service were utilising the resources of the service. This has been described as 'ethnic monitoring' of healthcare. Related to this is the idea that cultural groups may present with different rates of particular illnesses or disorders. The cross-cultural perspective is perhaps most obviously relevant to the concerns of health service managers.

Multicultural care

The third perspective is multicultural care. Multicultural care, while incorporating elements of transcultural and cross-cultural care, goes beyond these philosophies to provide both culturally appropriate and culturally sensitive care. Rather than focusing on the carer or the administration of caring services, multicultural care is concerned with the total systems of care within the community. Rather than fragmenting services it seeks to make systems of care more effective and applicable to a broader range of people. A key element in the multicultural perspective is recognising and addressing discrepancies between needs extant in the community and the agendas of organisations, institutions and professions that purport to serve the community. Often the conservatism and self-interest of those organisations, institutions and professions will mitigate against their recognition of the pluralism required in any health system that hopes to serve a multicultural community. It is the systemic aspect of the multicultural care philosophy that makes it particularly attractive as a model for healthcare.

Popular, folk and professional sectors of healthcare

Kleinman (1980) has suggested that there are three overlapping sectors of healthcare that constitute the healthcare systems of all societies. His point is that, although the content of these sectors differs across cultures, their structure is the same. Essentially the healthcare system is structured into popular, folk and professional sectors. Each of these sectors offers a particular approach to understanding the cause of, and prescribing treatment for, illness or disorder. Each sector also defines the sufferer and the healer in its own way and has its own rules for their interaction. This model for understanding healthcare systems across cultures has been very influential and so I consider each in turn.

The popular sector

This is the largest sector of the healthcare system. However, it is important to realise that it is not formally defined as a 'sector' and does not fit into an overall planned 'healthcare system'. Instead, the popular sector is where everyday ideas about health and illness are discussed by 'lay' or non-professional people. Healing knowledge and advice are passed on through informal discussions. This sector is where popular notions of health and illness live. It is in the popular sector that people first experience suffering. It is here that they label it and decide how to react to it. Thus, family, friends, colleagues and others whom one encounters in everyday life are part of this popular sector. These people will be sources of ideas about what gives you cancer, heart disease, 'piles', 'nerves', etc., how you know when you have them and what to do to get rid of them. The experience of suffering is often shaped through the beliefs extant in the popular sector.

As the popular sector is where suffering is first experienced, it is also this sector that usually determines whether someone seeks help from the folk or professional sectors. The popular sector is an expression of the community's beliefs about suffering and how to avoid suffering. Thus, jogging, eating raw eggs, taking cold baths, wrapping up tight in the winter and not sitting in draughts are all ideas salient to health and expressed through the popular sector. It can therefore be seen that this sector has perhaps the most influential contribution to make to the prevention of suffering. The popular sector should be the vehicle for the promotion of health because it not only reflects 'popular' beliefs, but also works through community mechanisms. I have argued elsewhere (MacLachlan, 1996) that health promotion, if it is to be successful, needs also to address and counteract 'anti-health promotion ideas' which are a part of the popular sector: 'There is nothing you can do to prevent

AIDS', 'Enjoy life while you can' or 'AIDS is just a new word for old problems.'

The popular sector of the healthcare system includes self-treatment, treatment based on the advice of family or friends, church groups, community groups, self-help groups and seeking out other people who have experienced similar forms of suffering. Part of this sector includes the commonly accepted ways to stay healthy and these beliefs about staying healthy will of course vary from culture to culture.

Professional sector

The professional sector is composed of the organised health professions. In Europe and North America the professional health sector has become dominated by scientific medicine. The medical profession has been successful not only in terms of making other approaches to healthcare subservient to the medical profession ('paramedics', 'professions allied to medicine', etc.) but also in terms of setting the health agenda. Thus western societies now tend to define, treat and evaluate suffering within a medical frame of reference. This is a substantial political 'achievement' by the medical profession when we consider the alternative models of suffering and healing that are available to us.

One function of professionalisation is to suggest that only certain individuals should be in positions of power or have control over particular resources. This is underwritten by the assumption that only some people have the right or ability to help with certain sorts of suffering. This sense of professionalisation has also been exported to less industrially developed societies. This has had some surprising and potentially challenging results for powerful professional groups in the west, e.g. in Malawi, which had a western trained medical doctor as its president for almost 40 years, there has been an attempt to develop a western system of healthcare. Resources have not, however, allowed for the range of professions that usually staff western hospitals.

Zomba Mental Hospital is the major in-patient psychiatric facility in the country. Except for occasional expatriate personnel on temporary contracts, the hospital is staffed by nurses, medical assistants and medical officers. In the early 1990s, when I had just a 'visiting' position there, the hospital has no western qualified medical practitioners, psychiatrists, psychologists, social workers, occupational therapists or physiotherapists. In fact, only a handful of the nurses had any western training. Nevertheless what is interesting about this situation is that, despite the lack of 'appropriate personnel', the hospital ran on a western medical model of psychiatric care, with the diagnosis, treatment (including drugs, electroconvulsive therapy and counselling), discharge and follow-up all being undertaken by nursing staff, clinical officers and/or clinical assistants (a grade mid-range between nurses and doctors). Such a situation would be unthinkable in most western European countries, not because nursing staff could not perform these same functions, but because we have been led to believe that they *should not*.

The exportation and 'expertation' of the western scientific biological model, with the dominating influence of the medical profession, may have come back to haunt the west because these alternative cadres of health workers may be just as effective, a possibility that needs to be explored by empirical research (MacLachlan & McAuliffe, 2005). It is not just in the sphere of mental suffering that our assumptions (you might want to be seduced into calling them 'standards'!) are being challenged. School leavers with two years' subsequent specialised training are in charge of surgical operations that we may believe require ten years of training. The point here is not to evaluate one system of healthcare against another (to my knowledge the effectiveness and 'value for money' of such systems has not been compared) but instead to emphasise that western healthcare is based on assumptions built into its system by different professional groups. There is nothing definitive or 'right' about the way that we do things, rather our systems of healthcare, like all others, reflect the society in which we live.

In western societies there are certain assumptions about who is in charge of a meeting between a health professional and a 'patient'. There are assumptions about the patient 'complying' with or 'resisting' treatment and 'accepting' or 'denying' the diagnosis. It is, of course, not only patients who are victims of this system, but clinicians too. Perhaps you, like myself, have experienced a sudden loss of respect and 'magical healing power' as a result of being so 'insensitive' as to consult a book in the presence of a patient! The assumptions built into western healthcare systems are a direct consequence of having a professional sector based on 'expert' knowledge around the ethos of biological reductionism. Other societies have professionalised alternative approaches to healing and they too have their drawbacks.

Folk sector

The folk sector combines some aspects of the popular and professional sectors. It is characterised as being non-professional (in the sense of formal qualifications), non-bureaucratic (in the sense of being immediately available and not constricted by 'rules') and specialist (in the sense of folk healers having expertise in particular problems and/or treatments). The folk sector includes sacred and secular healers. Although folk healers are more commonly associated with less industrialised countries, increasing internationalisation has resulted in urban communities having a plethora of indigenous and foreign folk healers.

Examples of folk healers traditionally found for instance in Britain, could include, faith healers, 'mediums', gipsy fortune-tellers and herbalists. It could also include a range of treatment approaches currently described as 'alternative' or 'complementary' medicine, such as homoeopathy, acupuncture and hypnosis. Homoeopathy, in Britain, is a particularly interesting example because, although it is seen as an 'alternative' therapy to 'modern' medicine, it was incorporated into the NHS, even to the extent of having specialist homoeopathic hospitals, staffed by medically qualified practitioners who have undergone further training in homoeopathy.

Increasingly, the folk sector, especially in urban areas, is incorporating healers from other traditional societies, including 'root doctors', 'witch doctors' and a great array of spiritual healers. Folk healers from whatever culture share and articulate the social meaning of suffering as understood in their own culture. Internationalisation, multiculturalism and a growing dissatisfaction with biological reductionism have combined to create an unprecedented situation. In the urban heartlands of those societies that consider themselves the most technologically and scientifically advanced in the world, we also have a wider choice of beliefs and treatments available to us than ever before. Many of these beliefs challenge the very assumptions on which technological advancement has been achieved, e.g. holism is preferred to reductionism, the involvement of family members is preferred to an 'expert' dictating the best treatment and a spiritual element to healing is sought.

Together these three sectors constitute a healthcare system that informally interlocks in some places and contradicts in others. Within each of these sectors the understanding of suffering is different and the means of removing suffering varies tremendously. Within any one society each of these sectors presents complex alternative understandings and offers a rich variety of explanatory combinations. Of course, whether or not the clinician is aware of them has no effect on their existence.

As an example, I recall once treating an agoraphobic woman in Dumfries, in the borders of Scotland. In the middle of our 'session' an ambulance passed by outside with the siren wailing. The woman caught hold of the collar of her jacket and smiled apologetically while at the same time indicating that we should continue. As we talked she kept staring out of my office window as though she was looking for something. The ambulance was long gone and the siren had faded 10 minutes previously. Finally, I asked 'Why are you holding your collar?' 'Because of the ambulance', she replied. I started to worry that I had misjudged the woman completely and responded 'Because . . . of the . . . ambulance?' 'Oh yes, don't you know, if you see an ambulance when you're out, you must hold onto your collar until you see three dogs, otherwise it will be going to your house, the ambulance I mean.' Then, she smiled warmly and said 'Well, some people round here believe that anyway.' Ten minutes later she left the clinic still holding on to her collar and laughing a smile. Before she let go of her collar, she later told me, she saw three dogs. When she arrived home there was no ambulance there.

Explanatory models

Kleinman (1980) has also addressed the issue of how people, including clinicians, explain suffering to themselves and to others. His idea is that people develop 'explanatory models' to understand their suffering. He describes this approach as 'ethnomedicine'. Essentially it is about understanding the interplay of cultural beliefs, the experience of suffering and curative methods. He argues that beliefs about illness are closely tied to beliefs about treatment. By understanding the way in which a person explains their suffering we should be able to present treatments to them more effectively. But people do not simply explain the cause of their suffering according to a model found in one of the sectors, rather each individual develops their own explanatory model for each episode of suffering, and each of these models may involve beliefs from the popular, folk and professional sectors, to a different extent. It should be emphasised that an individual's own explanatory models are important not only in the cross-cultural context, but also for understanding the illness models of people within one's own culture (Weinman et al., 1996).

Clinicians have their own explanatory models and in the professional sector these will generally relate to the substance of their professional training. However, even the explanatory models of professional clinicians will differ from each other and some will involve aspects of popular and folk beliefs. When the clinician and the client come together two different explanatory models are meeting. Communication involves understanding the other person's explanatory model. Sometimes the 'cognitive distance' between the models will be great and one of the parties (usually the client) will appear to modify their explanatory model and 'go along' with the understanding of the clinician.

This notion of explanatory models therefore includes the notion (albeit implicitly) that there may be some form of negotiation between the clinician and the patient. The logic for such 'negotiation' would be to come up with an explanatory model that both clinician and patient could 'work with' and which made sense to each of them. Presumably part of this idea of *making sense* is that, for instance, the cause of the problem should be related to its treatment. Thus 'cognitive distance' could be reduced by negotiation to produce a 'cognitively consistent' model.

Tolerance of pluralism

The ideas of popular, folk and professional systems of healthcare, of different explanatory models for each episode of suffering and of a multicultural system of healthcare all combine to present a daunting level of complexity that must appear beyond the grasp of just about anybody! To negotiate logically consistent explanatory models across all these levels of complexity must surely be beyond the time, knowledge and intellectual constraints of most of us. However, none of this is in fact necessary if we reject the notion that consistency is paramount. One problem is that in the western world people are so convinced of the absolute necessity of being scientific, logical and at all times consistent that it is hard for them to imagine how abandoning this ethos could be in any way helpful. They are so tied to it that psychologists have even come up with a term to describe the uncomfortable feeling that accompanies the realisation of inconsistency: 'cognitive dissonance'.

Cognitive dissonance (Festinger, 1957) is experienced when people become aware of inconsistencies in their beliefs and/or behaviour. As dissonance is an uncomfortable feeling, it is argued that people (in western cultures) try to impose consistency on their behaviours and/or beliefs in order to create 'cognitive consonance'. This drive towards consonance is so strong that sometimes they actually distort their beliefs in order to make them appear to 'fit' each other. This notion of things 'fitting' is also described by Kleinman who states (1980, p. 19): 'Thus, ideas about the cause of illness (as well as its pathophysiology and course) are linked to ideas about practical treatment interventions.' However, this need not be so. Ideas about what causes an illness may be quite different from ideas about how to treat the same illness.

In a series of studies conducted in Malawi we have found a lack of 'consistency' in ideas about suffering and how to alleviate it (MacLachlan & Carr, 1994a; MacLachlan, 1996a), e.g. although people may believe in a traditional spiritual cause for malaria they may nevertheless prefer a modern biomedical treatment for it. We have noted this lack of consistency or, to put it more positively, this *greater tolerance* for the ambiguity created by acknowledging different causal models across various illnesses in Malawi. We have also demonstrated how complex non-linear statistical regression techniques can predict apparently 'inconsistent' pluralistic beliefs about health (Carr, Watters & MacLachlan, 2002). If this is the case, we believe that there is a good logic behind such beliefs and that the strength of belief in any particular approach to health will be strongly influenced by the immediate context in which one is seeking help.

However, do not for a moment think that such 'inconsistency' is characteristic of only less industrialised or non-western countries. Similar inconsistencies are also found in the USA, Europe and many other more industrialised regions. In these cultures, for instance, when somebody is suffering from a virus, people often pray for them or give them a luck charm. Frequently nurses open a window in a room where someone has just died so as to 'let their soul out'. Also, people in western cultures may, for instance, take an aspirin for a headache, but this does not mean that they necessarily believe that the headache was caused by a lack of aspirin or by any other chemical deficit. On the contrary they may ascribe its cause to overwork, guilt, heat or whatever.

The point here is not that these actions do not make any sense. Of course they have their own therapeutic sense, but they also cross over explanatory models. Although we are often unaware of it, our ideas and behaviours about health are often inconsistent. This inconsistency can be viewed not as a problem but as a strength. To give it this positive connotation it may be referred to as 'cognitive tolerance'. However, it is clear that this tolerance is not restricted to any one geographical area. Its presence in the tropics is perhaps more obvious because many people living in these areas have confronted radically different systems of healthcare and have been able to do so without having to rubbish or reject all but one of them. However, this is also true elsewhere.

Bishop (1996), working in Singapore, has similarly described tolerance as an aspect of their health system. Singaporeans have access to traditional Chinese, Malay and Indian forms of healing as well as biomedical western healing. Singaporeans commonly seek help from more than one of these systems of healing at a time. Bishop (1996) has reported that compared with North American white students, Singaporean students use a greater number of cognitive dimensions to understand disease and synthesise eastern and western conceptions of disease to a greater extent. Jenkins et al. (1996) have reviewed the health-seeking behaviour of Vietnamese immigrants to the USA and concluded that, although these immigrants continue to have distinctive health beliefs and practices, these aspects of their Vietnamese culture have not acted as a barrier to them seeking western healthcare. It would seem that they are not being 'culturally doped', or forced into one exclusive category. Instead they are being pluralistic. Nevertheless, Kleinman's assertion that beliefs about illness influence treatment choice has also been supported by recent research (e.g. Brown & Segal, 1996). Of course these two positions are not incompatible and once again illustrate the complex interplay of individuals, cultures and health practices.

Tolerance is a strength that clinicians also need to develop because, living in multicultural societies, we are now confronting a broader range of explanations for suffering than perhaps ever before. The recognition of different cultural explanations is also giving life to the acknowledgment of multisectorial explanations from within our own healthcare systems. Multiculturalism may have liberated us to take our own subcultural and folk perspectives on health more seriously.

The professional sector of western healthcare systems is hung up on a dichotomy that other cultures do not even see as existing. Western healthcare has extracted mind from body, even to the extent of setting up separate hospitals to deal with 'mind suffering' and 'body suffering'. Despite it being difficult to imagine one without the other, this chasm has been driven into everyday experience, and is just one example of intolerance: 'If it's not one, then it's the other, but it can't be both!' Fortunately, in many western cultures there are now growing signs of this mentality diminishing (MacLachlan, 2004). This form of tolerance must be built on to develop a system of serving people's health needs, which is capable of responding to their own explanatory models of suffering. This does not necessarily mean agreeing with all alternative explanations, but it does mean treating them as alternative hypotheses worthy of investigation. It also means recognising that individuals may seek out alternative therapies because they believe that they offer something that mainstream services are lacking (Vincent & Furnham, 1996; see also the case study at start of Chapter 6 – Furnham & Vincent, 2001).

Functions of a healthcare system

The importance of developing tolerant health services becomes obvious when we face up to the challenge of providing health services that are culturally sensitive. A health service that reflects just one ethos of healthcare cannot possibly satisfy the needs of a multicultural community. Returning once again to

Kleinman, we can consider five functions that a healthcare system should perform:

- First, it should be able to explain the meaning of suffering within the sociocultural context of the patient or client (see Chapters 2 and 3).
- Second, a healthcare system ought to create order amidst the chaos of suffering. This ordering may include defining which problems are most serious, which require the most urgent attention, which resources should be allocated to which problems and to which people. Cultural relativism may well produce different priorities. Furnham, Hassomal and McClelland (2002) compared the allocation of scarce medical resources (a kidney dialysis machine), in England and Spain, according to a number of criteria. In each country they showed a preference for local people and women, but the two countries differed with respect to smoking behaviour, which the Spanish felt unimportant, whereas the English felt it made people less deserving.
- A third function is that of communicating (which was discussed in some detail in Chapter 6). Suffering should be classified and explained. How does the suffering relate to ideas about cause and treatment?
- A fourth function is to provide healing (see also Chapter 6), i.e. it should be able to alleviate suffering.
- Finally, the system should be capable of managing a range of different responses to its attempts to heal, including cures, contraction of iatrogenic illnesses, worsening of the suffering people presented with and ultimately death itself.

Healthcare systems should also include the function of promoting health. Without this function we are talking about a system that cares for illness and suffering rather than one that cares for health (see Chapter 8). A healthcare system based solely on scientific and medical knowledge cannot possibly hope to perform the above functions for people who do not share this ethos. A healthcare system that is culturally sensitive will need to reflect different meanings, order care in different ways, comprehend different ways of communicating, provide different methods of healing, manage different responses to its attempts to heal and use different mediums to promote health.

These are indeed ambitious aims, but they are the aims of a complete system, not of every individual within the system. Appropriate management of the system can provide the tolerance and plurality discussed above. Before describing some of the organisational features of a culturally sensitive healthcare system, I would like to focus on some of the misconceptions that can discourage individuals from embracing such an approach.

Barriers to multicultural healthcare

As health service providers have become more aware of the demands of multicultural communities, an array of exciting initiatives have been launched to meet such demands. However, a number of lores (as in folklore), or myths, have also characterised some of the thinking on developing multicultural community health services. In this section we consider some of these barriers, the rationales behind them and how they might be overcome. Some of this discussion is based on Masi's (1993) excellent paper on 'Multicultural health'.

'Positive discrimination is necessary'

It is now common to see advertisements for health or welfare positions that specify preference for applicants from a particular cultural minority. This is called 'positive discrimination' where there is an attempt to encourage applicants of a certain cultural background. There may be several reasons for this. Often ethnic minorities are under-represented and so, to provide health and welfare services more commensurate with the community that they seek to serve, people from such minority cultures are targeted in advertising campaigns. However, unless those responsible for selection are seeking specified ratios of, for instance, white Germans, Turks, Arabs, Chinese, simply increasing the number of non-white Germans may result in an equally unrepresentative service. This sort of positive discrimination has led to the now common quip that 'If you're white, male, middle aged and middle class, then you're soon going to be unemployable!' Of course this is an exaggeration based on a reduction in the employment privileges previously enjoyed by this section of western society. No doubt it also reflects some fear of, and resistance to, changing the privileged position of a powerful cultural group.

Many would argue that positive discrimination should take place at the level of opportunity rather than the level of selection. Thus different cultural groups should be given equal access to resources, including education. Members of the minority groups would then work their way through the system on the basis of merit rather than cultural preference. The drawback with this notion is that minority cultures, e.g. newly arrived immigrants, may not be able (because of language, economic or social reasons) to take advantage of available resources to the same extent that indigenous people can. The other drawback is that a 'work your way through the system approach' will necessarily have a time lag built into it before it bears fruit. Nevertheless, it may be that for workers from minority cultures to be accepted as equals among their co-workers they need to be seen as having equal merit. Positive discrimination is not necessarily beneficial, in the long run, either to the individual selected or to the minority cultural group being served.

'Like should treat like'

Related to the idea of positive discrimination is the idea that clinicians ought to be of the same cultural background as the people whom they are helping. Again there is a good rationale to this. It is argued that only a clinician of the same cultural heritage as the client can be sensitive to and understand the full cultural context of the client's suffering. However, several objections to this can be raised. First, simply because two people are from the same culture does not mean that they are able to understand each other's social context. They may be from different subcultures. Thus a French medical doctor from a well-off family who was educated at exclusive private schools, as well as university, may be no better able to empathise with the despair of a single parent housewife from a 'rough' Paris housing estate, than might an Indian doctor from a poor area of Mombai.

A second objection to the 'like should treat like' philosophy is that it fails to take account of the complexities of the therapeutic relationship. The key element in the selection of an appropriate clinician should be the ability to work effectively as a clinician. Although this ability can surely be tempered by the context in which one works, it should not be overshadowed by it. Sometimes a clinician's interest in people from a different culture will motivate them to perform very well. The 'like should treat like' philosophy thus has some points in its favour and some points against it.

'All or nothing'

This attitude implies that, if we cannot tailor healthcare to the idiosyncratic needs of each culture represented in a community, we should not tailor it to anyone. Certainly no individual practitioner can hope to understand how perhaps 20 different cultures relate to health and welfare, but it is not necessary that he or she should, if we can use the multicultural approach described above. This is concerned with developing *systems* of healthcare to accommodate the diversity of cultures that are the reality of many modern urban communities. It does not require each practitioner to be acquainted equally well with each culture; instead it requires a health system to have the capacity to deal equally well with the health and welfare problems that can be presented by members of different cultures within the community.

The approach that I have advocated confers the potential for understanding how different cultures see health. It does this by focusing on the process of gaining information rather than on the content of the information (see Chapter 2). To provide lots of 'facts' on Chinese ideas about health is simply to encourage fruitless stereotyping about what an ill Chinese person 'should' think is wrong with him. The essence of cultural sensitivity in the clinic is to learn about culture as it impacts on the person who needs one's help. This perspective always reminds us of the enormous variation between individuals of the same culture.

'"Culture" can be used to justify anything'

This barrier relates to an excessive degree of 'cultural relativism'. Cultural relativism is the doctrine that everything is relative and that if you truly understand a culture you will also appreciate the function of behaviours that might otherwise appear cruel, discriminatory or offensive. It is then extrapolated from this that one should not criticise the behaviour of people from another culture. Consequently people can use their culture to justify whatever they like: 'You don't understand my culture . . . and you shouldn't criticise what you don't understand . . . just because it's different from your culture'.

Such an extreme position need not be accepted. Presumably all cultures have some bad things about them, as well as some good things, e.g. it could be argued that it is part of the Irish 'culture' that Protestants and Catholics should dislike each other. Few would see this as a good characteristic and few, I believe, would object to finding ways to alleviate such sectarian tensions. If this was successfully done, indeed one could argue that the Irish culture had been changed, or interfered with. Clearly the same argument can be used with other cultures. The laws of a society will also determine what is and what is not acceptable. Occasionally these laws may take into account cultural differences (e.g. in Britain Sikh motorcyclists need not wear a helmet over their turbans) but in general they demand similar behaviour from across cultural groups. Thus the law can always be used as recourse.

Recall the case study of 'cultural asylum' concerning the culturally sanctioned initiation ceremony that Yoruba girls experience (Chapter 1). Rightly or wrongly the laws of one society were used to prevent the customs of another society being practised. The cultural relativism argument fails to recognise that cultures are dynamic, ever changing, social systems. They are not historical artefacts to be preserved at all costs. For a culture to 'survive' it must adapt to its environment.

'Cultural sensitivity: either you have it or you don't'

It is often thought that cultural sensitivity is a matter of personality type or communication ability. While some people are certainly more empathic and have better communication skills than others, cultural sensitivity is an ability that can be developed through training. Many large multinational companies now require their top executives to undergo cultural sensitivity training before letting them loose on clients in foreign countries. This requirement is not simply a philosophical commitment to a multicultural ethos; rather it is in recognition that people can be taught to interact more effectively with people from cultures different to their own. The same is certainly true with health professionals. This is especially so when we consider how culture can influence the cause, experience, expression and treatment of suffering.

These then are just some of the objections that are sometimes raised to the provision of multicultural health services. It is important to appreciate how they are weak objections. Healthcare professionals *can* be made more culturally aware and can develop skills that will increase their effectiveness as clinicians. In the next section we consider some of the ways in which this can be achieved.

Professional training

Although the rhetoric of 'pluralism', 'multiculturalism' and 'tolerance' is warm and positive, there are surprisingly few studies that provide evidence for the clinical value of this ethos. A recent study by Harmsen and colleagues (2002) studied Dutch parents and parents who were immigrants to the Netherlands (mostly from Turkey and Surinam), in terms of the understanding that they had of their children's illness and how this affected compliance with treatment. They also explored how this related to their general medical practitioner's (GP's) understanding and views. They found that communication in consultations between GPs and people from ethnic minorities was less effective than in consultations with Dutch people. There were not only more misunderstandings, but also a lower level of compliance. The authors concluded that mutual understanding between GPs and patients strongly predicted patient compliance (a finding that chimes with the discussion of therapist and client match and mismatch in Chapter 6).

Unfortunately many health professions continue to give scant attention to cultural sensitivity in their training requirements. Cultural sensitivity is perhaps seen as the 'software' of clinical skills rather than its 'hardware', which is perhaps thought of as being the factual knowledge and concrete skills generally assessed in professional examinations. However, the importance of cultural awareness extends beyond interpersonal and communication skills into the core of clinical practice. First let us consider how to conceptualise cultural sensitivity in clinical practice.

Conceptual awareness

Rogler and colleagues (1987) have described a pyramidal framework for conceptualising clinical innovations in the provision of culturally sensitive mental health services. Their framework need not be restricted to mental health and can be applied to all health services. At the bottom of their framework is *increasing the accessibility of treatment* to cultural minorities. In practice this may mean reducing the gap between professional and subcultural perceptions of health problems and needs. It is also likely to involve the modification of referral procedures, e.g. consultation with and/or inclusion of traditional cultural healers may help in this. It may also involve confronting linguistic barriers (see below).

The next level up the pyramid is the *selection of treatments to fit particular cultures*. In terms of modality of treatment this may, for example, mean physicians working with families rather than with individuals. For psychotherapists it could mean giving more emphasis to interpretation of dreams than usual. For psychiatrists it may mean appreciating that not all cultural groups respond to drugs in the same way (Casimir & Morrison, 1993). In addition it has been reported that the propensity to take home-made remedies in preference to prescribed medication is influenced by culture, poverty status and education, and the severity of the problem, as well as their perceived costs and benefits (Brown & Segal, 1996). Within any one particular cultural group the selection of treatments may also involve distinguishing between those who are acculturated (or pluralistic), to the extent of being able to accept conventional treatments, and those who wish treatments to be traditional in their culture of origin.

At the top of the pyramid is *modification of treatments to fit particular cultures*. In essence this is an extension of modifying treatments to fit the individual. It assumes that some treatment modalities may be more effective in some cultures than in others. As opposed to selecting the most appropriate treatment this approach calls for the development of new treatments. It is clearly the highest level of delivering culturally sensitive health services and deserves the considerable research interest that it is now attracting. Appreciating this sort of 'compartmentalisation' is an important aspect of professional training (Ho, 1985).

Mechanisms for encouraging cultural sensitivity in training

Casimir and Morrison (1993) have suggested various mechanisms for ensuring that cultural sensitivity is given a high profile in professional training. Unfortunately, I believe that many of these would be difficult to manage and/or very unpopular with staff. One notion is to offer salary differentials for staff who are 'culturally competent'. Such competence would be treated as a specialisation within the profession's domain. This would require making culture competence teachable and measurable so that it could constitute an aspect of certification or performance appraisal.

Another idea has been the use of paid 'minority mentors' who teach and supervise clinicians working with minority groups as part of their training. Related to this is the idea of pairing off clinicians with 'traditional' healers from the client's cultural group to work as co-therapists. Traditional co-therapists will have knowledge of culture-specific syndromes and treatments from which the 'contemporary' clinician may gain.

Although each of the above methods of transferring skills of cultural competence may be of some benefit, modifying the usual approach to professional training may also be important. The training programmes of most health professions do not acknowledge that health beliefs and practices vary across cultural groups. Instead, professional training seeks to achieve competence in universal principles. An emphasis on understanding the influence of socioeconomic status, gender and culture would better prepare clinicians to be sensitive to the needs of minority groups.

Defining culturally competent training

Bernal and Castro (1994) reviewed the extent to which clinical psychology training programmes in the USA prepared trainees for clinical practice and research with minority cultural groups. They compared the results of their survey with those of a previous survey, also carried out by Bernal ten years earlier. They reported a number of positive developments:

• The number of programmes offering modules on minority cultures had increased.
• The use of resource people from minority cultural groups (e.g. health professionals, community workers, lay people) had increased.
• The use of community mental health agencies serving minority cultural populations, as training placements, had also increased.

However, in contrast to this, 39% of clinical training programmes still had no minority-related courses, 40% of programmes did not use off-campus clinical settings serving minority cultural groups, and a third of programmes had no faculty (staff) member from a cultural minority. Bernal and Castro therefore concluded that the results revealed a 'mixed picture of progress'.

Bernal and Castro suggest that courses that train for 'cultural proficiency' be proactive and may be characterised as follows:

• Having a high regard and respect for cultures
• Including a knowledge base that exposes all students (i.e. not optional modules) to a standard cultural content relating directly to basic clinical competencies (e.g. assessment), and provides opportunity for in-depth understanding of specific health issues relating to minorities through specialty courses
• Continuing efforts to add to the knowledge base of culturally competent practice through the development and evaluation of new therapeutic and prevention approaches *based on culture*
• Planning and coordinating links between didactic course work and practical field experiences
• Paying careful attention to the dynamics of group differences in the training setting and in research and practice
• Provision of a continuous infusion of cultural knowledge and resources through regular evaluation of training curriculum.

Although these criteria for culturally competent training programmes have been developed with reference to clinical psychology doctorates, they are broad enough to be applicable to most health professional training programmes, and also clearly overlap with the ten considerations for culturally competent therapy discussed in Chapter 6. The extent to which such initiatives are proposed, encouraged and taken up often depends on the context in which health services are provided. Although many professions have addressed Bernal and Castro's recommondations over the last ten or so years, not all have done so sufficiently. Best practice in cultural training needs to be developed empirically and then taught through problem-based and participative methods.

Who treats black and who treats white patients?

It has long been recognised that black people in the USA generally receive a poorer quality of healthcare than white people. Bach et al. (2004) recently sought to compare the professional status of physicians who treated black or white patients, in order to explore the possibility that inequities in healthcare might be partly accounted for by inequities in those who provide healthcare services. One might have assumed that most medical doctors treat both black and white patients; however, this is not necessarily the case, perhaps because of geographical location or for other reasons. Bach and colleagues analysed records of over 150,000 visits by people aged 65 years or older to primary care physicians, paid for by Medicare, the largest healthcare insurance plan in the USA.

Although over 85% of white patients visited white physicians, fewer than 1% visited a black physician. In contrast, just under 60% of black patients visited a white physician, with over 22% visiting a black physician. Bach et al. noted that visits by black patients were highly concentrated among small subgroups of physicians. Moreover, a statistically significant lower proportion of this subgroup was 'board certified' and reported facing obstacles in gaining access to high-quality services for their patients. Thus, the possibility of differences in the training of physicians treating black or white patients, or differences in their access to resources, is a real one. As regards training differences, perhaps this may contribute to the finding that black patients receive less screening for most diseases than white patients, or more often receive a diagnosis at more advanced stages of disease progression (Bach et al., 2004). However, it is also important to acknowledge that simply because a physician is not board certified does not mean that she or he is ineligible for certification, or is less competent.

Bach et al.'s (2004) results are nevertheless of great concern and it is therefore important to understand their source. Fernandez and Goldstein (2004), while accepting that there may be training and resource discrepancies between physicians who primarily treat black and those who treat white patients, also argue that even within the same 'closed' healthcare system, such as the Department of Veteran Affairs (which provides free healthcare to current or former military personnel) – with the same resources and physicians – black patients still receive inferior care to white patients. They strongly argue that 'Interpersonal bias is a consequence of structural inequalities described by Bach et al., and yet bias itself partly explains our society's tolerance of these inequalities' (Fernandez and Goldstein, 2004, p. 2126). Their crucial point here is that the 'interpersonal bias versus structural inequalities' arguments are not competing accounts of the differences noted above; instead they are mutually reinforcing accounts, which are in practice often quite indistinguishable. They are also both accounts that need to be tackled at the broader policy level of healthcare delivery.

Healthcare policy and administration

When providing guidelines for the clinician it is important to remember the systems and contexts within which individual clinicians work. Community healthcare can be made culturally sensitive by incorporating certain ideas into the overall policies of community services. I end this chapter by considering some policy guidelines that can drive culturally sensitive community health services. In doing so I draw on a policy document of Ontario Province, in Canada, which has well-developed guidelines in this regard.

Who is in the community?

This issue relates mainly to the demographic 'shape' of the community and would include information on age, sex, education and socioeconomic status, in addition to the cultural mix within the community. The history of immigration into the community is also important to consider because cultural groups that have recently immigrated may have different health needs from those groups who are longer established. In addition to this some cultural groups will present with health requirements that are quite different from either the local population or other immigrants. An example of this would be sickle cell anaemia being much more common in west Africans than in other cultural groups. Thus demographic profiles must reflect cultural variations if they are to be of any use in planning a service to meet the needs of the community.

What is on paper?

The power of the written word is often overlooked by clinicians focused on action, at the 'coal face' of health service delivery. Yet a commitment in writing, in the dullest looking policy statement, can be an essential pivot for action. It is increasingly common these days for organisation within the health sector to issue 'mission statements'. These are essentially statements concerning what the service is trying to achieve and how it is trying to do it, e.g. 'We are committed to delivering quality health services to the population of . . . by focusing on the needs of individuals and families.' The mission statement is very important because the organisation is often run to achieve the aims described in it. Such statements should therefore make reference to cultural issues.

   Whether through the mission statement or other strategy documents certain principles should be documented. First and foremost there should be recognition of responsibility to provide health services that are equally accessible to all members of the community, including (explicitly) minority culture groups. Having equal accessibility is not, however, enough. All members of the community could have equal (and plentiful) 'access' to services for elderly people, on the one hand, and equal (and no) access to services catering for people with sickle cell anaemia, on the other. Thus health services must also be *equitable* in terms of providing equally for the health needs of each cultural group.

What are the mechanisms for empowerment?

Cultural groups within a community can be empowered by having their views fairly represented and by allowing for their participation in decision-making processes. This means having people from minority groups as members of the committees and boards that govern health provision and draw up health strategy. Sometimes, where a board is elected, minority groups will be under-represented (almost by definition). In this case having 'advisers' to the board can ensure that minority groups are still consulted as part of the decision-making process. Seeking feedback and surveying customer satisfaction are other ways of accessing minority opinion and this should be done on a continuous basis.

What operational contingencies are there?

Communication is one of the most obvious difficulties that a clinician faces in trying to understand the suffering of someone from a different culture. Empathy and accuracy are essential to the therapeutic encounter. Although having someone translate between the clinician and the client is never an ideal solution, it is often the only realistic way to communicate where neither speaks the other's language well. Policy statements should specify for which languages translation would be provided. In addition to this, policy statements should also specify how health services would be sensitive to different cultural norms and values. This must include religious and dietary considerations.

Is cultural sensitivity reflected in personnel policies and practices?

I have already discussed the importance of cultural minorities being recruited into community health services. Ideally the staff of community health services will be representative of the cultural mix within their community. However, the reality is that this ideal may be some way off for many communities, especially those with recently arrived immigrants. Furthermore, just because a community health service has a staff profile that reflects the cultural groups within its catchment area, this does not imply that the service is in any way culture sensitive. The management of personnel may still reflect biases in practices such as performance appraisal and selection for promotion.

Regarding the provision of health services to the community, each clinician, ancillary worker and manager should be required to undergo training in cultural awareness and sensitivity. Being a member of a minority group in no way exempts one from cultural insensitivity! Staff development courses should avoid the 'making us more sensitive to their needs' ethos and incorporate instead an approach that 'makes everybody more sensitive to the needs of different sectors of the community'. This latter ethos fits well with awareness of the needs of other minority groups such as people with physical disabilities, blind people, those with schizophrenia or alcoholism, all of whom also have special needs requiring the sensitive provision of services.

How is cultural sensitivity evaluated?

There are many ways in which the cultural sensitivity of health services could be evaluated. One approach would be to establish whether the health needs of different cultural groups were being served to an equivalent extent. Evaluation will always be a delicate issue and even though the focus may be on evaluating a service, individual clinicians will inevitably feel that they are themselves being assessed. However, although evaluation must address the extent to which an organisation is meeting its operational and strategic objects, it must also have a 'bottom-up' component, i.e. the grass roots concerns of the people being served should also influence the sort of evaluation undertaken.

Customer 'satisfaction' surveys may be one way of evaluating the cultural sensitivity of health services. Other forms of assessment and feedback might include special advisory committees, soliciting comments from community organisations that represent minority cultural groups, or seeking advice from 'cultural healers' about the extent to which they believe the needs of their own culture are being met. It should always be remembered that often minority groups coming to western countries experience their 'new' health service to be 'more advanced' than the one that they left behind. They may therefore feel that criticism would be either inappropriate or poorly received. In this sense getting accurate feedback from cultural minorities may be especially difficult. In this circumstance a strong argument can be made for the use of personal interviews (preferably by people from the same culture) as opposed to questionnaire assessment. A skilled interviewer will be better able to give the client 'permission' to be frank about how well their health needs are being met.

Standing back from culture

Before ending this chapter on culturally sensitive health services, let us briefly stand back from the detail of implementing it and consider how health systems may construct false assumptions about disorder, and how they may benefit from being more permeable to ideas from outside their own culture. Increasingly we recognise that healthcare policy needs to be evidence based: there should be good empirical reasons for doing what we do and for trying to achieve the goals that we have set. Many forced migrants have fled their country of origin following traumatic experiences. Those who have fled to western-oriented health systems came into a system of belief that traumatic experiences need to be 'worked through', especially if earlier intervention and 'debriefing' were not possible. The 'psychotrauma industry' arose primarily from the great mental distress that many American Vietnam veterans experienced, not only on active duty, but also, and some have argued particularly (Summerfield, 2005), on returning to a hostile or ambivalent 'welcome back' to the USA. The culture of acceptance of the value of immediate debriefing following trauma has now been widely discredited by the research reviewed by the National Institute for Health and Clinical Excellence (NICE, 2005) in the UK. However, they continue to support the value of psychological therapy for those with post-traumatic stress disorder (PTSD).

Even if psychological therapy is appropriate for some people with PTSD, is it appropriate regardless of cultural background? For many years now Summerfield (2005) has been arguing that 'no it isn't', and has noted the spread of the use of this diagnosis also among humanitarian aid programmes. Summerfield (2005, pp. 95–6) stresses that the diagnosis is used to capture and address the impact of 'events like wars regardless of the background culture, current situation, and subjective meaning brought to the experience by survivors'. The notion of personhood implied in such a diagnosis is of psychic conflict being dealt with internally and individually, and this is clearly not representative of many cultures and possibly undermines a community's natural rehabilitative potential to help people adapt by moving them on through ritual, necessities of survival or other means.

As with many assumptions within cultures, they may be seen as distortions through the lens of another culture. Furthermore, awareness of these different perspectives can cast the original cultural construction in a new light. Thus, reflecting on the emergence of PTSD in western cultures Summerfield (2005, p 96) states:

> An individualistic rights conscious culture can foster a sense of personal injury and grievance and thus a need for restitution in encounters in daily life that were formally appraised more dispassionately. Post-traumatic stress disorder is the diagnosis for an age of disenchantment.

Complementary to this view is Timimi's (2005) concern with the effects of globalisation on children's mental health in general. She argues that western value systems that promote individualism weaken social ties and create ambivalence towards children, potentially adversely affecting their mental health. Timimi (2005) argues that values such as duty, responsibility and a community orientation, which are emphasised in many non-western cultures, are health promoting. Consequently, the exportation of western child-rearing practices to many developing countries is undermining them and, in fact, these cultures may be able to provide new insights to enrich western psychiatric theory and practice.

In an attempt to play 'devil's advocate' and show the 'other side' of the coin, I close this chapter with one of my own cross-cultural clinical clashes!

Case study: the penis problem

Some years ago I assessed a man who sought my help as a clinical psychologist because his marriage was in difficulties. He had returned after 11 years working in another country, during the last two of which he had not been in contact with his wife and nine children, and previous to that had visited home infrequently and wrote only the occasional letter. Now that his work permit had been revoked he had decided to return 'home' and was distressed because the relationship between himself and his wife was 'very strained'. In fact, she had talked in anger of 'kicking him out'. He was, however, committed to making their marriage work and making up for time lost over the years, both with his wife and with his children.

As the assessment continued he confided that 'at my age, of course, I'm not able to . . . , ya know, any more'. For the past six months my client had been unable to sustain an erection. His erectile difficulties were, he understood, an inevitable consequence of getting older. He confidently stated that this was of no consequence to his wife, because since his return to her three months ago, there had been no physical side to their relationship.

Clearly in such a case there are many issues to be considered and it seemed to me that it would be appropriate to include his wife – if she would be willing – at the earliest possible stage. Summing up the assessment I recommended that his wife attend our next session. I also wanted to give him some hope for a positive outcome and indicated how some of the other issues that were causing him distress might be tackled. I then suggested that his inability to sustain an erection was most likely nothing to do with him getting older (he was in his late 40s) and that it was possibly related to the distress he experienced on learning that his work permit was not going to be renewed and the difficult atmosphere since he had come 'home'. I assured him that the vast majority of cases of erectile difficulties could be easily and relatively quickly treated.

My suggestion that the gentleman's penis could soon be back in working order greatly surprised him. He pondered for a moment, asked me if I was 'sure about that', pondered some more, and then suggested that we hold off bringing his wife along for the next session. My perplexity must have been quite apparent for he responded to my grimace thus: 'If that's the case, I will look for another, younger wife!' Now, sometimes it's hard not to be judgemental, and once again my non-verbals leaked out: 'It's alright, it's part of my culture . . . it is! I know lots of men who have done it!' After some discussion he encapsulated the issue nicely: 'Look you don't have to agree with my culture, but please help me get better.'

This case study clearly highlights the issue of 'Who has the right to decide on the appropriateness of health goals?' While this question may seem somewhat whimsical in this case study (no offence to my friend above), it is anything but whimsical when needing to decide which lives to try to save, with how the very scarce health resources that are available, particularly in many developing countries should be distributed.

Conclusion

The multicultural care philosophy of providing flexible systems of care that may be applied across different cultures has certain advantages over the transcultural and cross-cultural approaches. A multicultural framework, within the professional sector, may also be more able to accommodate contributions from the popular and folk sectors towards provision of comprehensive healthcare. It is always important to remember that people have different explanatory models of suffering, not just across different health sectors, but also within each health sector. One of the central features of culturally sensitive health services must therefore be tolerance of pluralism. If a healthcare system is to perform its many social functions then that system must allow for different interpretations of health, illness and suffering. The complexity of the challenge of providing culturally sensitive systems of healthcare has led to some erroneous assumptions, which have acted as barriers to their development. There is still insufficient priority given to cultural issues in the training programmes of many health professions. There is much that can be done to promote cultural sensitivity at the level of policy and administration. Rather than addressing cultural issues in isolation, they should be seen as part of a broader drive towards serving the needs of minority groups within the community. It is also important for mainstream healthcare to be open to learning from those outside mainstream culture.

Guidelines for professional practice

1. Clinicians should adopt a multicultural perspective in their work. This perspective goes beyond the comparison of different cultures, or communication in the clinician–client relationship to consider the total system of care within a community. It can be especially important for community clinicians to understand where they 'fit in' to the overall system of provision of a multicultural service.
2. Professionally qualified clinicians are but one part of the healthcare that is available to people. The popular and folk sectors also have an important

influence on health behaviour. Clinicians should try to establish the extent to which individuals draw from these different sectors in deciding on their health-related behaviour. Even clinicians working in a monocultural context will encounter influential beliefs, emanating from the popular and folk sectors, which may be significantly different to their own professional beliefs.

3. One of the predominant characteristics of western healthcare is that it has become heavily professionalised. This makes healthcare professionals suspicious and dismissive of people who have not been 'legitimised' by similar training. Consequently traditional cultural healers may not be taken seriously simply because they do not conform to our cultural expectations of (usually) academic achievement. Indigenous healers may be dismissed in the same fashion.

4. Although is seems reasonable that beliefs about the cause of a problem and beliefs about the solution to a problem should be on the same explanatory dimensions, this may not be the case. One of the keystones of a multicultural approach to health is for clinicians to show tolerance of pluralism. Research now supports the contention that many laypeople are able to tolerate more than one explanation for a disease or disorder. This is likely to be especially so in multicultural communities which present a diversity of explanations for certain problems. The clinician who precludes all explanatory models but his or her own is likely to be seen as narrow minded, defensive and conceited.

5. Healthcare systems can be understood as fulfilling a number of different functions such as explaining the meaning of suffering, being a medium of communication about suffering and providing healing. Individual clinicians or groups working together might benefit by assessing how well they provide for each of the functions outlined in this chapter, especially within a multicultural context.

6. A number of barriers to multicultural healthcare exist which can be characterised as myths. These include the belief that positive discrimination is necessary, that like should treat like and that 'culture' can be used to justify anything. Clinicians should examine some of the assumptions, or folklore, that may have built up through their own experience of working in a multicultural environment. They should ask 'What is the evidence for this assumption?'

7. Those who train health professionals have much work to do. Training should include not only conceptual awareness of multicultural issues, but also mechanisms for enhancing cultural competence and exposure to clinical problems occurring in cultural contexts different to that of the trainee. Training courses can uniquely legitimise multiculturalism by requiring this perspective through examinations and practical placements.

8. Healthcare policy makers and administrators also have a crucial contribution to enhancing truly multicultural healthcare, because it is they who set the context through which frontline clinicians operate. Appropriate policies and structures can do much to facilitate multiculturalism.

9. It has been argued that PTSD is a product of a particular cultural context, place and time. Practitioners should be aware that some cultural communities may have their own natural rehabilitative opportunities that allow people to 'move on' and that psychological therapy may not always be the best, or most appropriate, intervention even for people who have experienced very traumatic events.

10. Cultural sensitivity, while desirable, is not unproblematic. It can, at times, present practitioners with serious ethical issues and may even compromise patient care. Health systems and policies should be designed to minimise this and to give practitioners guidance when such situations do arise.

CHAPTER 8

Promoting health across cultures

In this chapter I consider the concepts of health promotion, risk reduction, and the prevention of disease and disorder from a cultural perspective. In the more industrialised countries, public health had been improving anyway throughout the last century and much of this improvement can be attributed to improved living conditions rather than biomedical innovations. However, access to good public health services is not equal and minority cultural groups, who often occupy the lower socioeconomic strata, have less exposure to, and therefore less opportunity to benefit from, health-promoting initiatives. Here I pay particular attention to recent recommendations for preventing mental disorders that incorporate the idea of 'cultural competence'. To give a more concrete example I return to the problem of depression, critically examining efforts to prevent depression and promote mental health across cultural minorities. I also examine the possibility that different cultures encourage different cognitions about the self and that some cultures can predispose its members to certain disorders, such as depression. This raises the possibility that culture can be a risk factor in itself. Subcultures may also constitute risk factors and to illustrate this I consider how disordered communities are being created by rural depopulation and international legislation. We conclude that health promotion may not be something that can be accommodated within existing social systems, but that, in some cases, it may work only through changing social systems.

The health promotion movement

Over the last century the leading causes of death in the more industrialised countries have changed dramatically. Although in the 1900s pneumonia/influenza, tuberculosis and diarrhoea were the most common causes of death, today diseases of the heart and cardiovascular system, and cancers, are the most common causes. This decrease in infectious diseases as a cause of death has gone hand in hand with a lengthening in average life expectancy from between 40 and 50 years in 1900 to over 70 years by the late 1980s. For a species that has been evolving for thousands of years, this flight into longevity is outstandingly dramatic and a testimony to the benevolent potential of modern life. However, what is it that has brought about this dramatic change?

The rate of innovation in biomedical technology has similarly increased exponentially over the past 100 years. From Alexander Fleming's accidental discovery of penicillin in 1929 we are now, on a daily basis, striding through the genetic landscape of humanity with the remarkable Human Genome Project, giving us a complete 'map' of the genetic make-up of *Homo sapiens*. That which was once sacred is now science. CT (computed tomography), MRI (magnetic resonance imaging) and PET (positron emission tomography) are modern imaging devices that allow us to look inside the human brain as it works away – souls and minds have been subverted by high-tech peeping Toms. 'Keyhole surgery' describes a degree of surgical precision undreamt of by nineteenth-century surgeons whose trade was so base and butcher like that they were not even dignified by the title 'doctor'. Today surgeons can 'cut' into internal organs without the need for a knife and without the blemish of a scar. We are indeed fortunate to live in such an age, where possibly our greatest challenge is to keep up with, and keep financing, the insatiable fast-forwarding of biotechnology.

It is therefore perhaps only 'common sense' to make a link between the remarkable increase in life expectancy, on the one hand, and the remarkable increase in biotechnological sophistication, on the other. What is surprising is that such a link is by no means clear. Figure 8.1 shows how the rate of death across a range of infectious diseases fell from 1900 to 1973 in the USA. It also indicates the point at which biotechnology presented an effective means of combating each disease. This illustrates that the decline in death rate cannot fully be accounted for by biotechnological innovations. If this is so, what can account for this improvement in health? Although there is some debate about the relative contribution of different factors, improved living conditions, reduced malnutrition, improved sanitation of food and water, and better systems of sewage disposal can probably take much of the credit for longer life. These factors, although not necessarily inconsistent with biotechnological innovation, are primarily concerned with the prevention of disease rather than with the high-tech treatment of disease.

This public health approach to disease emphasises the importance of preventing the conditions that cause disease. This notion of prevention is not, however, restricted to large-scale public health interventions such as improving sewage management or water supply. Psychological factors in the form of individual's health-related behaviours can have an equally dramatic effect on mortality. What about your own mortality? How many of the following health-related practices do you engage in?

1. Sleeping 7–8 hours daily.
2. Eating breakfast almost every day.
3. Never or rarely eating between meals.
4. Currently being at or near prescribed height-adjusted weight.
5. Never smoking cigarettes.

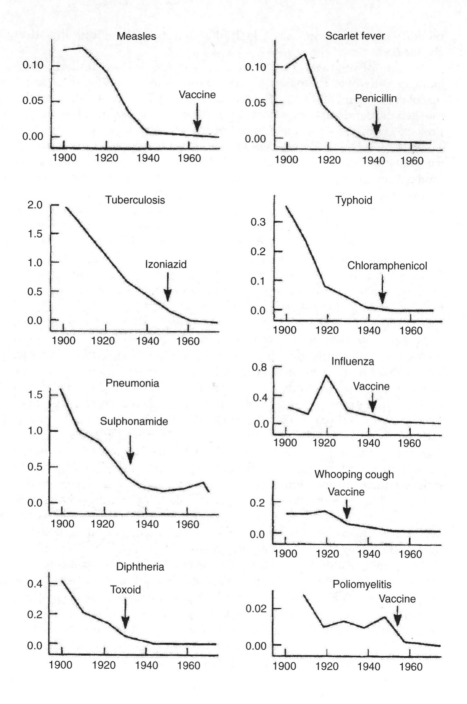

Figure 8.1 Standard death rate (per 100 population) for nine common infectious diseases in relation to specific medical measures in the USA (1900–73). (Reproduced from McKinlay and McKinlay, 1981, with permission.)

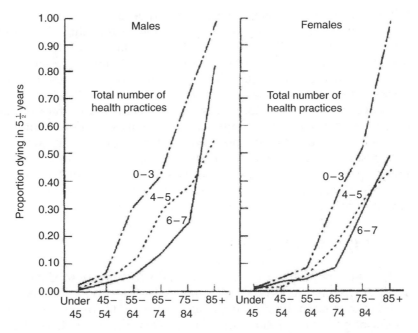

Figure 8.2   Age-specific mortality rates by number of health practices and gender. (Reproduced from Matarazzo, 1980, with permission.)

6. Moderate or no use of alcohol.
7. Regular physical activity.

Before reading any further make sure that you have a realistic idea of the number of these to which you can truly lay claim. In 1965 Belloc and Breslow (1972) asked the same question of almost 7,000 people who formed a representative sample of Alamede County in California. At the time of the survey, those in better health claimed to be engaging in more of the above health practices. However, the most interesting results came from their follow-up studies. Figure 8.2 shows the proportion of this sample surviving five and a half years later as a function of the number of health behaviours reported in the original survey, their age and sex. Once again the effects are clear and dramatic. Those people who reported engaging in a greater number of the seven health-related practices had a greater probability of being alive five and a half years later. For men this effect was particularly strong in the age range 55–75. The positive relationship between these rather innocuous, easily executed, health behaviours and subsequent mortality also held up in a subsequent follow-up study after nine and a half years (see Breslow & Enstrom, 1980). How many of these seven health practices did you endorse?

Although biotechnological innovation can greatly enhanced our capacity for treating life-threatening conditions, improvements in public health provision and the performance of simple health-related behaviours can also play a dramatic role in lengthening life. These preventive factors should contribute not only to the quantity of life but also to the quality of life. Preventive interventions are often directed at the context of people's lives, at the circumstances in which they live and at the way in which they behave. Once again it is cultures and communities that are the vehicles for the social context through which people live. Different contexts present different threats to health and welfare, but they will also present different opportunities for intervention and different barriers to interventions. Thus, effective preventive interventions in one context should not be assumed to be transferable across cultures, whether these cultures are in different parts of the world or different parts of the same city. The complexity of preventive intervention across cultures has recently been recognised in the field of mental health, to which I now turn.

Preventing mental disorders

In 1994, at the request of the US Congress, the Institute of Medicine produced a multidisciplinary report on 'Reducing risks for mental disorders'. This is an important document because it claims to speak authoritatively on the development of preventive interventions for mental disorders. One of the issues (briefly) dealt with in the report is how practitioners need to develop 'a set of skills and a perspective that have become commonly known as cultural competence' (p. 391).

Cultural sensitivity and cultural competence are conceptualised as existing along a continuum. Cultural sensitivity is about being aware of relevant issues. It therefore concerns an intellectual assimilation of relevant information. Cultural sensitivity is seen as necessary, but not sufficient, for cultural competence. At the other end of the continuum, cultural competence requires personal experience of working with different cultures, in order to be able to achieve a practical and appropriate match between intervention strategies and the cultural context of the intervention. Here the benchmark is not an intellectual fit but a pragmatic collaboration, wherein the recipients of the intervention will feel some ownership over the strategies employed and some real benefits from their participation.

The multidisciplinary Committee on the Prevention of Mental Disorders, which produced this report, highlighted ten points relating to the prevention of mental disorders where particular attention should be given to cultural competence. There now follows a brief interpretation of these points, several of which overlap and run into each other and are at times ambiguous.

Forging relationships between researchers and community

There is a real danger that much of the drive for preventing mental disorders will come from distant government ministries or academic institutions rather than from the communities that will be the sites for intervention programmes. Such a 'top-down' approach must be avoided at all costs. Communities must be allowed to define their own needs, their own targets and their own outcome measures. As such, health services will have to link into the appropriate extant networks of authority and communication in a given culture. Collaboration will have to be actual and active rather than a passive aspiration. For the health practitioner this may mean accepting the sharing of power, authority and knowledge with appropriate community members. Thus the content and process of intervention are likely to be the product of a negotiation process between the beliefs and aspirations of the community and those of the health practitioner(s).

Identifying risks, mechanisms, triggers and processes

Different cultural groups are likely to differ in what constitutes the risks, mechanisms, triggers and processes for mental disorder. Thus, in different cultures different causes may result in the same disorder or the same cause may result in different disorders, e.g. among the Hopi (Indians of North America) there is a increased risk of suicide among the children of parents who enter into traditionally disapproved marriages (e.g. between tribes). The children are stigmatised by the labelling of their parents as deviant and therefore encounter a series of accompanying social stressors. The same may be true of other cultural groups where colour, sect or religion presents a social barrier, the transgression of which may have harmful effects on the children of such marriages. The point here is that the specific social norms and lores of different cultures can be expected to impact, through unique risks, mechanisms, triggers and processes, on the health and welfare of its members.

Employing relevant theoretical frameworks

A relevant theoretical framework for a particular community will be one that the members of that community employ in their daily living. The way in which health and welfare are understood varies not only across cultures but also within them. Health practitioners may, for instance, be absolutely convinced by the theory that malaria is transmitted by the biting of mosquitoes, whereas those who are frequently bitten can easily dismiss it. Their own theory may be built on the immediacy of their own experience:

- 'Why when we are bitten ten times a day, should one mosquito bite, one day, cause such a dramatic reaction?'
- 'And even if a mosquito is somehow involved in the process, then why must it be such an arbitrary event, a biological game of Russian roulette, without any social meaning or significance?'

- 'Why rush out and buy mosquito nets when mosquitoes are only one vector at the disposal of malevolent spirits?'
- 'Why not instead go to the source of the problem and appease the spirits?'

Part of the challenge for the health practitioner is to employ a theoretical framework that makes enough sense to those whom they are trying to assist – *sense* being related to understanding a culture's way of existing in the world – while at the same time being able to deliver actionable ideas for practical interventions that will produce beneficial results.

Preparing the content, format and delivery of preventive interventions

In the light of what has been stated through the three previous points it follows that there is a need to ensure that the way in which preventive interventions are undertaken embrace rather than alienating cultural vehicles of communication. There needs to be a constant process of checking and re-checking the appropriateness of content, format and delivery of interventions. One practical way in which this can be done is to pay close attention to the lessons to be learned from pilot work and pre-testing.

Adopting appropriate narrative structures and discourse

Who is willing to discuss what, with whom and in what way? There are as many answers to this as there are customs of communication. Barriers to communication within a culture can include age, gender and status, e.g. issues about AIDS may be more openly discussed in single-sex groups than in mixed-sex groups. Particular metaphors may be used by some subcultures, but can be quite meaningless to others: 'My plates of meat are aching', 'I am feeling low' and 'I'm so tired I could fall asleep on a clothesline'! The essential point here is that across cultures not only do the rules of engagement differ but the way in which you engage another person also differs.

Tapping critical decision-making processes

The way in which decisions are made varies across cultures. In some cases one person decides, in others a council of elders may decide, whereas in some cultures the whole community or even the whole nation may be involved in the decision-making process. Some cultures invest authority in child rearing to mothers, others to fathers, and others to maternal uncles, etc. There is no one way of doing anything! Interventions that do not take these variations into account are unlikely to meet with success.

Determining points of intervention leverage

The decision-making processes within any culture will influence where those points of intervention are that can have greatest influence. Often the greatest leverage will be through recognised leaders; however, this need not exclude other conduits of change, as described in the next section.

Recognition of social networks and natural helpers

Within a cultural community there are also other types of authority and influence, working through a variety of formal and informal social networks. Thus, there may be several important points of leverage and conduits to which interventions can be addressed. Ignoring an influential group or an influential individual down the 'intervention line', and in doing so undermining their position, may be costly. Many cultures socially sanction certain types of people to do certain types of job. In Ireland, a well-off middle-class family may advertise for an au pair girl to help out with the housework and looking after the children, in exchange for 'bed and board' and an opportunity to learn English. However, to advertise for an au pair boy is definitely not the done thing! In Ireland foreign girls, but not foreign boys, are socially sanctioned for this task. It is important to recognise and empower the community's inherent social networks and 'natural helpers' in any intervention roles.

Seeking fidelity of implementation

This reads a bit like a 'jargon statement'. It refers to the desire that researchers have for real world interventions to 'keep faith' with the models upon which they are predicated. In reality, applying interventions across different cultures will require a degree of flexibility and adaptation of the methods used. The researcher's concern is that these modifications do not change the underlying basic nature of the intervention variables. The practitioner's concern may be focused more on whether 'it' works, rather than specifying exactly what the 'it' is. However, the researcher values a positive outcome only if she or he can attribute it to specific intervention variables. Without knowing what aspects of an intervention package have been responsible for a positive outcome, it is impossible to predict the success of a similar intervention in another context or even in the same context, but at another time.

Replicating interventions across diverse and changing populations

Although seeking fidelity of implementation is about being true to a model of intervention, the present point emphasises the practical difficulties, not only in standardisation, but also in matching the style of intervention across such a broad range of knowledge, skills, language, linguistic ability, etc. which

Table 8.1   Some generic risk factors for the development of psychological disorder.

Family circumstances	*Ecological context*
Low social class	Neighbourhood disorganisation
Family conflict	Racial injustment
Mental illness in the family	Unemployment
Large family size	Extreme poverty
Poor bonding to parents	
Family disorganisation	*Constitutional handicaps*
Communication deviance	Perinatal complications
	Sensory disabilities
Emotional difficulties	Organic handicaps
Child abuse	Neurochemical imbalance
Apathy or emotional blunting	
Emotional immaturity	*Interpersonal problems*
Stressful life events	Peer rejection
Low self-esteem	Alienation and isolation
Emotional dyscontrol	
	Skill development delays
School problems	Subnormal intelligence
Academic failure	Social incompetence
Scholastic demoralisation	Attentional deficits
	Reading disabilities
	Poor word skills and habits

Reproduced from Coie et al. (1993). (Copyright © 1993 by the American Psychological Association. Reprinted with permission.)

exists in many modern multicultural urban centres, e.g. it is estimated that the dozen or more distinct Asian–American groups – including Japanese, Chinese, Koreans, Vietnamese, Cambodians and Hmong – speak more than 75 different languages. Furthermore, depending on the particular group and how long they have been resident in North America, between one- and three-quarters do not speak English 'very well'. Such practical communication problems are certainly a challenge to those implementing intervention programmes.

The above points are therefore a sort of 'top 10' listing of salient issues in the process of prevention across cultures. Table 8.1 describes a series of risk factors for the development of psychological disorders. In previous chapters we have already noted that many of these risk factors may be particularly pertinent to minority cultural groups who are often marginalised socially, economically and politically. To think through how these factors apply to a particular disorder, and bearing in mind what has previously been said about depression, let us consider which risk factors are hypothesised to predispose to depression.

Risk factors for depression

The Committee on the Prevention of Mental Disorders review of the literature suggests the following five risk factors for the development of depression:

1. Having a parent or other close biological relative with a mood disorder: it is suggested that the risk of developing depression becomes greater the larger is the proportion of genes shared with a 'mood-disordered individual'. Thus, if your mother suffered with depression you would be more likely to develop depression yourself than if your uncle was the closest relation to you who had had depression. It is argued that the strength of hereditary influence diminishes with less severe (subclinical) mood problems and that even for the more severe disorders the mechanisms of genetic transmission remain unclear.

2. Having a severe stressor: examples of such stressors include a loss, divorce, marital separation, unemployment, job dissatisfaction, a chronic physical disorder, a traumatic experience or a learning disorder. Such stressors, especially when cumulative over time, are associated with an increased risk for a range of mental disorders including depression.

3. Having low self-esteem, a sense of low self-efficacy, and a sense of helplessness and hopelessness: a considerable literature from cognitive clinical psychology has illuminated a number of strong predictive relationships between these overlapping variables and the onset of depression.

4. Being female: it is well established that depression is more frequently diagnosed in females than in males. Adolescent females may be particularly 'at risk' because of the accumulation of stressors at a time of transition. Thus, if going through puberty, changing from primary to secondary school and family discord or break-up occur together, females may be especially at risk of developing depression.

5. Living in poverty: epidemiological studies have identified poverty as an important risk factor for the development of depression. This may be because it is related to other risk factors such as more frequently experiencing stressors, having low self-esteem, poor self-efficacy, etc.

In the light of previous discussions about the possible 'culture boundedness' of depression, let us acknowledge that the notion of 'depression', of biological and individual risk factors reflects 'western biological individualism'. However, being female and living in poverty suggest that contextual and environmental factors are also relevant to this North American idea of depression. It is therefore interesting to note that minority groups have been a target for intervention programmes specifically aimed at preventing depressive disorders.

North American estimates for the prevalence of clinical depression among the general population are generally between 9 and 14%. However, of these possibly only 20% receive professional help. The situation for members of minority cultural groups may be even worse, e.g. epidemiological research in California has found that only 11% of Mexican–Americans who met diagnostic criteria for the DSM (*Diagnostic and Statistical Manual of Mental Disorders* – American Psychiatric Association) disorders had sought mental health services, compared with 22% of similarly diagnosed non-Hispanic whites in the same catchment area. Such results suggest that minority groups may underutilise 'conventional' health services when it comes to mental disorder. If it is the case that minority groups underutilise treatment services, then greater emphasis might profitably be given to preventive interventions. An example of this would be Projecto Bienestar.

Projecto Bienestar targeted women who currently had no or only mild depressive symptoms, but who were nevertheless at high risk of developing depression of clinical severity. Emphasising the importance of environmental resources, the project sought to strengthen individuals' capacities for coping with stressors. Two types of intervention were used: first, replicating the cultural norm of natural helpers (*Servidoras*) found in low-income communities of southern California, was a one-to-one intervention to assist the at-risk women; second, there was a peer group intervention (*Merienda educativa*), which was organised and led by a *Servidoras*. Although the one-to-one intervention showed no positive effects in terms of preventing the onset of depression, the *Merienda* group intervention did. The effectiveness of the group intervention seems to have been accounted for by the benefits derived from it by women with relatively moderate depressive symptomatology, rather than those with relatively milder or greater symptomatology. These results, while encouraging in terms of the potential efficacy of preventive intervention, also warn of the probable complexities involved in matching preventive interventions to risk factors, especially across a range of migrant cultures at risk of developing a 'foreign' disorder, such as depression (see Vega & Murphy, 1990, for further details).

The interplay of risk factors

Coie and colleagues (1993), while supporting the risk factor approach, have also emphasised its complexities: there is no simple one-to-one relationship between a risk factor and a disorder. A particular risk factor – say family discord – can be a risk factor for many different disorders. A particular disorder may also have many different risk factors some of which may only occasionally be present. The salience of risk factors may also fluctuate developmentally. The idea of such 'sensitive periods' is that events occurring at one point in a person's life may have stronger effects on them than the same event occurring at other times in life. The redundancy of a father may have different effects on his son depending on whether the son is 4 or 14. As a final point, the accumulation of risk factors is likely to increase vulnerability to a disorder. The stressor that finally results in some form of breakdown may not be the most important stressor but simply the one that stretched the person beyond his or her coping abilities. Where risk factors and stressors relate to social norms, they are necessarily going to be a product of particular cultural beliefs. Risk factors may therefore show significant variation across cultures.

Schumaker (1996) illustrates this point by drawing our attention to the cultural assumptions that underlie theorising about depressive thinking.

Central to Beck's cognitive theory of depression is the idea that people who are depressed have a negative view of themselves, e.g. they attribute their failure to cope with stressors to faults within themselves when there may be other explanations of their failure. This model fits well the individualistic orientation of North American society for which it was developed. Within this context the attribution of negative events to personal shortcomings can be seen as a risk factors for developing depression. With increasing negative events exceeding a person's ability to cope the person may increasingly attribute failure to personal weaknesses, resulting in low self-esteem, self-depreciation, low mood and 'cognitive distortions' which can worsen into a state of clinical depression. This way of thinking reflects the individual who has not competed and won, who is not trying to 'develop' him- or herself, who is not a success. Arguably it is because western individualism encourages these ways of thinking that those who fail to make the grade are at risk of depression. It is difficult to emphasis the goodness of the successful individual without also emphasising the failings of the unsuccessful individual.

Research on postpartum depression has implicated the role of self-depreciatory cognitions in the disorder and some have advocated the use of cognitive therapy as an intervention. 'Dysfunctional cognitions' characteristic of a mother with postpartum depression might include 'I should always know how best to care for my baby' or 'I should always be available for my baby.' Such thoughts relate to the idea that women should be personally responsible for their children. The thinking patterns associated with feeling unable to fulfil such responsibilities may lead to depression. But how might women in cultures where the responsibility of child rearing is shared with other women react to stressful situations? The Kipsigis of Kenya are a culture in which there is no evidence of postpartum depression. In the Kipsigis childcare responsibilities are shared, especially after childbirth. In fact, at childbirth the mother is 'pampered' to such an extent that she is almost completely free of childcare responsibilities. In such a context it would make little sense for the mother to have negative self-directed cognitions concerning her inability to cope with her new child or her lack of availability to the child.

The above example illustrates how individual cognitions reflect cultural norms and that different cultures may have different norms operating through individuals as risk factors for (different or similar) disorders. Some cultures – particularly western cultures – have norms that promote individualism. Having a poor opinion of oneself (i.e. low self-esteem) is recognised as a hallmark symptom of the western experience of depression (MacLachlan, 1987). Thus, promotion of individualism as a way of being in the world has its particular costs as well as its particular benefits, its particular risk factors for disorder and its particular intervention methods.

By and large the ethos of risk reduction and prevention of disorder has much to recommend it and is certainly deserving of further research. However, these issues may be addressed in a rather narrow context. First, although the idea of prevention is a conceptual advance on treatment models, it can be argued that prevention does not go far enough. Second, the interventions being described are effectively attempts at social change; they usually aspire to change the health-related behaviour of target individuals or groups. We now turn to these two important issues.

Beyond prevention

Within the field of psychological disorder interest has traditionally focused on what goes wrong (psychopathology), the process by which things go wrong (pathogenesis) and how to fix what has gone wrong (psychotherapy). The idea of preventing things going wrong ('psycho-inoculation') is still oriented towards what makes for misery. An alternative approach is to consider what makes for health, what goes right, rather than what goes wrong. If we can identify the factors responsible for psychological wellness it should be possible to reach beyond the idea of preventing or avoiding a negative experience of disorder, to actively promoting a positive state of health. We have already seen how different cultures understand disease and disorder and therefore we should not be surprised if understandings of how to be healthy also vary across cultures.

Cowen (1994) has described five key pathways to wellness. Some of them reflect the western emphasis on individualism whereas others are possibly relevant outside that context. The pathways to wellness are:

1. *Forming wholesome early attachments*: this pathway recognises the long dependency period of human childhood and the need for children to form warm, loving and secure relationships with their primary caregivers. Such relationships allow for the development of a strong sense of self on which the infant can build throughout life. The opportunity to form such attachments may be restricted not only by the experience of adverse psychological environments but also by the experience of harsh physical living conditions. Thus poor shelter, nutrition and sanitation may all affect early attachments between children and caregivers.
2. *Acquiring age-appropriate competencies*: these competencies relate to cognitive and interpersonal skills, some of which may develop from sound early attachment relationships. In many societies the main contexts for the acquisition of age-appropriate competencies are home and school. Yet in other societies school is not freely available and collective community responsibility 'schools' the developing child, thus blurring the distinction between family and school. Incidentally, nor is the notion of adolescence universal. In some cultures children move from childhood to adulthood, a concept difficult for many westerners, quite literally weaned on the idea of adolescence, to comprehend. Different cultures often have the belief that their way of classifying human experience is based on some fundamental truth. In reality, different cultures not only respond to the world in different ways, but also make the world into different places to live in.

3. *Exposure to settings favouring wellness*: this pathway to wellness is very much to do with living in communities that foster the individual's development, both psychologically and physically. I have previously discussed the ways in which different cultures afford support to their members and the mechanisms that different cultures present for dealing with grievances, including how one expresses and responds to distress.

4. *Having a sense of control over one's fate*: this pathway essentially relates to empowering individuals so that they feel some sense of control over events in their lives. It could also easily relate to empowering groups or communities. As we have seen ethnic minority groups may often suffer from poor health partly because they are disempowered. Other disempowered groups might include poor, elderly, homeless and disabled individuals. They are disempowered by virtue of the fact that they have a weaker voice in 'mainstream society' and are therefore afforded a disproportionately small amount of resources. Those who have a sense of control feel that they can influence things that matter to them. Thus having a sense of control is a salient issue for wellness across cultures. It should, however, be recognised that trusting in the benevolence of a god may also give communities and individuals a sense of being in control. This may be the case even if they live in objectively unpredictable physical environments subject to earthquakes, drought or hurricanes.

5. *Coping effectively with stress*: this is the final pathway to wellness described by Cowen. Some people appear to respond well to stress in that it gives them an 'edge', they rise to the occasion and perform better than they might under less stressful circumstances. Others, at the slightest sign of stress, go to pieces. The concept of 'hardiness' refers to the extent to which an individual sees stressful situations as a positive challenge to their capabilities. Often this relates to the degree of control that they are able to assert over the situation. However, once again these findings come from western psychology where the ability of the individual to rise above his or her circumstances is seen as praiseworthy. In some cultures struggling against natural forces, or other people, might be seen as morally wrong. In other cultures the individual's ability to put his or her trust in a deity may be seen as praiseworthy. Yet again, elsewhere, the willingness of individuals to turn to the wider community might be the most valued response that an individual makes. Thus not only do sources of stress differ across cultures but the way in which stress should be dealt with also differs.

Not surprisingly this list of what makes for wellness overlaps with what is important for the prevention of disorder. Wellness and health are, however, more than just the absence of disorder. As we noted in Chapter 1 the World Health Organization (WHO, 1948) described health as 'a state of complete physical, mental and social well-being and not merely the absence of disease or infirmity'. A focus on wellness can be seen as a very positive approach to differing cultures in that it seeks to understand the social mechanisms that exist within a community to maintain stability, harmony and the well-being of its members. Cultural groups will offer different solutions to the problem of forming wholesome early attachments, to acquiring age-appropriate competencies and having a sense of control over one's own fate. In one culture individuals may achieve some sense of control over their fate through believing in a benevolent deity who can be pleased and who will grant favours contingent on the practice of certain religious ritual. Other cultures may achieve the same sense of being able to influence the future by promoting the idea of individual primacy, that 'nobody can be a victim without their own consent', that 'if you try hard enough you can achieve anything', that 'you've got to look after number one'. Although these are radically different belief systems they may well solve the same problem equally well and each may be valuable in promoting wellness within a particular context.

Serious fun

Although I have been at pains to point out the need for awareness of and sensitivity to cultural difference, I have also noted that sometimes these arguments can be 'overcooked'. Recently, Kiernan, Gormley and MacLachlan (2004) explored the outcomes associated with children's participation in a therapeutic recreation camping programme. These children came from 15 European countries, representing many different cultures and 12 different languages. Although most of these children were chronically ill (our study included a comparison group of ill children's siblings), it was hoped the camp would be therapeutic in the sense that it was health promoting through providing the children with opportunities to experience a sense of personal mastery, self-worth and self-sufficiency, but also giving them a break from their daily struggles. The serious intent of the camp was to give children a 10-day break that would be good fun!

What makes this programme of particular interest from a cultural perspective is that the 'model' of therapeutic recreation derives from specialised 'camping programmes' that originated in and continue to have a strong North American ethos. The American 'Hole in the Wall Gang Camps' were the inspiration for the Barretstown Gang Camp, located in Ireland, which we studied. The existing literature reports mixed findings about the outcomes associated with participation in such camping programmes, possibly because of the great variation in the camps and in the methodologies used to identify their outcomes. Our own research assessed children's self-reported physical symptoms, affect, self-esteem and quality of life; these measures were taken two weeks before coming to the camp, two weeks after its completion and again six months after completion.

While our study did find some benefits of participation (for instance, in specific sub-scales of the instruments we used, such as satisfaction with physical appearance, experience of certain physical symptoms, and quality of life), there were however, no benefits evident in many other aspects of children's functioning. Furthermore, the only variable that was influenced by participants' nationality was their rating of satisfaction with physical appearance. Thus of the many variables we measured all but one suggested that the 'Gang Camp' type of experience did not discriminate between children of different nationalities. This may be because of its strong activity-focus (sport, art, etc.), as opposed to linguistically focused nature, or because of other factors. From a cultural perspective we might consider this 'equality of effects' across nationalities to be a very good thing.

The contemporary creation of disordered communities

Albee, in his keynote address at the 1995 World Federation for Mental Health, emphasised that self-esteem, social support and stress management are important in preventing disorder and promoting health. As already noted, minority cultural groups, immigrants and peoples in transition immediately come to mind as groups who have their self-esteem challenged, social support mechanisms undermined and abilities to cope effectively with stress severely compromised. However one subcultural distinction that is rarely drawn is that between rural and urban dwellers within the same cultural group in the same country.

Where this distinction is drawn it is usually with reference to remote rural communities in the 'less developed' countries. An enduring belief is that such people are psychologically better off, because it is the stress of living in modern urban industrial societies that is responsible for much psychological and physical disorder. Epidemiological attempts to explore the extent of disorder in rural versus urbanised areas have been plagued by methodological problems such as the intensity of screening, the determination of what (severity) constitutes a case of disorder and the language of emotional distress (how problems are presented). However, a study by Mumford and colleagues (1996) reported that people living in isolated Chitral mountain villages in Pakistan, far from reporting stress-free lives had, in fact, higher rates of disorder than is found in most western societies. This was especially so for women, for those from lower socioeconomic groups and for less literate individuals.

In other countries too we must seriously question the assumption that psychological disorder is a 'disease of modern living'. Within Europe there are various factors that may lead to increased rates of disorder in rural communities. European agricultural policies may have many knock-on social effects in rural farming areas. For instance, for farms to be economic they will have to increase in size and/or productivity. Increased mechanisation, EU production quotas and the increasing cost of agricultural land (to name but a few factors) are likely to lead to the situation where fewer people are able to make a living off the land.

This may compromise the integrity of many rural communities. Already, post offices, police stations, schools and churches have closed in many rural areas. What are the likely social effects of such changes? Social support networks are being seriously undermined, as the number of venues for casual contact diminishes. Social contact with like-minded people may be seen as an empowering experience resulting in the maintenance of self-esteem through a self-belief in what one is doing. Farming has become a more isolating enterprise with increasing technology replacing the need for human labour and therefore human contact on a daily basis. It cannot be coincidental that the rate of suicide in for instance, young Irish farmers, is one of the highest for any occupational group. No doubt the effects of depopulation also impinge on the individual's perceived ability to cope with stressful situations as they arise. Such stress undoubtedly relates to trying to avoid going out of business and the shame of having to sell off a family's inheritance, perhaps of many generations.

This situation and many like it throughout Europe and elsewhere are examples of disordered communities in the making: communities that cannot effectively support their own members; communities denuded of their structural and functional integrity. Most tragically these disordered communities are often being legislated for, even unwittingly planned for. The idea of the 'country life' being the ideal and an escape from the rat race of urban living is not supported in studies of psychological disorder in rural and urban settings. However, we may well find that the 'country life' of the future will become increasing stressful for those dependent on farming for their livelihood and that the rates of psychological disorder and related problems, such as suicide, will be much greater than in inner city areas.

Psychology promoting public health

Although the role of psychology in community care has been recognised for some time, its contributions to health promotion, primary care and public health have only recently begun to make an impact. Here we need not think of psychology as a profession, but rather as an active part of the professional life of most practitioners. Vinck (1994) has recently outlined how health psychologists can contribute to the promotion of public health. Most of the points that he has made also generalise to other professions, although psychologists may be particularly well placed to carry out some of the functions. Vinck's suggestions include the following:

- Forming a coalition with particular communities and collaborating with the community at every stage of their attempt to enhance their well-being.
- Translating data from large-scale epidemiological studies in terms of everyday behaviour.
- Monitoring behaviours in the population that are of particular interest (e.g. high risk or protective behaviours).

- Translating data gathered from monitoring into objectives for action.
- Establishing the determinants of relevant behaviours.
- Describing relevant aspects of the community's structure and function (e.g. subgroups, communication channels, leaders, values, resistances).
- Designing and executing 'multi-modal, multi-level' interventions.
- Designing and applying health education programmes.
- Designing, executing and evaluating project work.
- Mobilising financial, social and political support for action.

These points may be particularly useful when applied in a cross-cultural context. Yet in a sense what Vinck is arguing for is that each community should be treated as if it were a separate culture. It is to be hoped this is also an emerging theme to the reader of this book: that communities cultivate different ways of living depending on the resources available to them, their geographical, social, political and economic context. No two communities are the same and these differences are often simply of greater degree when we compare communities across cultures. It is also apparent that, for example, urban and rural, military and civilian, religious and secular, rich and poor communities all differ and all are made up of differing combinations of the above variables.

An important debate within the health promotion field is whether interventions should be directed at the individual or at the system and context within which individuals live. In fact, psychology is usually identified with intervention at the individual level because of its concern with what motivates individuals to engage in or avoid certain health-related behaviours. The ethos of focusing on 'lifestyles' and choice is probably embedded in the Euro-American value of individual freedom. However, in this book I have repeatedly noted the importance of looking beyond the individual to the context in which behaviours occur. In reality the focus of health promotion should not be the individual or the context, but the relationship between the individual and the context. In practice most health-promotion efforts work at both levels.

Take the example of an advertisement that warns against the dangers of cigarette smoking by presenting an image of a cigarette in the form of a coffin. At what level is this advertisement intended to work? At the individual level people may be made aware of an association between smoking and death, and this awareness may scare them so that they reflect on their own smoking behaviour. Although this mechanism is theoretically possible I suspect that it is not an important factor in discouraging people from smoking. At the contextual level the same advertisement may reinforce non-smoker's beliefs that smoking is bad for you. When a smoker enters the company of such people he or she may be given very negative feedback about smoking, and particularly smoking in the company of non-smokers. Thus, although the advertisement may have made smoking a salient topic, it may be the social pressure from others that has the greatest impact on smoking behaviour. Such pressure may result in the changing of norms and customs to the extent of certain areas being determined as 'smoke-free zones'. This is not to deny that efforts should be directed at promoting the effectiveness of health messages at the level of individuals or market segments (MacLachlan, Ager & Brown, 1997). Health-promotion interventions should be seen as working at both the individual and the contextual level. Changing social contexts is the next issue addressed.

Health promotion as social change

Given that health behaviours occur in the much broader context of society, it is often the case that attempts to change health-related behaviours are attempts at social change. Yet there are often good reasons why communities may resist attempts to change them and there are also different ways of producing the change process. Intervention programmes are all too often aimed at achieving dramatic changes, the process of which does not take into account, or build upon, the social structures that already exist in a community or culture. Although it is tempting to produce sweeping changes quickly, such attempts at change are often unsustainable because they fail to ignite the social forces that can integrate them into the life of the community. An alternative approach, which I now explore, is to seek incremental improvement by integrating small-scale changes into the sociocultural fabric of community life (MacLachlan, 1996b).

Within any community, traditional knowledge, attitudes, beliefs and behaviours reflect a degree of equilibrium between forces that promote change and those that inhibit it. Customs relating to health have evolved, sometimes over thousands of years, in order to serve the well-being of the community and its members. If certain beliefs or practices have existed for hundreds of years, it is probably because they offer acceptable solutions to problems in living. Seeking to change people's health behaviour may therefore have ramifications that reach far beyond the ken of the health practitioner. Health service interventions may challenge not only a way of thinking about health or specific health behaviours, but also a complete way of understanding how the world works and one's place in it. Lewin's (1952) field theory describes how a balance exists when forces for change (driving forces) are equal to forces against change (restraining forces). Changing this balance therefore requires either an increase in driving forces or a decrease in restraining forces.

So, for example, the situation of many immigrant minorities into western cities is that they encounter powerful driving forces (in the form of the dominant biomedical health care system) to change their ideas and practices regarding health. At the same time they may experience a weakening of the restraining forces (in the form of 'loosening' of the social context for traditional beliefs and practices). Unless this 'decoupling' of their familiar belief system is effectively resisted, or the transitional process is carefully negotiated (through a health system that is tolerant of pluralism), individuals may be catapulted into a nihilistic state where they cannot accept either approach to health. This may result in their rejection of any coherent system of beliefs or practices regrading their health and/or other important aspects of their life (see also Chapter 4).

This calamitous outcome is not, however, inevitable. According to field theory, the first stage of (successful) change involves 'unfreezing', or dismantling, existing patterns of behaviour. Among immigrant groups this process may occur simply because there is insufficient social support for their traditional ways of living. In the second stage, 'change', new patterns of behaviour are adopted, hopefully ones that are adaptive to managing the imbalance brought about by the increase in driving forces and/or decrease in restraining forces. The third and final stage, 're-freezing', occurs when people are able to integrate their newly acquired knowledge, attitudes, beliefs or practices into their previously existing repertoire. A crucial issue in this whole change process will be the magnitude of change required. The term 'required' is used here to suggest that, e.g. in the case of an immigrant group, their new environment will require some degree of adaptation if they are to function successfully. The smaller the change required the more readily it can be assimilated into the existing repertoire of skills. There are great difficulties when the message from health practitioners is not only that 'The way you're treating your child's measles is wrong', but 'Your whole system of understanding health and illness is wrong'!

We have already considered the situation where people have migrated to a country in which they are lacking sufficient social support for their customary way of dealing with life, illness and well-being. What of the situation where immigrants find a place in a large and well-established community with similar cultural origins and practices to their own? Here there is sufficient social support to maintain traditional customs, health beliefs and practices. If members of this community are presented with requests to make large changes to their way of life their most likely recourse will be to reject the need for change. The strength of support to resist such change may well exist in their new community. More than this, rejecting 'mainstream' healthcare services may even be seen as an important way of establishing your credentials as a committed member of your new community. Your allegiance to traditional values and willingness to reject 'neocolonial' ideas of health and wellbeing may well earn you a 'place' and status in your new community. Indeed such a strategy can be seen as a very sensible way of managing the transition, because it reduces the degree of change required of you in adapting to your new environment.

Whether the health practitioner is attempting to intervene in promoting the health of an individual from a marginalised minority culture group or from a well-established subculture, the magnitude of the change being suggested will be of paramount importance. The smaller the proposed change, the less the upheaval and adaptation that it will require. The problem with this rationale is that, to be realistic, sometimes the health practitioner will feel that it is not a small change that is required, but a big one. It may be that health practices, which were thought to be adaptive at a certain time and/or in a given place, are not adaptive in the presenting context. It is suggested that, where significant changes in health behaviours are sought, these should be driven through a series of complementary incremental steps in the direction of the desired change. This incremental improvement philosophy argues for the integration of new ideas and behaviours into an existing repertoire, before the next increment in the change process. However, here the change process is not directed by the health practitioner as such, but by the ease with which the community can integrate new ideas, i.e. by the rate of the unfreezing–change–re-freezing process. The practitioner, once having indicated an initial small change, is then reactive to the community's rate of change. The fact that the practitioner is not proactive does not reduce his or her potency because he or she remains the facilitator of the community's change process.

Incremental improvement is essentially a strategic approach to community change, operationalised through a series of small steps in the desired direction. However, it is also a learning process for the practitioner because he or she may not know either the best way forward, or the ultimate destination of the change process. Ultimately the way in which a community negotiates the change process, through umpteen unfreezing–change–re-freezing cycles, is a journey into the unknown. For the health practitioner this uncertainty can be a frustration, as can the slow pace of change. Nevertheless, these may be acceptable costs of a process that can enhance the community's ownership of positive changes in health behaviour. The notion of attempting to achieve modest incremental improvements has also been emphasised by Leviton (1996) in her review of the ways in which psychology can be integrated with public health.

Incremental improvement through leaning from the community

Social institutions offer vectors for promoting health. The workplace is a context in which a community atmosphere can be utilised to enhance interventions. Community groups, social clubs and schools are also alternative modes of intervention. Let us briefly consider a health-promotion project that used the community school as the site for intervention. In the initial stage of this intervention, we set out to learn from the community, before trying to 'teach' to it (MacLachlan, Chimombo & Mpemba, 1997). Although this research took place in a Malawian government secondary school, the general principles of the intervention would probably be applicable in many schools, in many countries. The focus of the intervention was to explore and, where appropriate, to change unhealthy knowledge, attitudes, beliefs and practices relating to HIV/AIDS.

The project, which extended over three years, began with a qualitative search for existing ideas about HIV/AIDS. This search included published written sources of information such as newspaper reports, short stories, official government statistics and press releases. The search also considered feedback from trainee teachers and their pupils, on lessons about HIV/AIDS. Our search put particular emphasis on the short story medium of communication that is very popular in Malawian newspapers. Although this source would be ignored by many conventional methods of research we felt that it was an important aspect of cultural learning for secondary school students. Many of the stories are clearly prescriptive and moralistic. Whether or not one agrees with the prescription or morals is not the point; what is important is to recognise that this medium was feeding potentially influential messages into the school community. Having identified these local understandings of HIV/AIDS and related sexual behaviour, we checked them out with a panel of local 'experts' (lecturers, medical practitioners, counsellors working with AIDS sufferers) asking them to add other important points that we may have missed. Consequently, by removing and adding items through several iterations, we derived 40 statements covering HIV/AIDS and sexually related behaviour.

These statements covered a variety of themes including the presentation of the disease (e.g. 'Everyone who loses a lot of weight in a short time has AIDS', 'Some people who get AIDS become mentally disturbed', 'All babies of mothers infected with HIV are born with HIV'), its transmission (e.g. 'You can get AIDS from a mosquito if it bites you shortly after biting an AIDS victim', 'You can get AIDS from hugging', 'You can get AIDS from sharing a cup with an AIDS victim'), folklore (e.g. 'Ministers of religion cannot get AIDS', 'A woman cannot get HIV/AIDS if she has sex only once with an infected man', 'You cannot get AIDS if you have sex standing up') and treatment ('At present there is no cure for AIDS', 'AIDS victims can benefit from counselling'). Other items referred to methods of prevention and protection, sex education and statistics on AIDS/HIV (see MacLachlan, Chimombo & Mpemba, 1997). The pupils were required to give 'yes' or 'no' answers to each of these statements. However, we were keen that this should not happen in a didactic teacher-to-pupil manner. We wanted to create a learning environment in which pupils were actively involved in the learning process and, ideally, where they could learn from each other.

We achieved this active mutual learning by presenting the information in the format of a board game – based on Snakes and Ladders – which pupils played in groups of four to six with a facilitator (in this case a university student). Over four weekly sessions of playing the board game, the percentage of correct responses significantly increased. This mode of intervention and our emphasis on the qualitative collation of local information are described as a modest example of how a community intervention to promote health knowledge can be undertaken. The importance of first learning from the community is underlined by some of the statements that were identified for the board game – statements that we certainly could not have foreseen as being an aspect of the pupil's understanding of AIDS and sexually related behaviour. Furthermore, although some health beliefs can be similarly constructed in different cultures (e.g. coping strategies – see Ager & MacLachlan,

1998), the relevance of others may differ substantially across cultures (e.g. health locus of control – see MacLachlan et al., 1997). Identifying exactly what people think before a health promotion intervention is possibly the most important stage of the whole intervention process. It is the bedrock on which further ideas and behaviours must take root with behaviour change being the ultimate outcome of interest (see later in this chapter).

The benefits of community health-promotion programmes

There have now been a number of large-scale health-promotion programmes that focus on the community as the mechanism of intervention. The outcomes of these projects have generally been quite impressive and recent Japanese research suggests that investing financial resources in health promotion subsequently reduces the demand for (and cost of) medical care (Nakanishi, Tatara & Fujiwara, 1996). One of the first major health-promotion projects was the North Karelia Project, conducted in northern Finland, which focused on reducing the unusually high incidence of death from cardiovascular diseases in Finland. The interventions were focused on schools (e.g. healthy heart lifestyle programmes), community centres (e.g. low-fat cooking classes), work sites (e.g. smoking cessation courses), etc. A five-year follow-up study compared the citizens of Karelia State with those of a neighbouring state that did not experience the intensive health promotion intervention. The risk of cardiovascular diseases decreased by 17% in men and 11% in women and these improvements were maintained over a 10-year follow-up period. The North Karelia Project, initiated in 1973, thus demonstrated that community interventions could be effective in combating serious diseases and so reducing mortality.

Another ground-breaking, community, health-promotion initiative was the Stanford Three-Community Study, which was undertaken by Stanford University in three small communities in northern California. The primary aim of the project was to assess the influence of a mass media programme on, once again, cardiovascular diseases. Two of the communities received the same mass media programme, which included television, radio, mailing of information sheets, newspaper reports and stories, and billboards. In addition one of these communities also received an intervention programme (including smoking cessation, weight loss, diet enhancement and physical exercise), which was targeted at high-risk individuals, identified by questionnaire assessment. The third community received only the initial risk assessment and neither the media programme nor the behavioural intervention programme. The risk of cardiovascular diseases significantly decreased in the first two communities, but not the third. In the community that received the additional behavioural intervention, the rate of decrease was greater, but over time each community achieved a reduction in risk for cardiovascular disease of between 25 and 30%. The significance of this project is that it demonstrated that health promotion programmes could be targeted at relatively small communities and that the improvement in health could be community wide rather than restricted to a few high-risk individuals.

Many other community-based health-promotion programmes have subsequently been undertaken in different parts of the world and this seems to be a mode of intervention that is increasingly recognised as valuable. However, probably the majority of such programmes target a geographical community without taking into account the different cultural groups that may constitute the larger, geographical community. As such the means of health promotion employed may favour certain sections of the community over members of minority groups. It is therefore important to consider what these factors might be and to think through health promotion techniques that can be sensitive to the needs of different cultures.

Douglas (1995) has described the importance of developing 'anti-racist health promotion strategies'. Writing about the development of health promotion in Britain, she identifies three phases of racist social policies since the early 1960s. The assimilation phase was characterised by health-promotion information being given to cultural minorities to encourage them to conform to British lifestyle norms. This was actioned through a proliferation of health-promotion literature on family planning, the diets of Asian families and tuberculosis (TB). An implicit goal of this phase was the modification of 'deviant' ethnic minority lifestyles in order to allow for assimilation into the British way of life.

The next phase was one of social integration where minority groups did not need to abandon their cultural heritage completely. Thus, in the late 1960s, a greater sense of tolerance was emerging towards differences between mainstream British society and minority groups within it. A greater emphasis was put on physical and cultural differences, an example of this being the increased interest in hereditary conditions such as sickle cell anaemia. However, this sort of 'tolerance' reflected a move away from integration. The 1970s and 1980s were associated with a concern to compare the behaviour of individuals from one culture with that of individuals from another (usually mainstream British) culture. Much of the research at this time reflected a medical model concerned with how illness and disease (such as TB, rickets, mental illness, perinatal mortality and low birthweight) affected minority cultural groups.

The model of health promotion based on this third phase attempted to 'educate' individuals to adopt more 'appropriate' lifestyles. As such they could be seen as targeted at 'deficit behaviours' where the individual or their culture was 'blamed' for their poor health. An often quoted example of this is the rickets campaign of the early 1980s which was the first health education campaign specifically targeted towards ethnic minority communities. As we have previously discussed, a poor diet, particularly one lacking in vitamin D, and the custom of covering almost all of the body, thereby preventing exposure to sunlight, have been implicated in the cause of rickets in Britain. The rickets campaign therefore emphasised the importance of the Asian community changing its diet in order to have a higher intake of vitamin D. Critics have pointed out that there was quite a different emphasis in combating rickets in the British (mainly white) population during the Second World War, where the problem was addressed through the supplementation of particular foods with vitamin D (e.g. margarine). This later strategy reflected the assumption that rickets was caused in the British population by poverty, yet 40 years later it was seen as being caused in Asians by cultural styles of living, including diet.

Douglas's (1995) critique of British health promotion and social policy emphasises that illness among minority cultural groups is often attributed to their alternative cultural practices rather than to the relative poverty in which many minority communities live. She also stresses that the illness targets for health-promotion interventions are often those of concern to (predominantly white) health professionals rather than members of the minority culture groups themselves. Douglas's main point appears to be that the position that minority cultures are 'put in' by mainstream society should be a major interest of health promoters and more generally of social policy (see also Ahmad, 1996). Thus experiences of poverty, broader aspects of socioeconomic position, racial discrimination, etc. should be recognised. These are indeed important points but, at the same time, there is also a risk of placing too much emphasis on the broader sociopolitical and economic context and subtracting from the value of a cultural level analysis.

It is clear that some cultures engage in behaviours detrimental to their health, despite being relatively 'comfortable' on a broad range of social, economic and political indicators. One comparison might be between the islanders of the Western Hebrides of Scotland and the inhabitants of the Norfolk Broads of England. The exceptionally high rates of alcoholism in the former group could be attributed to some aspects of social disadvantage. It would generally not be attributed to aspects of Hebridian islanders' relative advantage. However, the difference might more appropriately be attributed to the different heritage of Celtic and Anglo-Saxon peoples and to the particular ways in which these two cultures encourage socialising.

A major concern with regard to promoting health in different cultures should not only be to avoid 'blaming the victim' of disadvantage but also to avoid the well-known psychological actor–observer effect. In the present context this is demonstrated by illness being observed in a particular cultural community and the 'observers' (those looking on, in this case 'mainstream society') attributing its cause to the behaviour of the minority cultural group – the actors. At the same time the actors (those immediately experiencing the problems) attribute the cause of it to the context in which they are acting out their lives. The focus of the actors and observers is on each other as the cause of the problem. Racism is usually thought of as coming from the observer and being directed at the hapless actors. Yet by this formulation it could also come from the actors and be directed towards the hapless observers. My point is therefore that the context and the culture interact in complex ways to define how any group of people live.

Changes in social, economic, geographical or political contexts may also require cultures to change if the culture is going to remain an adaptive medium through which its members can live in the world. The situation in relation to all cultures and their broader context is therefore complex (involving many interrelated variables) and dynamic (in a process of continual change for the purpose of adaptation). It would indeed be a fallacy to believe that some cultural practices are not maladaptive in certain contexts. Anyone who doubts this need only observe the after-effects of the first days of sun-bathing by English tourists on the Spanish Costa del Sol – ouch! On a more serious note, the high incidence of skin cancer among white Australians may be a result of the failure of their cultural practices to adapt to their present environment. It could be argued that health promotion directed at getting white people to cover up, spend less time in the sun, wear protective creams, etc. are directed at 'deficit' behaviour. However, this 'deficit', as with the case of vitamin D and rickets among British Asians, should not be seen as intrinsic to a particular cultural group as such, but particular to certain behaviours in certain contexts, which may put one cultural group at greater risk than another.

The benchmark of culturally sensitive – but not racist – health promotion must be treating different cultural groups with the same integrity and respect. There can be nothing racist in recognising that different groups of people, living in the world in different ways, may have different needs for maintaining their health. However, such a recognition must in no way distract our attention from the health consequences of living in poverty and experiencing racial discrimination. It is a travesty that in many of the world's so-called 'developed' countries minority cultures are treated opportunistically as cheap labour and do not have the same social welfare rights as the majority of citizens. What sort of host culture allows such a situation to persist? This is as much a moral question as it is a psychological, sociopolitical or economic one. It is, nevertheless, a question that we should all address in our efforts to promote health within all cultures, and reduce discrimination. More recent research suggests the potential for new methods of communication in promoting health particularly in stigmatised and socially isolated groups.

Homosexual subculture and HIV in China

Gao (2005) undertook research into HIV/AIDS in Chengdu city, Sichuan Province, China. Sichuan, with a population of just under 10 million, is in the interior basin of south-west China. It is a large province with 39 minority groups. Chengdu is renowned not only for its historical and cultural traditions, but also for its large gay community, with an estimated 200,000 plus gay men, and men-having-sex-with-men (MSM), living in Chengdu. They are attracted there partly by its large population and commercial traditions, and partly by its reputation for more liberal attitudes and practices.

China has been described as 'economically and culturally backward' by no less a person that its new Party Secretary General. The recent relative relaxation of central political control and the ideology of class struggle has led to greater individual flexibility, at least in some regards, such as more freedom in social life and greater integration with foreign cultures. In the 1980s the *Beijing Review* noted that homosexuality (*tongxinglian*) and casual sex are 'illegal and contrary to Chinese morality' (Gao, 2005, p. 11) and this oppressive attitude naturally led to a lack of attention to the problem of sexually transmitted infections (STIs) and HIV in this section of the population. Contrast this with Health Minister, Zheng Wenkang's, public acknowledgement of the seriousness and complexities of the HIV/AIDS epidemic in China in 1999, and his statement that:

> Under the leadership of the Communist Party Central Committee and the State Council and each level of the Party and government organisation, we must not miss any opportunity to implement all HIV prevention and control policies and measures. We must strive to build and complete this long-term social system project so as to reduce to the greatest extent possible the harm that HIV causes to the people and society.

> Cited in Gao (2005)

The most important clause there is perhaps the idea of 'a long-term social system project' because it recognised both that the effects of HIV/AIDS are not just an immediate health issue but also a longer-term strategic issue for the government, and that it is a problem of social systems – how people relate – not just a biomedical pathogen.

The importance of a subculture being at particular health risk in China has also previously been recognised, but not necessarily a 'sexual orientation subculture' – more an 'economic entrepreneurial' subculture. So, for instance, in the context of China, Wang and Keats (2001) have explored the relative risk of living in different sectors of the dual employment system: the more morally and financial conservative State system of employment, compared with the more recent, more morally liberal and economically unreliable, *Getihu* (self-employed) system, where the incidence of HIV is notably higher. Their research strongly suggests that the social networks and contexts of each system constitute quite distinct subcultures, with characteristic health risks that are also woven through the fabric of historic cultural customs and economic circumstances.

Gao's (2005) research addresses the gay and MSM community in Chengdu as a similarly meaningful and distinct Chinese subculture, overlapping with, but distinct from, the *Getihu* subculture, and no doubt many other subcultures too. Doubting the value of conventional western models of health behaviour (e.g. the health belief model or the theory of reasoned action) she adopted more of a social constructivist approach – the idea that people seek to construct meaning out of their lives through their interaction with others – and a culturally informed approach. She argued that China broadly emphasises collectivist and family values and is a 'high-context' culture (as opposed to a low-context culture which assumes little inside knowledge and where all terms of communication are fully explained – where they do not use much jargon or 'in' words).

Gao (2005) developed an intervention based on an integration of several communication-based theories. The *diffusion of innovation model* (Rogers, 1982), concerning how new ideas are communicated through social systems, emphasises, for example, that unique population groups should be targeted through the 'socio-economic, cultural and linguistic terms which characterise those special groups. It also recognises the importance of activating opinion leaders and social networks in the unique population group in order to affect behaviour change' (Bowles & Robinson, 1989, p. 559). The *empowerment* model, also adopted by Gao, emphasises the value of disadvantaged people working together to take control of those factors determining their own health and lives (Israel et al., 1994). Finally, embracing the *participatory methods* of the visionary Brazilian educator, Paulo Freire (e.g. 1972), Gao also sought to 'go to the people' and to learn from them before presuming to 'teach' them. Combining facets of these approaches through *edutainment* (education through entertainment – Tuft, 2002), Gao used an innovative participatory approach and people-centred communication theory, in the form of multilevel interventions. This included mini-dramatic presentations, small-media materials, internet chat rooms, hotlines and opinion leaders, and many other interventions based in the venues where gay and MSM met and related to each other. Although admittedly it is difficult to distinguish which of these methods may have been the most important among the plethora of interventions used, Gao's results were nevertheless impressive.

Following the interventions, and relative to a comparison group, Gao (2005) reported significant increases in HIV/AIDS-related knowledge, attitudes towards safe sex, increased condom use and reduced number of sexual partners, e.g. the affirmative response rate to the item 'always using a condom for anal sex with casual sexual partners' rose from 4.3% before the intervention to 76.8% after it; whereas in the comparison group there was no significant change (2.9% to 4.2%). Although condom use for oral sex also increased (from 1.4% before the intervention to 15.9% after the intervention), this change, although statistically significant, was much more modest and more worrisome. To place these figures in the context of the actual sexual behaviour itself, in the total sample of 180 men, 3.8% reported having only one male sexual partner in the past 6 months, whereas 19.4% reported having between 11 and 20 male partners and another 19.4% reported having 20+ male partners in the past 6 moths. Of these men 50% also reported having one or more female sexual partners during the same period.

Culture, subculture and stigma

Li (1998) reported that, whereas in the west only about a fifth of male homosexuals are in heterosexual marriages, in China most of them are. According to Li (1998), this is because of pressure from cultural norms that emphasise the importance of family and of carrying on the family name. The Confucian philosophy of ordered family and social relationships is apparent here. An extract from the interviews conducted by Gao (2005) with Gong, a 33-year-old serviceman, conveys the great distress that many homosexual men in China live with today:

> Why did I want to come out and play with gay men? I felt that I looked down on myself; I was annoyed and lived like rubbish. In ten years time I attempted suicide three times. Nobody, including my parents, knew why I wanted to kill myself. They always thought, maybe the pressure of my studies. Actually, I felt bored of living and kept asking myself why I was this type of person. . . . Why? I believed in Buddha so I thought that my previous life did not do good things otherwise I wouldn't look like this. . . . I was discovered by my elder brother the last time I attempted suicide. When I woke up, I saw how miserable my mother was, I swore that I would live even like a dog afterwards, just for my mother.

Gao (2005, p. 143)

This terribly sad quotation illustrates how cultural and spiritual beliefs can exert very strong role expectations as well as germinating stigma. Furthermore, in as much as society represents a social mirror of ourselves (the 'looking-glass' mirror theory of self perception), it produces an image of the self that may be internalised, and produce such low self-esteem as to make one feel as if existing is to 'live like a dog'.

Of particular interest from a cultural and subcultural perspective is Gao's analysis of those segments of the personal interviews that she undertook, where the men discussed subcultural language of sexual positions, with relative ignorance of their associated HIV contraction risks. Gao argues that 'Anal sex is the symbolic centre of gay identity having a high level of interpersonal meaning, such as love, trust and intimacy' (Gao, 2005, p. 184).

Homosexual relationships between men are expressed through a subcultural slang, e.g. a '419' is sex with someone 'for one night', whereas '2p', '3p', etc. is used to refer to having sex with two or three, etc. sexual partners. Slang confers linguistic demarcation and a distinctive identity, and may eschew more pejorative 'mainstream culture' terminology. It may make something that society at large regards as unacceptable into something that is 'cool'. In recognising and (re)naming a subcultural norm it has the potential to help people feel 'OK' about their behaviour. Several of the people interviewed by Goa referred to a specific instance of this and illustrate that within such subcultural constructions there remain inequalities that are related to the risk of contracting HIV. (2005, pp. 147–50):

> In Chengdu we use '0' and '1' to represent the positions of anal sex. '0' represents receptive position; and '1' represents insertive. (Xi)

> I think this kind of fixed saying related to our tradition. In Western countries people are more equal, but here people who are more feminine

may depend on those who are more masculine. So those who are more feminine are to be '0'; those who are more masculine are to be '1'. . . . In our circle this type of thinking is rooted deeply. They don't think that '0' and '1' are equal, on the contrary' '1' should look after '0'. . . . Some '0' can be one '1', but they don't want to, they are afraid to take the responsibility. . . . (Xi)

I always act like a '1', I feel happier being a '1' when having sex with men than women. My friend suggested to me to be a '0' when I turned 30, he said that I have been a '1' for half my life, I should try to be '0'. So I tried once but felt very unhappy, it was very painful . . . I don't know why most people I met would like to be '0', especially for those younger ones who just joined our circle. 8 out of 10 of them are '0'. . . . (Gong)

You can just about tell from their appearance, if they are very 'sissy', they would be '0', otherwise they would be '1'. (Wu)

Although not all participants felt that there was such an absolute distinction between being a '1' and a '0', one participant linked these roles to the sort of reception one would get from a doctor:

If you were infected you go to the hospital. If you were a '1', the doctor can treat you as a normal STD patient, but if you were infected as '0', they would get to know that you are homosexual, you would be discriminated against right away. (Gong)

The social construction of the '0' role within the Chengdu homosexual community is therefore one of it being stigmatised relative to '1', not only within their own subculture, but also by those outside it and crucially by those who would be in a position to treat STIs. Being a '1' rather than an '0' not only confers this perceived advantage, but is also related to the likelihood of developing STIs including HIV, the '0' receptive position being at greater risk than the '1' insertive position, a fact of which most of Gao's participants were quite unaware. Interestingly, and reflecting the complex interface between broader cultural and subcultural ideas, Gao (2005) argues that the dichotomous influence of yin and yang theory is played out in the relatively fixed '0' or '1' roles. The yin and yang philosophy suggests that all material, and the inner world, is made up of two elements, forces or principles. Yin is negative, passive and weak, whereas yang is positive, active and strong. 'He Yin-Yang', a harmonious state of development, is seen to result from a balance between the elements of yin and yang. Other aspects of Chinese heritage are possibly relevant: the Confucian emphasis on family has already been cited, but Gao also notes the attribution by some gay people of their sexuality to their (poor) conduct in previous lives, according to Buddhist beliefs.

The sort of contextually and culturally driven intervention described by Gao chimes with other advances in the area of primary care and STIs, e.g. the UNAIDS suggested a new framework for addressing behaviour change in relation to HIV/AIDS. This framework draws attention to five key contextual domains: government policy, socioeconomic status, culture, gender relations and spirituality. Although these domains may lie outside the control of individuals, it is recognised that they do nevertheless have a significant influence on their HIV/AIDS-related health behaviours. This implies a moving beyond individual level theories to more multilevel and contextual explanations and interventions, in which culture and subcultures play a much greater part (www.comminit.com/roundtable2). Resonating with the notion of culture being a conduit to health promotion rather than a barrier (MacLachlan, 2001), Gao (2005) also notes that the Rockefeller Foundation (www.rockfound.org) contrasts approaches to HIV where people are seen as *objects* of change, with those where people are seen as *agents* of change. The theme of a different approach, and one much more culturally centred, that is needed to address the global problem of HIV/AIDS is developed further in Chapter 9.

Guidelines for professional practice

1. The dramatic increase in the health of citizens of most industrialised countries can be attributed to improvements in public health, such as safe drinking water, efficient sewage systems and better nutrition, rather than to biotechnological innovations in treatment. Clinicians should be proactive in identifying the ways in which health can be promoted, rather than being solely concerned with reactively treating problems as they arise.

2. The relatively poor health of many minority cultural groups may be attributed to their lower access to health-promoting initiatives rather than to a relatively higher intrinsic incidence of disease or disorder. With equal access to health-promoting initiatives and with the provision of similarly health-promoting environments, the health of minority cultural groups can be equal to the health of majority cultural groups. However, clinicians may need to work with different mediums for promoting health in different cultural groups.

3. Relatively simple behaviours (e.g. eating breakfast daily, moderate use of alcohol, sleeping 7–8 hours daily) have been shown to be significantly associated with longer life spans. It would therefore seem that certain behaviours are strongly health promoting, whereas others are strongly health threatening (e.g. physical inactivity, smoking cigarettes, eating between meals). Clinicians should not, however, assume that the same 'package' of health-promoting or health-demoting behaviours will have identical effects across cultural groups. Presumably the effects of some of these behaviours depend on what else you do and there may be some cultural practices that are especially effective or defective in promoting health. This is an empirical issue.

4. Although cultural sensitivity (awareness of cultural issues) is important for clinicians, it is not sufficient. Clinicians must also be culturally competent and this requires personal experience of working with different

cultural groups. This book is intended to enhance cultural sensitivity and to encourage clinicians to strive towards cultural competence.

5. Although health promotion has historically focused on physical health, its value in mental health is now well recognised. A recent US report has highlighted 10 issues to be considered when clinicians are working with different cultural groups and seeking to prevent mental disorders. These points in themselves constitute guidelines and may be used to help individual clinicians or clinical teams review their interventions across cultures.

6. Specific risk factors can be identified for particular disorders. Sometimes these risk factors may be particularly prominent in a cultural group, e.g. experiencing a severe stressor, having low self-esteem and living in poverty have been identified as risk factors for depression. Recent immigrants often experience stress as a result of their transition. They may find that the minority cultural group of which they are a member is discriminated against, with the result that many of them feel undervalued and have low self-esteem. Furthermore immigrant groups are often economically disadvantaged such that they will be living in poor housing and possibly without employment or full access to social services. In such cases whole communities may be at risk of developing 'depression'. Thus minority cultural groups may deserve special efforts to be made in preventing disorder and promoting health.

7. Culture influences the way in which people think. Many western cultures emphasise the primacy of the individual and of the individual achieving success. Such an emphasis may predispose people in these cultures to react negatively to the realisation that they are not, in fact, the outstanding individuals that they (and their friends) would like them to be. A loss of belief in the self is a central 'symptom' of depression. Thus western cultures may be seen to predispose to this experience of depression. Cultures emphasising other values may predispose to different reactions. In some sense, then, culture itself can be thought of as a risk factor.

8. Clinicians should analyse different cultures in an attempt to identify how each seeks to solve certain common problems: how to deal with stress, how to acquire age-appropriate competencies or how to form wholesome early attachments. These pathways to health are the routes that clinicians must work through even though they may be foreign to the clinician.

9. A widespread assumption is that life in urban communities is more stressful than life in rural communities. Recent research does not support this belief. Furthermore, the urbanisation of many societies may result in rural life becoming more stressful through, for example, the reduction in available social support networks. Contemporary government and international policies may place people in rural and urban areas at greater risk of developing disorders. The health implications of such policies deserve the attention of clinicians who wish to facilitate health promotion.

10. Health promotion will often require clinicians to work with communities, not as leaders, but as facilitators of social change. In this role clinicians

can be catalysts for better health by empowering people to take charge of their own well-being. This role may involve monitoring behaviour, translating data, mobilising resources, etc., rather than being seen as the agent of change.

11. Incremental improvements to health is a philosophy of change where the magnitude of change that occurs at any given time is determined by factors within the community that the clinician is seeking to serve, rather than by the aspirations of the clinician. Often it will require the clinician to be prepared to learn from the community before attempting to assist it.

12. There is now strong evidence that community health-promotion programmes can be effective in reducing serious diseases and mortality, that health gains need not be restricted to high-risk individuals but can be community wide, and that they can specifically target minority cultural groups. It is important that we learn from past mistakes and do not see minority cultural lifestyles as deviant or deficient. However, it is equally important not to cocoon minority or majority cultural behaviours in 'cultural relativism'. It is reasonable to assume that some behaviours relate more strongly to health than to disorders and it is the clinician's responsibility to identify and advise on these, treating each cultural group differently, but with equal respect.

13. HIV/AIDS is truly a pandemic, now reaching into virtually every community in the world. Within some communities marginalised groups are particularly stigmatised because of the relatively high incidence of the disease among them. When these groups are also stigmatised because of intrinsic differences between their own beliefs and/or behaviours, and those of mainstream society, their marginalisation can be magnified and society's fear of them increased. Particularly among these groups, 'mainstream' messages about infectious diseases such as HIV/AIDS may have little penetrance, and subcultural norms and trustworthy sources and contexts need to be recruited into attempts to protect and promote health.

CHAPTER 9

Global health

According to Nussbam we must develop:

> an ability to see [ourselves] . . . not simply as citizens of some local region or group but also, and above all, as human beings bound to all other human beings by ties of recognition and concern because the world around us is inescapably international. Issues from business to agriculture, from human rights to the relief of famine, call our imaginations to venture beyond narrow group loyalties and to consider the reality of distant lives.
>
> Nussbam (1997, p. 10)

Global health is about 'the reality of distant lives'. This reality is hauntingly brought home to us by Mallaby (2002, p. A.29) when he writes:

> A century from now, when historians write about our era, one question will dwarf all others, and it won't be about finance or politics or even terrorism. The question will be, simply, how could our rich and civilised society allow a known and beatable enemy to kill millions of people?

That killer is of course HIV/AIDS and it is perhaps one of the most distressing exemplars of the global reach of human suffering and illness.

In Chapter 1 we noted that McAuliffe (2003) defines global health as an attempt to address health problems that transcend national boundaries, may be influenced by circumstances and experiences in other countries, and are best addressed by cooperative actions and solutions. Within this perspective the world's health problems are seen as shared problems and are therefore best tackled by shared solutions. An implicit aspiration is to work towards removing inequalities and privileges in accessing health, i.e. to establish health as a human right.

Global health disparities

The Global Forum for Health Research (GFHR) is dedicated to helping correct what they refer to as the '10/90' gap (2004, p. 1), i.e. of the US$ 73 billion invested annually in global health research 'only about 10% of the global funding on health research from all sources is devoted to 90% of the world's health problems'. However, even this 10% is not used as effectively as it could be and needs to be used better. The world's health problems can be conceived of as a 'global disease burden' and is measured by disability-adjusted life years (or DALYs). It has been argued that many of the factors that account for the high level of disease burden in terms of morbidity and mortality have very low levels of research funding (Murray & Lopez, 1996), particularly acute respiratory infections, diarrhoeal diseases, tuberculosis (TB), tropical diseases, prenatal conditions, and even HIV/AIDS. Although the inclusion of HIV/AIDS in this list of under-funded research may be surprising, remember that the issue being addressed here is whether the investment in health research reflects the burden of specific diseases – the burden of HIV/AIDS is even more massive than the proportion invested in health research on it.

For the non-communicable diseases that occur with similar prevalence in both rich and poor countries (e.g. cardiovascular disorder, hepatitis B, diabetes) there is a relatively high intensity of research, compared with those diseases that occur predominately, or exclusively, in poorer countries (e.g. malaria, schistosomiasis, Chagas' disease). GFHR (2004) reports that, of the 1233 drugs that reached the global market between 1975 and 1997, only 13 (i.e. 1%) were for use in combating tropical infectious diseases, which mainly affect the poor. In view of the fact that 85% of the world's population live in low- and middle-income countries, this is a cause for concern.

So how does culture relate to the problems of global inequality and health? As argued in Chapter 1 we have to 'loosen up' our thinking on what 'culture' is and how it can affect health (see Table 1.2). We noted that globalisation constitutes a new force that is powered by various concerns, with economic growth being prominent amount them. Although it is common to talk about certain diseases, e.g. malaria, being carried by a 'vector' (in this case mosquitoes), Lee (2004) has described globalisation as the vector for deaths as a result of tobacco smoking. She notes that the 4.9 million annual tobacco-related deaths currently constitute more than one in ten adult deaths world wide, a figure that will inevitably rise: thanks to globalisation, the tobacco industry is again looking at growing markets, particularly around middle- and low-income countries.

We have previously noted that globalisation is 'led from the West, bears the strong imprint of American political and economic power, and is highly uneven in its consequences' (Giddens, 1999, p. 4). Giddens goes on to say that we 'must find ways to bring our runaway world to heel' (p. 5). Although there are many facets to globalisation (technological, cultural, political, economic), some of which may be quite positive, there are also many victims, especially of economic globalisation, e.g. in 1989 the poorest fifth of the world's population had 2.3% of global income, whereas by 1998 this had dropped to an alarming 1.4%, and in sub-Saharan Africa 20 countries now have lower per head incomes in real terms than they had 30 years ago (Giddens, 1999).

World Bank loans to developing countries had become virtually conditional on the recipient country's agreement with the International Monetary Fund

(IMF) on a fund programme (Cassen, 1994). Often countries were required to invest in cash crop production to be traded on the world market under 'free trade' regulations. This created bizarre situations such as that during the height of the 1984 Ethiopian famine, oilseed, rape, linseed and cottonseed were being grown on prime agricultural land to be exported as feed for livestock to Europe (Corner House Briefing, 1998). Similarly, in 1997 the UN Development Report stated that, in Africa alone, the money spent on annual debt repayments could be used to save the lives of about 21 million children by the year 2000. Debt has been seen as *the new colonialism* (see, for example, George, 1988; Sommers, 1996) and recent efforts to cancel it must be warmly welcomed.

Sommers (1996, p. 174) quotes the following emotive statement from UNICEF:

> Hundreds of thousands of the developing world's children have given their lives to pay their countries' debts, and many millions more are still paying the interest with their malnourished minds and bodies.

So, for instance, Somers reports that in Nicaragua overall budget spending on health was less than half the level of the early 1980s and infant mortality rates increased after declining steadily for more than a decade. The same is now true in many other 'third world' countries that have had to cut back spending on health and social welfare, liberalise their markets and invest in cash crop production – all in order to compete on the global market, to meet the requirements for structural adjustment loans (SALs) from the World Bank. The 'cultural' element being examined here is the selling of globalisation (with all its political and economic baggage) as if it is synonymous with 'development.' Economists can be justly criticised for adopting a simplistic and unsympathetic 'black box' mentality to Africa in the 80s and 90s: money in, debt out, and goodness knows what goes on inside.

Some of the ways through which the process of globalisation works include what has been referred to as the 'digital divide' and the 'knowledge divide'. The digital divide describes the inequality of access to information and communication technologies (ICTs), whereas the knowledge divide refers to inequity in knowledge flows, where the richest countries and multinationals tend not to share knowledge with the poorer populations that might have an even greater need for it. We might add to this nomenclature of division the idea of a 'pharmaceutical divide', where the research and production of pharmaceuticals are targeted at the rich world with the fewest health problems and not at the poor world with the greatest health problems.

Each of these 'divides' reflects a set of shared values by those propagating them. But are they really shared, or are they more pursued in the face of the majority's indifference? Whatever the correct answer to this, it is apparent that the result still reflects a position adopted by people in some parts of the world towards the plight of others in a different part of the world. However, at a multilateral and intergovernmental level, there has been a move to establish a set of public health goals that could be aimed for – globally – in the near future. The millennium development goals (MDGs) represent a partnership between the 'developed' countries and the 'developing' countries determined, as the Millennium Declaration states 'to create an environment – at the national and global levels alike – which is conducive to development and the elimination of poverty'. The 8 MDGs may be broken down into 18 public health targets with 48 indicators for their achievement. These goals are to be taken in the context of other salient indicators of development and are primarily focused on low income countries. The MDGs, and associated targets, arose from the Millennium Declaration, signed by 189 countries, including 147 heads of state, in September 2000. Table 9.1 gives the MDGs with associated targets.

Health and development

One issue that has attracted much attention recently is how we should see the relationship between health and development (Sachs, 2005). Labonte (2004) has suggested that health has been presented variously as a prerequisite to economic development, as a human right and as a matter of security. In terms of health as a *prerequisite for development*, it has been argued that health represents one of the best investments, in terms of return on money, by producing a workforce that is more economically produce and competitive. Although the hard-headed financial facts of this case are well supported (Commission for Macroeconomics and Health, 2004), it also has overtones of the provision of a labour force for the benefit of global capitalism, as opposed to primarily being a benefit for the poor themselves. Sachs (2005) has, however, argued that once the poor are helped onto the first run of the 'economic development ladder', market forces (in a mixed economy) can 'kick in', such that capitalism and social development become mutually reinforcing.

The idea of health being key to *global security* has also been used to justify increased funding of health, based on the assumption that an unhealthy population is more problematic and unstable than a healthy one. In particular, the politically and economic destabilising effects of HIV/AIDS in sub-Saharan Africa are seen as a real concern as an increasing number of adults spend long periods in illness and subsequently die, leaving behind a larger proportion of traditionally less economically productive children and elderly people.

A third argument sees health as a *human right*, in the same way as people tend now to see education as a human right. Just to be clear, the 'right' here is not necessarily a right to health itself, but to have access to resources and services that allow for the provision of health, just as people may have access to resources and services that provide for education. This right to health should not, however, be subordinate to trade agreements or other international agreements that undercut the possibility of health being achievable (see McAuliffe & MacLachlan, 2005). Furthermore, the right to health is seen as extending to underlying health determinants, such as clean water, sanitation, maternal/child programmes and health education. This conception of the *right* to health implies that development is also a right and that assistance to

Table 9.1   The United Nation's indicators for the millennium development goals (MDGs).

Millennium Development Goals (MDGs)

GOALS AND TARGETS	INDICATORS
GOAL 1: ERADICATE EXTREME POVERTY AND HUNGER	
Target 1: Halve, between 1990 and 2015, the proportion of people whose income is less than 1 US$ a day	1. Proportion of population below US$1 per day 2. Poverty gap ratio (incidence × depth of poverty) 3. Share of poorest quintile in national consumption
Target 2: Halve, between 1990 and 2015, the proportion of people who suffer from hunger	4. Prevalence of underweight children (under 5 years of age) 5. Proportion of population below minimum level of dietary energy consumption
GOAL 2: ACHIEVE UNIVERSAL PRIMARY EDUCATION	
Target 3: Ensure that, by 2015, children everywhere, boys and girls alike, will be able to complete a full course of primary schooling	6. Net enrolment ratio in primary education 7. Proportion of pupils starting grade 1 who reach grade 5 8. Literacy rate of 15–24 year olds
GOAL 3: PROMOTE GENDER EQUALITY AND EMPOWER WOMEN	
Target 4: Eliminate gender disparity in primary and secondary education preferably by 2005 and to all levels of education no later than 2015	9. Ratio of girls to boys in primary, secondary and tertiary education 10. Ratio of literate females to males of 15–24 year olds 11. Share of women in wage employment in the non-agricultural sector 12. Proportion of seats held by women in national parliament
GOAL 4: REDUCE CHILD MORTALITY	
Target 5: Reduce by two-thirds, between 1990 and 2015, the under-5 mortality rate	13. Under-5 mortality rate 14. Infant mortality rate 15. Proportion of 1-year-old children immunised against measles
GOAL 5: IMPROVE MATERNAL HEALTH	
Target 6: Reduce by three-quarters, between 1990 and 2015, the maternal mortality ratio	16. Maternal mortality ratio 17. Proportion of births attended by skilled health personnel

Table 9.1   Continued

Millennium Development Goals (MDGs)	
GOALS AND TARGETS	INDICATORS

GOAL 6: COMBAT HIV/AIDS, MALARIA AND OTHER DISEASES

Target 7: Have halted by 2015, and begun to reverse, the spread of HIV/AIDS	18. HIV prevalence among 15–24-year-old pregnant women 19. Contraceptive prevalence rate 20. Number of children orphaned by HIV/AIDS
Target 8: Have halted by 2015, and begun to reverse, the incidence of malaria and other major diseases	21. Prevalence and death rates associated with malaria 22. Proportion of population in malaria risk areas using effective malaria prevention and treatment measures 23. Prevalence and death rates associated with tuberculosis (TB) 24. Proportion of TB cases detected and cured under DOTS (directly observed treatment short course)

GOAL 7: ENSURE ENVIRONMENTAL SUSTAINABILITY*

Target 9: Integrate the principles of sustainable development into country policies and programmes and reverse the loss of environmental resources	25. Proportion of land area covered by forest 26. Land area protected to maintain biological diversity 27. GDP per unit of energy use (as proxy for energy efficiency) 28. Carbon dioxide emissions (per capita) (Plus two figures of global atmospheric pollution: ozone depletion and the accumulation of global warming gases)
Target 10: Halve, by 2015, the proportion of people without sustainable access to safe drinking water	29. Proportion of population with sustainable access to an improved water source
Target 11: By 2020, to have achieved a significant improvement in the lives of at least 100 million slum dwellers	30. Proportion of people with access to improved sanitation 31. Proportion of people with access to secure tenure (Urban/rural disaggregation of several of the above indicators may be relevant for monitoring improvement in the lives of slum dwellers)

GOAL 8: DEVELOP A GLOBAL PARTNERSHIP FOR DEVELOPMENT*

Target 12: Develop further an open, rule-based, predictable, non-discriminatory trading and financial system Includes a commitment to good governance, development, and poverty reduction – both nationally and internationally	Some of the indicators listed below will be monitored separately for the least developed countries (LDCs), Africa, landlocked countries and small island developing states Official development assistance (ODA) 32. Net ODA as percentage of DAC donors' GNI (targets of 0.7% in total and 0.15% for LDCs) 33. Proportion of ODA to basic social services (basic education, primary health care, nutrition, safe water and sanitation)

Target 13: Address the special needs of the least developed countries

Includes: tariff and quota free access for LDC exports; enhanced programme of debt relief for HIPC and cancellation of official bilateral debt; and more generous ODA for countries committed to poverty reduction

Target 14: Address the special needs of landlocked countries and small island developing states

(through Barbados Programme and 22nd General Assembly provisions)

Target 15: Deal comprehensively with the debt problems of developing countries through national and international measures in order to make debt sustainable in the long term

Target 16: In cooperation with developing countries, develop and implement strategies for decent and productive work for youth

Target 17: In cooperation with pharmaceutical companies, provide access to affordable, essential drugs in developing countries

Target 18: In cooperation with the private sector, make available the benefits of new technologies, especially information and communications

34. Proportion of ODA that is untied
35. Proportion of ODA for environment in small island developing states
36. Proportion of ODA for transport sector in land-locked countries

Market access
37. Proportion of exports (by value and excluding arms) admitted free of duties and quotas
38. Average tariffs and quotas on agricultural products and textiles and clothing

39. Domestic and export agricultural subsidies in OECD countries
40. Proportion of ODA provided to help build trade capacity

Debt sustainability
41. Proportion of official bilateral HIPC debt cancelled
42. Debt service as a percentage of exports of goods and services

43. Proportion of ODA provided as debt relief
44. Number of countries reaching HIPC decision and completion points

45. Unemployment rate of 15–24 year olds

46. Proportion of population with access to affordable essential drugs on a sustainable basis

47. Telephone lines per 1,000 people
48. Personal computers per 1,000 people

Other indicators TBD

GDP, gross dosmetic product; GNI, Gross National Income; HIPC, Highly Indebted Poor Countries; OECD, Office for Economic Co-operation and Development.

achieve this right is not presented as assistance through charity, but, rather, assistance as an *obligation*.

Each of the arguments above concerning the need to invest more in health will appeal to different constituencies. However, although economic growth may be necessary to achieve greater investment in health, it is not in itself sufficient; the benefits of economic growth need to be distributed with equity, the fruits of such growth need to be spread in such a way that it encourages the attainment of health by all (Cassels, 2004). Although it is natural to assume that the increasingly sophisticated achievements of the wealthier countries over the past 10 years are reflected in a similar, if less dramatic, improvement in poorer countries, this is not the case, e.g. in sub-Saharan Africa, the incidence of under-5 child mortality has increased in 16 countries, in comparison to 10 years ago (Cassels, 2004).

The millennium development goals

A human rights approach to health advocates for people's rights not only to receive appropriate health services, but also to participate in identifying their own health needs and the ways in which these might be addressed. Thus, while the MDGs represent a range of laudable and internationally relevant public health goals, these goals may not reflect the priorities of local communities. There is therefore a tension between the imposition of health goals from 'above' and the identification of health needs and initiatives more locally. It is evident that the identification of such health needs will be influenced by cultural priorities, beliefs and values.

Although knowledge of the MDGs is valuable in terms of understanding the international context of public health promotion, it is important that their pursuit does not stifle local initiatives or overlook local strengths relevant to their achievement, so that health is not something 'done unto' others, it is important that it be rooted in local priorities, strengths and existing capabilities. Let us consider an example of how cultural factors may influence the attainment of one of the MDGs: to reduce by two-thirds the under-five mortality rate.

Mortality rates are of course often associated with morbidity rates. Sometimes, e.g. in cases of severe undernourishment, the physical state of the child will be very obvious. At other times problems that predispose to eventual mortality will need to be observed at a behavioural level, a level where cultural differences can express themselves more easily, e.g. motor development should proceed through a series of 'motor milestones', the achievement of which augers well for the health of the child, and the delay of which may be the first signs of disability. However, although well-nourished black African infants tend to show precocity in psychomotor development (in comparison to other children), the ability of a three year old to ascend a flight of stairs (which is used in the Bayley scales as an indicator of psychomotor development) is not necessarily appropriate to an environment where rural three year olds rarely need to negotiate such obstacles. Pointing this out, Dawes et al. (2004) argue that, although there is a need to develop standards in this domain in order to address threats to survival, they must also be locally sensitive. They also note that, in areas where children are at risk of cerebral malaria, mothers pay especial attention to motor development, and so this awareness should be cultivated and extended for its broader value too.

Perhaps one of the essential conduits for culture is language, and in South Africa the right to be educated in your 'own' language has now been established ('where possible'). Literacy is probably the major health-promoting intervention that can aid children's increased awareness and understanding of health problems and how to protect themselves against them. Again, the idea of standards here is important, but there are no measures of literacy that have been developed across the numerous South African languages. More generic pictorial tests (e.g. the Peabody Picture Vocabulary Test – you show a child a picture and ask him or her to name it) assume an equal exposure to the items pictured, an eventuality that is unlikely because culture and language are still conflated with poverty and access to educational resources in South Africa, and indeed in many other countries.

Dawes et al. (2004) also emphasise that decrements in motor, cognitive and social development can be indicators of underlying neurological, nutritional, health or mental health problems, and so some way of measuring this broad range of behaviours in a culturally meaningful way is important. Of course, the measurement of cognitive development ('intelligence') in different cultural groups is something of a psychologically political minefield. But indicators of memory, attention, decision-making, etc. are surely important in all cultures. As Dawes et al. (2004, p. 37) state:

> The challenge for a standards approach [which allows for comparisons] in South Africa is to make the tests sufficiently child-friendly, language appropriate and culture-fair so that children are able to show their real potential rather than their reaction to a strange and somewhat threatening demand.

The point being made here is that there are difficulties in measuring the progress of different cultural groups with regard to achieving the MDGs, and yet such a comparison is necessary if we are to be sensitive to cultural differences in their achievement. However, above and beyond that, the MDGs are a powerful political tool to hold governments accountable for achieving the goals to which they have signed up. Nevertheless, it is important to realise that they are averages, and that there remains the possibility for a country or region to be appearing to being doing well, whereas in fact these gains are unevenly distributed across cultural or income groups, and between genders (Cassels, 2004). Before returning to the theme of HIV/AIDS, I want briefly to consider three factors that along with culture contribute to diversity in healthcare, and that interact with culture to influence people's sense of dignity: gender, disability and caste (or class).

Gender inequalities

In Chapter 1 I noted how gender inequality can be seen as seriously compromising the human rights of women and girls. One of the most distressing facets of this is to be found in the 2001 Indian census report that there are only 933 females per 1,000 male births, whereas normally women outnumber men in most societies (perhaps because of sex-linked recessive disorders being more rarely expressed through a XX, as opposed to XY inheritance). Khanna and colleagues (2003) sought to explore the extent to which this finding could be accounted for by sex discrimination, antenatal selection and termination of female pregnancies. Indeed this concern has been so real that it led to the Pre Natal Diagnostic Techniques Act 1994 prohibiting sex determination in India.

It also appears that afterbirth mortality is higher in girls than in boys, with girls being 30–50% more likely to die between their first and fifth birthdays (Claeson et al., 2003). Reviewing the relevant literature Khanna et al. (2003) conclude that in India girls are often brought to health facilities in a more advanced stage of illness, are taken to more poorly qualified medical practitioners when they are ill, and have less money spent on their medication, compared with boys. In their own study Khanna et al. found a similar rate of death for infants of both sexes from diseases with a usually 'grave prognosis' (e.g. asphyxia, septicaemia or congenital abnormalities), but, for the preventable and treatable disease of diarrhoea, there were twice as many deaths among girls compared with boys. Furthermore, under the category of 'unexplained deaths' there were three times as many girls as boys, leading the authors to ask the distressing question: 'Could such deaths be an extension into the early neonatal period of female feticide?'

Although some might imagine that these finding could be explained to some extent by poverty or poor education, the fact that such sex discrimination is known to be more common among families with higher incomes argues against this interpretation (Booth, Verma & Beri, 1994). In Khanna et al.'s (2003) study, the income of families where infants died of unexplained causes was higher than in those families where they died of diarrhoeal diseases. It is highly likely that the preponderance of deaths under suspicious circumstances among the financially better off reflects a cultural value for boys that is greater than that for girls. Although the above findings are certainly not restricted to India, the World Health Organization (WHO) has reported that sex discrepancies in health and education are higher in south Asia (including India) than anywhere else in the world. Thus the cultural background here is not of one 'pathological' or 'cruel' culture, but rather a general discrimination against one gender, across many cultures, an effect that is of course also seen, albeit in a much different form, in most western countries.

Sometimes discriminatory practices travel with migrant groups and their inhumanity may become even more apparent in societies where there is not such explicit subjugation of women. So-called 'honour killings' are an example in point where a woman may be killed by a family member, or spouse, in order to uphold the supposed 'honour' of her family. Although these sad and outrageous cases are not uncommon among immigrant groups in many western countries, a recent book by Souad (2004) tells of her own experience of surviving an attempted 'honour' killing, some 30 years ago. Souad was raised in strict Islamic doctrine as a Palestinian on the West Bank, where eye contact with a man earned a girl the label of *charmuta*, or whore. When she fell pregnant at 17 she thought her likely punishment would be death.

A few days after her family learnt of her pregnancy her brother-in-law poured petrol over her and set her alight in the courtyard of her house. She managed to escape into the street where local women beat out the flames and arranged for her to be taken to hospital. With severe burns and excruciating pain, Souad was ultimately saved by an aid worker who arranged for her to be flown to Switzerland. Souad's account also recognises the pressures on parents to comply with such traditions, for fear of being ostracised by their community. She describes how in her community 'being born a girl is a curse' and how her brother was educated, but not her sisters or herself. In hospital the staff sympathised, not with her, but with her family. Although Souad survives, living in continental Europe, she still fears revealing her full name in case she becomes a target for extremists. With over 5,000 'honour' killings reported each year (and who knows how many go unreported) there seems to be a lot of extremists.

We must challenge cultural traditions that inflict pain through circumcision, cause death through feticide or purposeful neglect, or tacitly condone murder. We must not be 'culturally sensitive' to traditions that deny people their human rights and, when such rights are denied on the basis of biological sex, we must cultivate new and equitable relationships that promote health as well as healthy respect of difference.

Disability

Disability is another contributor to our experience of diversity. Here I briefly consider cultural variations with regard to attitudes towards intellectual disability (also referred to as learning disability, developmental disability, mental handicap or mental retardation), and cultural aspects of just one type of acquired physical disability, spinal cord injury. This brevity cannot hope to do justice to the range or complexity of issues regarding disability, and is intended simply to raise awareness of the salience of cultural factors in disability. My discussion highlights cultural differences regarding stigma and social inclusion in intellectual disability, and in the cause and consequence of an acquired physical disability.

Recently Siperstein et al. (2003) published a multinational study of attitudes towards individuals with intellectual disabilities. This study was commissioned by the Special Olympics and involved between 400 and 1,000 members of the public in each of the countries involved. The motivation for the study was for better understanding of the attitudes and practices that prevent many of the 170 million individuals around the world with intellectual disability from fully participating in society. The stigma that public attitudes towards

Table 9.2 Public's perceptions of the abilities of persons with intellectual disabilities (selected capabilities).

	Brazil (%)	China (%)	Egypt (%)	Germany (%)	Ireland (%)	Japan (%)	Nigeria (%)	Russia (%)	USA (%)
Sustain friendships	88	53	33	93	88	88	41	86	93
Wash and dress	59	71	13	84	75	81	47	92	85
Tell time	65	73	19	87	81	80	47	83	83
Understand news event	41	22	5	44	53	41	27	46	46
Handle emergencies	18	18	8	32	20	17	16	14	28

Based on Siperstein et al. (2003).

disability present is of course the ultimate social handicap that those individuals must endure. Table 9.2 shows the countries surveyed and the percentage of respondents from each country that endorsed the likely abilities of intellectually disabled people. There are huge differences between the countries.

Within the social domain, the ability of intellectually disabled people to sustain friendships, for example, varied from 33% of Egyptian respondents endorsing this, up to 93% of German and US respondents endorsing it. Obviously one's estimation of the ability of a person to sustain a social relationship is going to influence one's inclination to invest in such a relationship, and so such an attitude can be expected to be salient to intellectually disabled people's degree of social inclusion, and ultimately their quality of life. Table 9.2 also shows great variation in ratings across countries for ability to engage in instrumental activities, such as washing and dressing, and telling the time, as well as more abstract activities, such as understanding the news, and stress-related experiences, such as handling emergencies.

Although 92% of the Russian public surveyed thought that people with intellectual disabilities could wash and dress themselves, only 13% of Egyptians thought likewise. Clearly the social barriers to inclusion, to access to self-esteem-enhancing activities and to opportunities to provide a contribution to society are important mechanisms through which intellectual disability is stigmatised. Cultural constructions of disability (reflected in Table 9.2) must be challenged where they preclude the opportunity for intellectually disabled people to participate in their own society meaningfully. Only though participation can stereotypical negative images be countered and dismissed.

According to the National Spinal Cord Injury Statistical Centre (2000) approximately 200,000 individuals in the USA are living with spinal cord injury (SCI), with 10,000 new cases occurring each year. The cause of these injuries varies across cultural groups with African–Americans and Native Americans being over-represented. However, they are over-represented for different reasons. Native Americans have the highest motor vehicle SCI incidence rates, accounting for upwards of 67% of new injuries, and among the lowest violence-related SCI rates, accounting for only 9%. Motor vehicle accidents account for 27% of African–American SCIs, whereas violence-related incidents account for over 40% (Neville, 2000). Neville also notes that SCI is patterned by a much higher incidence among men (82% on the US National SCI Database) and among the urban working class. Interactions between culture and cause of SCIs may of course influence social attitudes regarding responsibility and rehabilitation potential.

Historically, pressure sores were the condition that received most research attention in the SCI population. Now emotional reactions are receiving increased attention. This consequence of SCI also seems to be patterned by culture, e.g. Krause, Kemp and Coker (2000) found that cultural minorities, particularly women, were more likely to develop depressive reactions to SCI than members of the majority cultural groups. Although differences in education and level of income largely mediated the relationship between culture and depressive reactions, a small effect remained independent of these. Thus in SCI, and many other forms of acquired physical disability, there is a cultural patterning to cause and consequence, but much of this is interwoven with the social and economic standing of different cultural groups. Culture is important and distinctive, but not necessarily independent, of the other factors relevant to disability.

Caste

At the opening of the World Conference on Racism, held in South Africa in 2001, one protester demonstrated with a placard: 'Racism excludes, restricts, discriminates . . . So does Caste'. Caste systems are traditional in parts of Africa and Asia. They commonly include a degree of physical segregation (e.g. not being able to drink from the same cup, or water source, as higher castes), social segregation (e.g. a prohibition on intercaste marriages), restricted work opportunities (usually in traditional work occupations associated with death or filth), low wages and bonded labour, and high levels of illiteracy, poverty and landlessness. Perpetrators of crime against lower caste communities may often go unpunished, and these communities are discriminated against based on ideas of 'purity' and 'pollution'. According to the National Campaign for Dalit Human Rights (2005, www.dalits.org) under the *devdasi* system thousands of Dalit girls living in the southern states of India, are 'dedicated to a deity or temple: unable to marry and forced to become prostitutes for upper-caste men, they are eventually auctioned into brothels'. Although many countries have specific laws against class discrimination, they are rarely enforced. Mahatma Gandhi talked of the 'calculated degradation' to which the 'depressed classes' had been assigned for centuries by Hinduism, a travesty that continues today. Why?

Thekaekara (2005a) suggests that the caste system originated as a means of dividing labour, exercising social control and maintaining order. The power and broad acceptance of the system derive from its apparent religious sanction from the 4,000-year-old *Manu Sashtra* (laws of Manu) which divided society into four broad orders (or *varnas*), each arising from a part of the creator's body. The *Brahmins*, priests and teachers, the most pure, came from the head. The *Kshatriyas*, warriors and rules, came from the arms. The *Vaishyas*, traders and merchants, came from the lower limbs. The *Sudras*, the lowest caste, came from the feet, and were destined to serve the other three higher castes, as labours and artisans. Within these castes there are also many sub-castes. But below all of these were the '*Untouchables*', who were excluded from Manu's system because they were considered unacceptably impure and polluting. Not only were they 'untouchable', they were also excluded from society, living on its absolute margins: not being allowed to talk to other castes or to walk on the same ground as them. Today in India, these Untouchables refer to themselves as *Dalits*, or 'broken people'. Today their exclusion continues; they may not be served food in many eateries, or they are asked to sit outside or at a distance from other customers. They may need to use a special 'Untouchable' cup to drink from, and then wash it before returning it to the proprietor (Thekaekara, 2005a).

Although the caste system is perhaps strongest in India, it also persists in the Indian diaspora. Thekaekara (2005a) notes that as Hindu communities have grown in the west caste distinctions have in fact become more pronounced. She also suggests that the rise of Hindu fundamentalism has promoted what she describes as the 'be proud of your culture' syndrome, where caste is read as 'culture'. This has led to increased segregation between castes. CasteWatch UK was established in Britain in 2003, in an attempt to combat caste discrimination. Van der Gaag (2005) cites some examples of such discrimination in Wolverhampton, England. In one case a customer in a shop insisted that their change be placed on the counter in order to avoid contact with the person serving them who was of a lower caste. In another case, women from a higher caste refused to take water from the same tap as women from a lower caste, even though they all worked on the same 'factory floor'.

Despite this shocking stigma and discrimination, KR Narayanan was the first *Dalit* to serve as India's president, from 1997 to 2002. When asked by Thekaekara, about the paradox of India's achievements in regard to some of the most sophisticated IT in the world, on the one hand, and a feudal caste system, on the other hand, Narayanan responded thus:

> Fifty years is a miniscule period for the caste system which has survived for thousands of years. The caste system has fundamentally been attacked by very few people. Even the lower castes found it convenient, a kind of safety system to manage, mingle in society. Everyone had someone to exploit. Though there were many challenges, no fundamental revision was ever attempted. . . . The opposition was basically related to land struggles and the feudal economic system in existence. Morally only Gandhi shook the system, but the economic foundations were too strong. . . . Today caste is being perpetrated by politics and politicians. . . . Revolution has to come from below – through education and through protests from the oppressed people.
>
> Thekaekara (2005b, p. 17)

It is perhaps demoralising that 'revolution from below' is the conclusion of someone who broke out of the caste mould and made it to 'the top'. It does, however, point to the potential collective power of oppressed people when they are mobilised and focused. Perhaps one of the lessons for global health here is that much could be gained through local community groups coming together into collective action and pressure groups to establish, promote and maintain their own right to health.

It is nonetheless important to end this section by emphasising that the *potential* power of the oppressed should not exempt those from 'above' taking action. In her research with sex workers in Calcutta, Cornish (2004) has sought to identify how rather broad societal phenomena, such as those in which we are interested here, become active in mediating health-related behaviours. She notes that identification of the 'reflected mediating moment' of fatalism, regarding how women are sexually exploited by the structures and values of society, may indeed constitute insight, but may not in fact be particularly empowering: conscientisation (becoming aware of your oppression) is not, in itself, liberation.

HIV/AIDS

Throughout this book we have emphasised cultural differences with regard to specific diseases and disabilities, and we have noted the significance of stigma in the previous three sections as an affront to an individual's dignity and quality of life. Westbrook, Legge and Pennay (1993) investigated the degree of stigma attached to 20 different diseases and disabilities, across six cultural groups. They found a remarkably consistent pattern across all cultural communities: people with asthma, diabetes, heart disease and arthritis were the least stigmatised, whereas those with AIDS, intellectual disability, psychiatric illness and cerebral palsy were the most stigmatised. Comparing their own research with research over the previous 20 years, the findings appeared remarkably consistent across time also. Although AIDS had not previously been included in such studies, Westbrook et al. (1993) found it to be the most stigmatised condition across all cultures. As a pandemic, HIV/AIDS is perhaps the major health challenge of our time, and how we – globally – respond to it will define our generation – our morals and our sense of compassion and responsibility, for generations to come. What will be our legacy?

The human immunodeficiency virus (HIV) is perhaps the clearest exemplar of the interplay of cultures, communities and health. It has given rise to paranoid reactions towards 'gay communities', drug users, immigrants, people with haemophilia and cultural minorities. It is often a fatal disease contracted through a variety of activities. High-risk behaviour for HIV/AIDS transmission varies in different places and among different groups, but includes sexual relations (particularly through multiple partners, casual relations, violent intercourse and prostitution), mother-to-child transmission (during pregnancy, at birth or through breast-feeding), intravenous drug use (through infected needles) and contaminated blood (encountered during sexual intercourse, in certain initiation ceremonies, unhygienic excision or circumcision, tattooing and skin piercing).

As of the end of 2004 WHO and UNAIDS, through their AIDS epidemic update, estimated that there were 39.4 million people living with HIV, and 3.1 million people had died from HIV. In 2004 alone, an estimated 4.9 million people became infected with HIV. A staggering 25.4 million of those living with HIV live in sub-Saharan Africa. With a prevalence of around 7.4% across sub-Saharan Africa, this represents close to one in every 12 people being HIV positive, with pockets of much higher prevalence to be found throughout the region. However, the steepest increases in the rate of HIV infection have been in east and central Asia and eastern Europe. The number of people living with HIV in east Asia rose by almost 50% between 2002 and 2004, an increase largely attributable to China's 'swiftly growing epidemic'.

Although differences in the reporting of cases – as opposed to their actual occurrence – may account for some of the differences observed between countries, it is clear that significant differences actually do exist. Equally there are significant differences regarding the number of people who are estimated to be HIV positive, but who have not yet developed symptoms of AIDS. In this section we explore why it has taken the scientific community so long to take culture seriously in the fight against HIV/AIDS. This is of particular concern given some excellent early anthropological research on the problem, and the subsequent relative neglect of culture over the last 15 years. It is only relatively recently that it has been incorporated through innovative programmes, such as that reviewed in Chapter 8 (Gao, 2005) and work in Singapore, where they helped local sex workers develop negotiation skills to encourage condom use and worked with brothel keepers to create a context that would support this.

AIDS in Hispanic communities in the USA

In 1994 the USA had the highest number of reported AIDS cases of any country in the world. In fact with 411,907 cases reported by June 1994, the USA not only had more cases than any other country, but also had more reported cases than any continent, including Africa. Singer and her colleagues (1990) from the Hispanic Health Council, Hartford, Connecticut gave a detailed account of the Hispanic AIDS crisis in the USA. Although the Hispanic community constituted 8% of the population, it accounted for 15% of AIDS cases reported in the USA in 1988. More recent accounts of AIDS confirm its high prevalence among cultural minorities both in the USA and in other industrialised countries. Initially the medical model of the disease focused attention on the individual, rather than on cultural variables and the social, economic and political reality of marginalised communities. Now these realities are beginning to be addressed.

Table 9.3 Cumulative incidence of AIDS cases through April 1989, USA: percentage of adult/adolescent cases in each exposure category by culture.

Exposure category	Hispanic (%)	White (%)	Black (%)	Asian/Pacific Islander (%)	Native American (%)	Total (%)
Male homosexual/ bisexual contact	42	77	37	75	51	61
Intravenous drug use (heterosexual: male and female)	40	7	38	4	16	20
Male homosexual/ bisexual contact and intravenous drug use	7	7	7	1	14	7
Haemophilia/ coagulation disorder	0.5	1	0	2	6	1
Heterosexual contact	5	2	11	3	6	4
Receipt of blood products or tissue	1	3	1	8	3	2
Other/undetermined	5	2	5	7	5	3

Reproduced from Singer et al. (1990). (With permission of the American Anthropological Association.)

Hispanic communities in the USA are not homogeneous. Nevertheless, when statistical averages are compared, e.g. with white communities, they live in significantly more poverty and are less well educated. They suffer disproportionately more infectious and parasitic diseases, higher rates of infant mortality and lower life expectancy. Research conducted in the late 1980s found that the rate of HIV infection in Hispanic communities was almost twice as high as that in non-Hispanic communities. Furthermore, the ways in which AIDS is contracted also appears to be different across cultural groups. Table 9.3 gives a breakdown of 'exposure category', or route of contraction, by culture. It is clear from these figures that male homosexual or bisexual contact accounted for a much greater percentage of cases among white, Asian and Pacific Island communities than it did among Hispanic and black communities.

Likewise there was a dramatic difference across the cultural groups in the extent to which intravenous drug use had been a route of contracting HIV. Comparisons such as these attest to the degree to which culture, through a variety of social processes and social disadvantages, is pathoplastic (shapes the development) in physical diseases.

Table 9.4 breaks down different possible preventive activities with regard to AIDS undertaken by Hispanic, African or white Americans (Singer et al.'s terms). Table 9.5 shows variations in sexual practices across these groups. In both cases there were significant differences among the three groups.

Table 9.4   Reported preventive activities during the previous 12 months: percentage of affirmative responses for each cultural group.

	Latino (%)	African–American (%)	White (%)	All (%)
Discussed AIDS-preventive behaviour with sex partner	35	49	65	47
Avoided sex with prostitutes	62	90	84	78
Limited number of sex partners	74	85	84	81
Used condoms more frequently	34	43	36	38

Reproduced from Singer et al. (1990). (With permission of the American Anthropological Association.)

Table 9.5   Sexual practices and condom use in the past year: percentage of affirmation responses for each cultural group.

	Latino (%) (n = 117)	African–American (%) (n = 100)	White (%) (n = 73)	All (%) (n = 290)
Vaginal intercourse with condoms	37	54	33	42
Vaginal intercourse without condoms	69	81	86	78
Anal intercourse without condoms	17	16	28	19
Oral sex without condoms	28	53	67	46
Oral sex with condoms	11	20	20	16

Reproduced from Singer et al. (1990). (With permission of the American Anthropological Association.)

Interventions that seek to promote low-risk AIDS behaviours need to take into account the reasons for such differences and to build them into prevention programmes, e.g. the traditional cultural stereotypes of male *machismo* (being authoritarian within the family, having extramarital sex, drinking heavily, physically abusing family members, etc.) and of female *marianismo* (women being chaste before marriage, submitting to their husband's authority, enduring suffering, being morally and spiritually pure, etc.) could easily be seen as providing a context for transmission of HIV through 'hot-blooded' Hispanic men chasing Hispanic women. However, heterosexual contact may have accounted for only about 5% of cases, whereas intravenous drug use and homosexual contact may each have accounted for over 40% of cases. This sort of initial anthropological research has been supported by subsequent psychosocial research, which is now briefly considered.

Psychosocial interventions for HIV/AIDS

It now seems clear that awareness about HIV/AIDS and its primary routes of infection are high in most countries, but high-risk behaviours continue to be practised to varying degrees in different countries. Much research has focused on the determinants of sexual risk (e.g. sex with multiple partners) or protective behaviours (e.g. condom use) using general health behaviour theories (e.g. theory of planned behaviour) or those that are specifically developed to address HIV/AIDS-related risk (e.g. AIDS risk reduction model). According to recent report on the epidemic of the joint UN Programme on HIV/AIDS (UNAIDS), sexual risk taking or inconsistent condom use is closely intertwined with a variety of personal and interpersonal psychosocial factors, including poor knowledge, low sense of threat of infection, high sensation seeking, strong need to comply to social norms, and group or community level risk factors such as poverty, migration and pervasive norms that perpetuate women's subordination within sexual relationships (UNAIDS, 2002). In the context of sub-Saharan Africa, negative attitudes towards sex with condoms, female sexual compliance to ensure economic security, lack of negotiation skills to implement condom use, desire for children and an external locus of control have been identified as potential obstacles to condom acceptance and use (Campbell, 2002).

Although the effectiveness of interventions varies by type, length and other characteristics of the intervention, the most efficacious HIV prevention programmes have specifically been directed at groups at risk of infection, focused on relationship and negotiation skills, involved multiple sustained contacts and used a combination of culturally appropriate media of delivery (MacLachlan & Mulatu, 2004). Despite the fact that most intervention studies have not explicitly studied the role that cultural variables play within cross-cultural contexts, those that integrated cultural factors into their HIV prevention themes and contents have confirmed the pervasive influence of culture in risk perception, risk-taking behaviours and adoption of protective behaviours (Wilson & Miller, 2003).

When considering interventions targeted at persistent pain and psychosocial consequences associated with HIV/AIDS, there is strong evidence that culturally appropriate interventions that take into account sociocultural resources, explanatory models and contextual factors are more likely to effectively to reduce persistent pain, psychosocial distress and negative disease outcomes, e.g. the use of traditional healers, midwives and indigenous social support systems in developing countries, and 'alternative and complementary therapies' in the west have been found potentially useful interventions to manage pain and to mitigate the psychosocial impacts of HIV/AIDS (Swanson et al., 2000; UNAIDS, 2002).

Although almost all health conditions can lead to stigmatising experiences, diseases that elicit fear of illness, contagion and death, and those with uncertain origins and their limited treatments tend to cause more stigmatisation than those that do not (Taylor, 2001; Brown, Macintyre & Trujillo, 2003). Patients with such diseases as leprosy and TB have historically evoked fear and revulsion in others. Although advances in knowledge and treatment have increased acceptance of such patients, as we have already noted, the 'new' illness of HIV/AIDS has now become perhaps the most stigmatising health condition around the world.

Among HIV-infected individuals, stigma manifests itself in many ways. HIV-infected individuals may refuse to disclose their status to others for fear of negative reactions from their partners, family members, employers and members of their communities. This has been found to be a major obstacle to preventive efforts in many sub-Sahara African countries. They may also refuse to receive the necessary health services because of potential negative reactions of healthcare providers or for fear of being discriminated against by others. HIV-infected people who belong to some sectors of society, such as commercial sex workers in sub-Saharan Africa and injecting drug users in western countries, may face an extra layer of stigmatisation simply because of their association with 'deviant' or 'immoral' behaviours. These and other stigmatising experiences lead to negative effects on test-seeking behaviour, willingness to disclose HIV status, health service-seeking behaviours, quality of healthcare received, and social support solicited and received (Taylor, 2001; Brown et al., 2003;). Having returned to the theme of stigma, it would indeed be remiss of me not to recall the shameful scientific pursuit of the racist source of AIDS.

AIDS, Africans and racism

Describing the cultural or racial aspect of a disease can be a tricky business. Focusing on the differences between cultural groups can, whether intentionally or otherwise, promote racism, ignorance or naivety. Such allegations are usually made when it is felt that one culture or cultural group is being negatively compared with another group. And such comparisons, although not necessary, are nevertheless inevitable. If a disease is found more often in one cultural group than in another it is reasonable for people to ask why and how this should be. However, the ascribing of disease origin to a particular group, which is then understood to have infected other peoples, is a potentially explosive situation. From a social psychological standpoint the search for an origin or source of disease can take on the function of scapegoating certain social groups or nations. In the case of AIDS some have argued that the fear aroused by the disease has compelled people to project its source into things that they also fear and/or denigrate. The unspoken rationale goes something like this: 'What is different is dangerous and things that are different from us and dangerous to us go together.' This sort of 'witch hunt' can certainly be fuelled by the popular media, but, in the case of AIDS, scientists and clinicians have also been caught up in, and become a key part of, the process. Although 'we are all human' it is necessary to be aware that the collective forces of 'inhumanity' can draw clinicians in as well.

In their book *AIDS, Africa and Racism* Chirimuuta and Chirimuuta (1989) catalogue explicit examples of racism in ascribing the source of the AIDS epidemic to people of African origin:

> The widespread, uncritical acceptance of the AIDS from Africa hypothesis by the normally sceptical scientific community is most disturbing. It would be comforting to believe that this was a simple mistake or an unfortunate result of an excess of enthusiasm. It seems to us far more likely that the AIDS researchers, the medical "experts", the media and the public at large are affected by the insidious and frequently unrecognized disease of racism.

> Chirimuuta and Chirimuuta (1989, p. 136)

How many times have you heard people (perhaps including yourself) say that 'research suggests AIDS started in Africa'? The Chirimuutas' point is that there is good evidence to suggest that this may not be the case and that, regardless of its origin, African peoples are seen as a more fertile 'culture' in which the virus can 'grow'.

When AIDS first appeared in white male American homosexuals, they became obvious scapegoats. However, the Chirimuutas argue, this meant that the disease was still American. Another source was desirable:

> Given the racist stereotyping of black people as dirty, disease carrying and sexually promiscuous it was virtually inevitable that black people, on the first sight of the disease among them, would be attributed with its source. ... Racism, not science, motivated the search for the origin of AIDS.

> Chirimuuta and Chirimuuta (1989 p. 128)

By 1982, 700 cases of AIDS had been reported in the USA; 34 of these were Haitian immigrants. Haiti is a small island off the Florida coast mainly inhabited by the descendants of African slaves. On the basis of these statistics, it was quickly suggested that gay American tourists visiting Haiti had contracted the disease from the Haitians. These American tourists had then passed on the disease to other Americans (generally homosexuals) on their return to the USA.

This notion, generated by statistics and derived from 'scientific speculation', was zealously promoted by the American media, which gelled together the idea of 'AIDS' with the idea of 'Haitian'. The result was that Haitians resident in the USA were sacked from their jobs and evicted from their homes, and Haitian prisoners were quarantined. Fortunately within a few years the idea that one country (Haiti) was responsible for the suffering of another country (USA) did not hold up to closer scrutiny. It transpired that although there did appear to be a link between Haiti and the USA, it was in the opposite direction. Apparently it was the Americans who had brought AIDS to Haiti and not the other way round. The search for the 'true' source of AIDS shifted again, this time to the 'dark continent'.

With the Haitian hypothesis debunked the 'steaming jungles' deep within the 'hidden interior' of central Africa presented fertile ground to search for the source of AIDS. Research scientists jetted in, swooping down from the skies, to collect precious blood samples, swiftly returning to their technological lairs 'back home' for analysis. One of the notions that arose from this flurry of activity was the 'monkey hypothesis'. This was the idea that monkeys had transmitted an AIDS-like virus to humans when Africans were bitten by them, ate them, gave their children dead monkeys as pets, injected monkey blood as a sexual stimulant or as I have heard on more than one occasion 'had sex with a monkey'! What could distance the western world more from the cause of AIDS than it coming from a monkey in Africa committing an 'unnatural act' with somebody deep in the centre of that disease-ridden continent? Help!

The tragedy of AIDS illustrates the often complex interplay between culture and disease. It is a worldwide scourge; it does show different rates of prevalence across ethnic groups, it is transmitted through specific behaviour patterns, and it is so 'bad' that there is a strong desire to 'externalise' its cause and project our fears and anger onto an identifiable target. This way of dealing with a fearful disease is not new, e.g. in the Middle Ages the English ascribed syphilis to the French. Later the French described it as the 'Italian disease'. There will surely be future epidemics on to which society will graft its racial insecurities. The challenge for clinicians is to be aware of the extent to which they, their colleagues or leading 'authorities' are caught up in their culture's way of dealing with such threats. A key element in being able to do this is to understand the sociocultural symbolism and the function of explaining a disease in a particular way compared with another.

Culture and HIV/AIDS again!

For over a decade governments, international agencies and non-governmental organisations (NGOs) have put great efforts into changing people's high-risk behaviour regarding HIV/AIDS. Despite this the infection continued to spread and serious questions began to be asked about the methods of prevention used. Many information, education and communication (IEC) strategies focused too strongly on imparting knowledge and not enough on bringing about behaviour change; they were too general and not specific enough to people's lived contexts, and were too individualistic, rather than taking into account broader community issues. Also, there was insufficient credence given to underlying value systems regarding sexuality, communication procedures were unidirectional and artificially didactic and traditional media were not well identified and poorly used (UNFPA Evaluation Report, 1999).

In this context UNESCO and UNAIDS have proposed taking a much more explicitly cultural approach to encouraging behaviour change:

Taking a cultural approach means considering a population's characteristics – including lifestyles and beliefs – as essential references to the creation of action plans. This is indispensable if behaviour patterns are to be changed on a long term basis, a vital condition for slowing down or for stopping the expansion of the epidemic.

UNESCO (2001, p. i)

The Declaration of commitment on HIV/AIDS, adopted by the Special Session of the UN General Assembly on HIV/AIDS (June 2001), makes clear the importance of:

emphasizing the role of cultural, family, ethical and religious factors in the prevention of the epidemic and in treatment, care and support, taking into account the particularities of each country as well as the importance of respecting all human rights and fundamental freedoms. (paragraph 20)

More recently UNESCO has stated that:

the difficulty in establishing effective HIV/AIDS programmes comes from a lack of openness, in many societies, regarding sexuality, male–female relationships, illness and death, taboo subjects deeply rooted in cultures. Understanding what motivates people's behaviours, knowing how to address these motivations appropriately, and taking into consideration people's cultures when developing programmes address-ing HIV/AIDS are essential to changing behaviours and attitudes towards HIV/AIDS. (UNESCO, 2005)

UNESCO recommends that culture should be taken into account in three respects:

- *Context*: i.e. the environment in which HIV/AIDS communication takes place
- *Content*: local cultural values and resources that can influence prevention education, whereby culturally appropriate content of sensitisation mes-sages is crucial for them to be well understood and received
- *Method*: enabling people's participation, which helps to ensure that HIV/AIDS prevention and care are embedded in local cultural contexts in a stimulating and accessible way.

UNESCO also recommends that HIV/AIDS projects, programmes and strate-gies must fulfil the following five criteria, in order to be effective:

1. Cultural appropriateness
2. Fully respectful of universally agreed human rights
3. Gender responsiveness
4. Age responsiveness

5. Involvement of people living with HIV/AIDS at every stage.

These criteria promise the possibility of a more culturally enlightened era for combating the causes and consequences of HIV/AIDS. It was perhaps unnecessary to take quite so long to get to these criteria, but now that we have arrived at this point, there is no time to waste. One of the barriers that remains is, however, people's broader attitudes to cultural difference and harmony.

Racial hygiene and ethnic cleansing

Throughout this book we have largely focused on how the interplay between culture and health can be developed for the good of all peoples. However, we have also just noted cultural 'scapegoating' with regard to AIDS/HIV. Perhaps the most horrific example of the destructive interplay between culture and medicine was the 'racial hygiene' practised by the Nazis in World War II. Proctor (1988) describes the ethos of racial hygiene as initially promoting the benefits, for all races, of encouraging breeding within well-educated civilised families but controlling it among criminals, illiterates and the insane. This ethos then developed into suggestions that medical care should not be given to the 'weak' because it might encourage the continuation of 'weak' genes in the racial gene pool. Diseases such as TB and leprosy were described as 'our racial friends' because they attacked and 'weeded out' the weak.

When the Nazis came to power in Germany in the 1930s they promoted the goal of achieving 'purity' of the Aryan race. Genetic courts ruled on what sorts of people should be sterilised. This philosophy of racial purity extended to racial superiority, culminating in the mass murder of millions of people who were judged to be of 'inferior race', such as Gypsies and Jews. The holocaust is a haunting example of how one culture – the Nazi culture – saw illness and culture and how it was dealt with. The 'ethnic cleansing' in the former Yugoslavia and in and around Rwanda are poignant reminders that horrific ways of dealing with cultural differences cannot be dismissed into history, but that they are part of our present and will undoubtedly be part of our future too. Without a serious commitment to multiculturalism and tolerance of different ways of understanding human health and suffering, clinicians will not be well equipped to prevent humanity from picking away at and re-opening its horrific racist wounds. Health and health education cannot be divorced from the challenge of cultivating a positive sense of global citizenship, with all the challenges that it throws up.

Towards global citizenship

Carr (2002) uses the term 'glocality' to describe the interaction between local beliefs and global systems, pointing out that each interaction produces a distinctive local resolution. This sense of multiform connectivity it put quite succinctly in a recent report of the UK's Department for Education and Skills

(2005): 'We live in one world. What we do affects others – and what others do affects us – as never before' (p. 3). The report, entitled 'Putting the world into world-class education' emphasises the importance of life-long learning in a global context. I hope that it is now clear that the interaction between culture and health is braided through people's understandings of their world and so education (formal and informal) constitutes the crucial context in this inter-play. The document recommends that education (from primary to tertiary, and beyond) needs to provide an understanding of eight key concepts:

1. *Citizenship*: gaining the knowledge, skills and understanding of concepts and institutions necessary to become informed, active, responsible global citizens.
2. *Social justice*: understanding the importance of social justice as an element in both sustainable development and the improved welfare of all people.
3. *Sustainable development*: understanding the need to maintain and improve the quality of life now without damaging the planet for future generations.
4. *Diversity*: understanding and respecting differences, and relating these to our common humanity.
5. *Values and perceptions*: developing a critical evaluation of images of other parts of the world and an appreciation of the effect these have on people's attitudes and values.
6. *Interdependence*: understanding how people, places, economies and envi-ronments are all inextricably interrelated, and that events have repercus-sions on a global scale.
7. *Conflict resolution*: understanding how conflicts are a barrier to develop-ment and why there is a need for their resolution and the promotion of harmony.
8. *Human rights*: knowing about human rights and, in particular, the UN Con-vention on the Rights of the Child.

We might also add to the last category, the *right to health*, which I have already argued for. I hope that the above list of key concepts for living in a global society also resonates with some of our earlier discussions, particularly around the 'types' of relationship between culture and health, as outlined in Chapter 1, Table 1.2. This is as good a prescription for cultivating a positive interaction between culture and health as I have seen, even though that was not its primary target.

Conclusion

The importance of culture is braided through the ethos of global health. Global health recognises the interconnectedness of health problems and health solu-tions, acknowledges the broader social, political and economic contexts that give rise to many health inequities, and recognises the importance of devel-oping strong and resilient health delivery systems, in contrast to narrowly focusing on individual treatments regimes. In that global health brings the 'social' into the mainstream of health, it inevitably encounters different social perspectives and socially constructed meanings. Taking into account inequities in health that are patterned by gender, disability, class and many other social categories is inseparable from a concern with the relationship between culture and health.

Guidelines for professional practice

1. Global health is a movement that sees many of the world's major health problems as being interconnected, either through common themes of disadvantage (gender, disability, class), through the effects of globalisation (e.g. knowledge flows and mobility of health professionals away from where they are most needed), through common diseases (such as HIV/AIDS) or though developing common solutions, such as strengthening overall health systems, empowering oppressed groups or encouraging people to play a more active part in their own health.
2. There are huge disparities in the allocation of health resources globally with approximately 90% of the world's health spend being allocated to 10% of the world's disease burden.
3. The problems of health and poverty are interlinked and for many of the poorest countries it is unrealistic to expect them to trade their way out of their current situation, in a global 'free' marketplace.
4. The value of investing in the health of impoverished people can be justified on at least three grounds: it is a prerequisite for development; it is important for global security; and health is a human right. Although these are not mutually exclusive, the global health movement puts greater emphasis on the human rights argument.
5. The millennium development goals seek 'to create an environment – at national and global levels alike – that is conducive to development and the elimination of poverty'. The eight MDGs may be broken down into 18 public health targets with 48 indicators for their achievement. Even if these targets are achieved in some countries, these averages may hide large regional, cultural or gender variations.
6. The achievement of the MDGs will require culture-sensitive measures of need and progress, for at least some of their aims.
7. Gender inequalities remain a major obstacle for the attainment of health and dignity. Female feticide, infanticide and 'honour' killings are among the most horrific instruments of discrimination against girls and women.
8. There are different cultural attitudes towards the ability and inclusion of intellectually disabled people. There are also different causes and consequences of acquired physical disability in different cultural groups.
9. The caste system in India continues to be strongly discriminating against lower castes and 'Untouchables', greatly diminishing their quality of life and access to health resources. Intercaste prejudice has also been

'exported' with the Indian diaspora, to other areas of the world where they have settled in larger numbers.

10. Stigma is a major obstacle that is often directed towards women and girls, disabled people, people of low caste and cultural minority groups, among others. Stigma greatly reduces people's quality of life, self-belief and ability to mobilise resources to protect and promote their health.

11. HIV/AIDS is perhaps the major health challenge of our time and how we respond to it will define our generation.

12. Despite early research showing the importance of culture in understanding HIV/AIDS, the value of a cultural approach is only now being fully taken on board and 'mainstreamed' by international health and development agencies.

13. The relationship between culture and health can be abused by those who wish to discriminate against others: they may use concepts such as 'racial hygiene' or 'ethnic cleansing'. These ideas promote the supposed inherent superiority and need for purity in one group in relation to others.

14. Our multicultural world presents us with the challenge not only of valuing local identities while tolerating cultural difference, but also of being committed to an expansive conception of global citizenship. The values inherent in such a conception are perhaps one of our strongest levers to cultivating health on the basis of equity and human rights.

Postscript

"May you live in interesting times"

Chinese Proverb

In times now past the study of different cultures was the exotica of social sciences. Incomprehension of another culture was taken as confirmation of the legitimacy of ethnocentric world views. Now the study of culture is an imperative for human existence. In evolutionary terms we have been catapulted into a multicultural hot-house. We kick and struggle with each other and occasionally, and too frequently, betray our universal virtues with murderous rampages through humanity. These rampages often have an explicit cultural or racial element and where they may not, then these are often grafted on. It is everyday experience that multiculturalism is a big problem for a small planet.

This book has set out a path through the complexity of culture and health. Culture affects health even for those unaware of their cultural heritage and unconcerned about their health. It is an inescapable interplay even when you resist being a player. Many clinicians resist being players. They crouch behind a glace of scientific objectivity which 'objectifies' the patient. Patients (or clients) ought not to be the 'object' of our activity but the *subject* of our concern, and we must be concerned with how their experience of the world contributes to the problems which they present.

Some of the themes emphasized in this book have included: an interdisciplinary perspective; dynamic tension between keeping the individual foreground and their cultural background in perspective; considering the social, economic and political context in which different cultural groups operate; seeing the communities which people live in, especially immigrant groups, as resources for promoting health; recognising the wholeness of health and illness rather than splitting it into mind and body; developing tolerance for pluralistic approaches to health; and viewing health as a human right and inequity in access to healthcare as intolerable.

The guidelines at the end of each chapter have tried to give practical suggestions for action. Only through such action can you set out on your own path through this most perplexing and fascinating forest of human health and culture. From a cultural perspective, no time in human history has been more interesting than these times. However, only by positively embracing the undeniable challenges of multiculturalism can the whole of humanity be greater than the sum of its parts. Those who deny complexity may live in a simpler world, but also one more prone to prejudice and more threatening to the virtue of humanity.

References

Abbotts, J., Harding, S. & Cruickshank, K. (2004) Cardiovascular risk profiles in the UK-born Caribbeans and Irish living in England and Wales. *Atherosclerosis* **175**: 295–303.

Ager, A. (1999) Perspectives on the refugee experience. In: Ager, A. (ed.) *Refugees: Perspectives on the Experience of Forced Migration*. London: Pinter.

Ager, A. & MacLachlan, M. (1998) Psychometric properties of the coping strategy indicator (CSI) in a study of coping behaviour amongst Malawian students. *Psychology and Health* **13**: 339–410.

Ager, A. & Young, M. (2001) Cultivating the psychosocial health of refugees. In: MacLachlan, M. (ed.) *Cultivating Health: Cultural Perspectives on Health Promotion*. Chichester: Wiley.

Ahdieh, L. & Hahn, R.A. (1996) Use of terms 'race', 'Ethnicity' and 'National Origin': A review of articles in the American Journal of Public Health, 1980–89. *Ethnicity and Health* **1**: 95–8.

Ahmad, W.I.U. (ed.) (1996) *'Race' and Health in Contemporary Britain*. Buckingham: Open University Press.

Airhihenbuwa, C.O. (1995) *Health and Culture: Beyond the Western paradigm*. Thousand Oaks, CA: Sage.

Alarcon, R.D. & Foulks, E.F. (1995) Personality disorders and culture: contemporary clinical views. *Cultural Diversity & Mental Health*, 1, 3–17.

Allen, T. (1992) Taking culture seriously. In: Allen, T. & Thomas, A. (eds) *Poverty and Development in the 1990s*. Oxford: Oxford University Press.

Allen, W.R. & Farley, R. (1986) The shifting social and economic tides of Black America. *Annual Review of Sociology* **12**: 277–306.

Althusser, L. (1999) Ideology and ideological state apparatuses. In: Rivkin, J. & Ryan, M. *Literary Theory: An anthology*. Oxford: Blackwell pp. 294–305.

American Psychiatric Association (1994) *Diagnostic and Statistical Manual of Mental Disorders*, 4th edn. Washington: APA.

Andary, L., Stolk, Y. & Klimidis, S. (2003) *Assessing Mental Health Across Cultures*. Bowen Hills, Queensland: Australian Academic Press.

Anderson, A.E. (2002) Eating disorders in males. In: Fairburn, C.G. & Brownell, K.D. (eds) *Eating Disorders and Obesity*, 2nd edn. New York: Guilford Press.

Anderson, A.E. (1987) Preoperative preparation for cardiac surgery facilitates recovery, reduces psychological distress, and reduces the incidence of acute postoperative hypertension. *Journal of Consulting and Clinical Psychology* 55: 513–520.

Antonovsky, A. (1987) *Unraveling the Mystery of Health: How people manage stress and stay well*. San Francisco, CA: Jossey-Bass.

Asad, T. (1973) *Anthropology and the Colonial Encounter*. London: Ithaca Press.

Asano, S. (1994) Unrelated bone marrow donor registry in Japan. *Bone Marrow Transplantation* **13**: 699–700.

Bach, P.B., Pham, H.H., Shrag, D., Tate, R.C. & Hargraves, L. (2004) Primary care physicians who treat blacks and whites. *New England Journal of Medicine* **351**: 575–84.

Baider, L., Kaufman, B., Ever-Hadani, P. & De-Nour, A.K. (1996) Coping with additional stresses: comparative study of healthy and cancer patient new immigrants. *Social Science and Medicine* **42**: 1077–84.

Bandawe, C.R. (2005) Psychology brewed in the African pot: Soaking in indigenous philosophies in the quest for relevance. *Higher Education Policy* in press.

Baumeister, R.F. (1991) *Meanings of Life*. New York: Guilford Press.

Baumeister, R.F. (2002) Religion and psychology: Introduction to the Special Issue. *Psychological Inquiry* **13**: 165–7.

Beautrais, A.L. (2000) Methods of youth suicide in New Zealand: trends and implications for prevention. *Australian and New Zealand Journal of Psychiatry* **34**: 413–19.

Becker, E. (1962) *The Birth and Death of Meaning*. New York: Braziller.

Becker, E. (1968) *The Structure of Evil: An essay on the unification of the science of man*. New York: Braziller.

Becker, E. (1973) *The Denial of Death*. New York: Free Press.

Belloc, N.B. & Breslow, L. (1972) Relationship of physical health status and health practices. *Preventive Medicine* **5**: 409–421.

Berman, A.L. (1997) The Adolescent: the individual in cultural perspective. *Suicide and Life-Threatening Behaviour* 27: 5–14.

Bernal, M.A. & Castro, F.G. (1994) Are clinical psychologists prepared for service and research with ethnic minorities? Report of a decade of progress. *American Psychologist* 49: 707–805.

Berry, J.W. (1990) Psychology of acculturation: understanding individuals moving between cultures. In: Brislin, R.W. (ed,) *Applied Cross-Cultural Psychology*. Newbury Park: Sage.

Berry, J.W. (1994) Cross-cultural health psychology. Paper presented at International Congress of Applied Psychology, Madrid, July, 17–22.

Berry, J.W. (1997a) Cultural and ethnic factors in health. In: Baum, A., Newman, S., Weinman, J., West, R. & McManus, C. (eds) *Cambridge Handbook of Psychology, Health and Medicine*. Cambridge: Cambridge University Press, pp. 98–103.

Berry, J.W. (1997b) Immigration, acculturation and, adaptation. *Applied Psychology: An International Review* 46: 5–68.

Berry, J.W. (2003) Conceptual approaches to acculturation. In: Chun, K.M., Organista, P.B. & Marin, G. (eds) *Acculturation: Advances in theory, measurement, and applied research*. Washington, DC: American Psychological Association.

Berry, J.W. (2005) How shall we all live together? Alternative visions of intercultural relations.

Berry, J.W. & Kim, U. (1988) Acculturation and Mental Health. In: Dasen, P., Berry, J.W. & Satorious, N. (eds) *Health and Cross-Cultural Psychology*. London: Sage.

Berry, J.W. & Sam, D.L. (2003) Accuracy in scientific discourse. *Scandinavian Journal of Psychology* **44**: 65–8.

Berry, J.W., Poortinga, Y.H., Segall, M.H. & Dasen, P.R. (2002) *Cross-cultural Psychology*. Cambridge: Cambridge University Press.

Bhopal, R. (2004) Glossary of terms relating to ethnicity and race: for reflection and debate. *Journal of Epidemiology and Community Health* **58**: 441–5.

Bhugra, D. (2003) Migration and depression. *Acta Psychiatrica Scandinavica Supplementum* **108**(4): 67–72.

Bhugra, D., Hilwig, M., Mallett, R. et al. (2000) Factors in the onset of schizophrenia: a comparison between London and Trinidad samples. *Acta Psychiatrica Scandinavica* **101**: 135–41.

Bishop, G. (1996) East meets West: Illness, cognition and behaviour in Singapore. Paper presented at the 10th European Health Psychology Society Conference, 4–6 September, Dublin.

Black, J. (1989) *Child Health in a Multicultural Society*. London: BMJ Publications.

Bloche, M.G. (2004) Race-based therapeutics. *New England Journal of Medicine* **351**: 2035–7.

Bochner, S. (1982) The social psychology of cross-cultural relations. In: Bochner, S. (ed.) *Cultures in Contact: Studies in cross-cultural interaction*. Oxford: Pergamon Press.

Bogin, B. & Loucky, J. (1997) Plasticity, political economy, and physical growth status of Guatemala Maya children living in the United States. *American Journal of Physical Anthropology* **102**: 17–32.

Bond, M.H. (1988) Finding universal dimensions of individual variation in multicultural studies of values: The Rokeach and Chinese Values Survey. *Journal of Personality and Social Psychology* **55**: 1009–15.

Bond, M.H. (1991) Chinese values and health: a cultural-level examination. *Psychology and Health* **5**: 137–52.

Booth, B.E., Verma, M. & Beri, R.S. (1994) Fetal sex determination in infants in Punjab, India: correlations and implications. *British Medical Journal* **309**: 1259–61.

Bowles, J. & Robinson, W. (1989) PHS grants for minority group infection education and prevention efforts. *Public Health Report* **104**: 552–9.

Boyd, J.H. & Weissman, M.M. (1981) Epidemiology of affective disorder. *Archives of General Psychiatry* **38**: 1039–46.

Brady, M. (1995) Culture in treatment, culture as treatment: A critical appraisal of developments in addiction programmes for indigenous North Americans and Australians. *Social Science and Medicine* **41**: 1487–98.

Branscombe, N.R. & Wann, D.L. (1992) Role of identification with a group, arousal, categorization process, and self-esteem in sports spectator aggression. *Human Relations* **45**: 1013–33.

Breslow, L. & Enstrom, J.E. (1980) Persistence of health habits and their relationship to mortality. *Preventive Medicine* **9**: 469–83.

Brislin, R., Cushner, K., Cherrie, C. & Yong, M. (1986) *Intercultural Interactions: A practical guide*. Newbury Park, CA: Sage.

Brown, C.M. & Segal, R. (1996) The effects of health and treatment perceptions on the use of prescribed medication and home remedies among African American and white American hypertensives. *Social Science and Medicine* **43**: 903–17.

Brown, G. & Harris, T. (1978) *The Social Origins of Depression*. London: Tavistock Publications.

Brown, L., Macintyre, K., & Trujilla, L. (2003) Interventions to reduce HIV/AIDS stigma: what have we learned? *AIDS Education & Prevention* **15**(1): 49–69.

Campbell, C.A. (2002) Prostitution, AIDS, and preventive health behavior. *Social Science and Medicine* **32**(12): 1367–70.

Carr, S.C. (2002) *Social Psychology*. Chichester: Wiley.

Carr, S.C., McAuliffe, E. & MacLachlan, M. (1998) *Psychology of Aid*. London: Routledge.

Carr, S.C., Watters, P.A. & MacLachlan, M. (1996) Beyond cognitive tolerance: towards the edge of chaos. European Health Psychology Society Conference, Dublin, 4–6 September.

Casimir, G.J. & Morrison, B.J. (1993) Rethinking work with 'multicultural populations'. *Community Mental Health Journal* **29**: 547–59.

Cassels, A. (2004) The challenges in global health: an overview. Global Health – The Challenges, Inaugural Conference of the Irish Forum for Global Health, Trinity College Dublin, 7–8 July.

Cassen, R. (1994) *Does Aid Work?* Oxford: Oxford University Press.

Chavez, L.R., Hubbell, F.A., McMullin, J.M., Martinez, R.G. & Mishra, S.I. (1995) Structure and meaning of models of breast and cervical cancer risk factors: A comparison of perceptions among Latinas, Anglo women and physicians. *Medical Anthropology Quarterly* **9**: 40–74.

Cheng, S.T. (1994) A critical review of the Chinese Koro, International Congress of Applied Psychology, Madrid, 17–22 July.

Cheng, S.T. (1996) A critical review of Chinese Koro. *Culture, Medicine and Psychiatry* **20**: 67–82.

Chirimuuta, R. & Chirimuuta, R. (1989) *AIDS, Africa and Racism*. London: Free Association Books.

Chowdhury, A.N. (1998) Hundred years of Koro: The history of a culture bound syndrome. *International Journal of Social Psychiatry* **44**: 181–8.

Church, A.T. (2000) Culture and personality: towards an integrated cultural trait psychology. *Journal of Personality*, **69**: 651–703.

Claeson, M., Bos, E.R., Mawji, T. & Pathmanathan, I. (2003) Reducing child mortality in India in the new millennium. *Bulletin of the World Health Organization* **78**: 1192–9.

Cockerham, W.C. (2001) *Medical Sociology*, 8th edn. New Jersey: Prentice Hall.

Coie, J.D., Watt, N.F., West, S.G. et al. (1993) The science of prevention: A conceptual framework and some directions for a national research program. *American Psychologist* **48**: 1013–22.

Collett, P. (1982) Meetings and misunderstandings. In Bochner, S. (ed.) *Cultures in Contact: Studies in cross-cultural interaction*. Oxford: Pergamon Press.

Commission for Macroeconomics and Health (2001) Macroeconomics & Health: Investing in Health for Economic Development. Geneva: World Health Organisation.

Cornish, F. (2004) Making 'context' concrete: A dialogical approach to the society–health relation. *Journal of Health Psychology* **9**: 281–94.

Cornish, F., Peltzer, K. & MacLachlan, M. (1999) Returning Strangers: The children of Malawian refugees come 'home'? *Journal of Refugee Studies* **12**(3): 264–83.

Corson, P.W. & Andersen, A.E. (2002) Body Image issue among boys and men. In: Cash T.F. & Pruzinsky, T. (eds) *Body Image: A handbook of theory, research, and practice*. New York: Guilford Press.

Cowen, E. (1994) The enhancement of psychological wellness: challenges and opportunities. *American Journal of Community Psychology* **22**: 149–79.

Critser, G. (2003) *Fat Land: How Americans became the fattest people in the world*. London: Penguin.

Curran, M.J., Bunting, B. & MacLachlan, M. (2002) Health and acculturation of the Irish diaspora in Britain. *Irish Journal of Psychology* **23**: 222–33.

Dawes, A., Kvalsvig, J., Rama, S. & Richter, L. (2004) Going global with indicators of child well-being: Indicators of South African children's psychosocial development in the early childhood period: Phase 1 Report to UNICEF, South Africa. Cape Town: Human Sciences Research Council.

Department for Education and Skills (2005) *Putting the World into World-Class Education: An international strategy for education, skills and children's services*. London: DfES.

Dick, L. (1995) 'Pibloktoq' (Artic Hysteria): a construction of European–Inuit relations? *Artic Anthropology* 32: 1–42.

Dizmang, L., Watson, J., May, P. & Bopp, J. (1974) Adolescent suicide at the Indian reservation. *American Journal of Orthopsychiatry* **44**: 43–9.

Dollard, J. (1935) *Criteria for the Life History: With analysis of six notable documents*. New Haven, CT: Yale University Press.

Dona, G. & Berry, J.W. (1994) Acculturation attitudes and acculturative stress of Central American refugees. *International Journal of Psychology* **29**: 57–70.

Douglas, J. (1995) Developing anti-racist health promotion strategies. In: Bunton, R., Nettleton, S. & Burrows, R. (eds) The *Sociology of Health Promotion: Critical analyses of consumption, lifestyle and risk*. London: Routledge.

Draguns, J. (1990) Applications of cross-cultural psychology in the filed of mental health. In: Brislin, R.W. (ed.) *Applied Cross-Cultural Psychology*. Newbury Park: Sage.

Dubow, S. (1995) *Illicit Union: Scientific racism in modern South Africa*. Johannesburg: Witwatersrand University Press.

Durkheim, E. (1897) *Le Suicide*. Paris (translated by J.A. Spaulding & C. Simpson, 1952) as *Suicide: A Study of Sociology*. London: Routledge & Kegan Paul.

Earleywine, M. (2001) Cannabis-induced Koro in Americans. *Addiction* **96**: 1663–6.

Early, K.E. & Askers, R.L. (1993) 'It's a White thing': An exploration of beliefs about suicide in the African American community. *Deviant Behaviour* **14**: 227–96.

EchoHawk, M. (1997) Suicide: The scourge of the Native American people. *Suicide and Life-Threatening Behaviour* **27**: 60–7.

Eisenbruch, M. (1990) Classification of natural and supernatural causes of mental distress: development of a mental distress explanatory model questionnaire. *Journal of Nervous and Mental Disease* **178**: 712–19.

Fernandez, A. & Goldstein, L. (2004) Letter re primary care physicians who treat blacks and whites. *New England Medical Journal* **351**: 2126.

Festinger, L.A. (1957) *A Theory of Cognitive Dissonance*. Stanford, CA: Stanford University Press.

Fish, J.M. (1995) Why psychologists should learn some anthropology. *American Psychologist* 50: 44–5.

Flanagan, J.C. (1954) The critical incident technique. *Psychological Bulletin* **51**: 327–58.

Foster, G.M. & Anderson, B.G. (1978) *Medical Anthropology*. Chichester: Wiley.

Frank, J.D. & Frank, J.B. (1991) *Persuasion and Healing: A comparative study of psychotherapy*, 3rd edn. Baltimore, MD: John Hopkins University Press.

Freire, P. (1972) *Pedagogy of the Oppressed*. London: Penguin Books.

Freud, S. (1927/1989) *The Future of an Illusion*. New York: Norton.

Furnham, A. & Bochner, S. (1986) *Culture Shock: Psychological reactions to unfamiliar environments*. London: Methuen.

Furnham, A. & Vincent, C. (2001) Cultivating health through complementary medicine. In: MacLachlan, M. (ed.) *Cultivating Health: Cultural perspectives on promoting health*. Chichester: Wiley.

Furnham, A., Hassomal, A. & McClelland, A.G.R. (2002) A cross-cultural investigation of the factors and biases involved in the allocation of scarce medical resources. *Journal of Health Psychology* **7**: 381–91.

Gao, M.Y. (2005) Participatory communication research and HIV/AIDS control: A study among gay men and MSM in Chengdu, China. Unpublished doctoral dissertation, University of Newcastle, NSW, Australia.

Garcia-Campayo, J., Campos, R., Marcos, G. et al. (1996) Somatisation in primary care in Spain II: Differences between somatisers and psychologisers. *British Journal of Psychiatry* **168**: 348–53.

Garfinkle, H. (1967) *Studies in Ethnomethodology*. Cambridge: Polity Press.

Garner, D.M. & Garfinkle, P.E. (1980) Sociocultural factors in the development of anorexia nervosa. *Psychological Medicine* **10**: 647–56.

Gaw, A.C. (2001) *Concise Guide to Cross-Cultural Psychiatry*. Washington: American Psychiatric Association.

Geertz, H. (1968) Latah in Java: A theoretical paradox. *Indonesia* **3**: 93–104.

Gelfand, M.J. & Holcombe, K.M. (1998) Behavioural patterns of horizontal and vertical individualism and collectivism. In: Singelis, T.M. (ed.) *Teaching About Culture, Ethnicity and Diversity*. Thousand Oaks, CA: Sage.

George, L.K., Ellison, C.G. & Larson, D.B. (2002) Explaining the relationship between religious involvement and health. *Psychological Inquiry* **13**: 190–200.

George, S. (1988) *A Fate Worse Than Debt*. London: Pelican.

Gibson, K. & Swartz, L. (2001) Psychology, social transition and organisational life in South Africa: 'I can't change the past – but I can try'. *Psychoanalytic Studies* **3**: 381–92.

Giddens, A. (1999) *Runaway World: How globalisation is reshaping our lives*. London: Profile Books.

Giger, J.N. & Davidhizar, R.E. (1999) *Transcultural Nursing: Assessment and intervention*. St Louis, MO: Mosby.

Gillespie, A., Peltzer, K. & McLachlan, M. (2002) Returning refugees: Psychosocial problems and mediators of mental health among Malawian returnees. *Journal of Mental Health* **9**(2): 165–78.

Global Forum for Health Research (2004) *The 10/90 Report on Health Research, 2003–2004*. Geneva: Global Forum for Health Research (www.globalforumhealth.org).

Goldie, N. (1995) *Sociology in Practice: Health for all?* London: Distance Learning Centre.

Gordon, R.A. (2000) *Eating Disorders: Anatomy of a social epidemic*, 2nd edn. Oxford: Blackwell.

Gordon, R.A. (2001) Eating disorders east and west: A culture-bound syndrome unbound. In: Nasser, M., Katzman, M.A. & Gordon, R.A. (eds) *Eating Disorders and Cultures in Transition*. Hove: Brunner-Routledge.

Gordon, T., Garcia-Palmieri, M.R., Kagan, A., Kannel, W.B. & Schiffman, J. (1974) Differences in coronary heart disease in Famingham, Honolulu and Puerto Rico. *Journal of Chronic Disease* **27**: 329–44.

Gray, R. (1998) Four perspectives on unconventional therapy. *Health* **2**: 55–74.

Halliday, A. & Coyle, K. (eds) (1994) The Irish Psyche. Special Issue. *Irish Journal of Psychology* **15**: 243–507.

Halpern, D. (1993) Minorities and mental health. *Social Science and Medicine* **36**: 597–607.

Halpern, D. & Nazroo, J. (2000) The ethnic density effect: Results of a national community survey of England and Wales. *International Journal of Social Psychiatry* **46**: 34–46.

Hancock, T. & Perkins, F. (1985) The Mandala of health: a conceptual model and teaching tool. *Health Promotion* **24**: 8–10.

Harmsen, H., Meeuwesen, L., van Wieringen, J., Bersen, R. & Bruijnzeels, M. (2002) When cultures meet in general practice: intercultural differences between GP's and parents of child patients. *Patient Education and Counseling* **51**: 99–106.

Harris, M. (1980) *Cultural Materialism: The struggle for a science of culture*. New York: Vintage Books.

Haviland, W.A. (1983) *Human Evolution and Prehistory*, 2nd edn. New York: CBS College Publishing.

Health and Welfare Canada (1986) *Achieving Health for All*. Ottawa: Government of Canada.

Heller & Monahan (1977) cited in Winett et al. (1989).

Helman, C.G. (2000) *Culture, Health and Illness*, 4th edn. London: Arnold.

Ho, D.Y.F. (1985) Cultural values and professional issues in clinical psychology: Implications from the Hong Kong experience. *American Psychologist* **40**: 1212–18.

Hobfoll, S.E. (2001) The influence of culture, community and the nested-self in the stress process: Advancing conservation of resource theory. *Applied Psychology: An International Review* **50**: 337–421.

Hofstede, G. (1980) *Culture's Consequences: International differences in work-related values*. Beverly Hills, CA: Sage.

Hofstede, G. (1986) Cultural differences in teaching and learning. *International Journal of Intercultural Relations* **10**: 301–20.

Hofstede, G. (1991) *Cultures and Organizations*. London: HarperCollins.

Holdstock, L. (2000) *Re-examining Psychology: Critical perspectives and African insights*. London: Routledge.

Hopkin, J. (2002) Development – the basics: Making sense of the world. In C. Regan (ed.) 80:20, development in an unequal world. Bray, Co. Wicklow, Ireland: 80:20 Educating and Acting for a Better World (email: info@8020.ie).

Hubble, M.A., Duncan, B.L. & Miller, S.D. (1999) The *Heart and Soul of Change*: What works in therapy. New York: APA.

Hughes, C.C. (1985) Culture-bound or construct-bound?: The syndromes and DSM-III. In: Simons, R.C. & Hughes, C.C. (eds) *The Culture Bound Syndromes: Folk illnesses of psychiatric and anthropological interest*. Dordrecht: R. Reidel, pp. 3–24.

Ilechukwu, S.T.C. (1989) Approaches to psychotherapy in Africans: do they have to be non-medical? *Culture, Medicine and Psychiatry* **13**: 419–35.

Ilola, L.M. (1990) Culture and health. In: Brislin, R.W. (ed.) *Applied Cross-Cultural Psychology*. Newbury Park: Sage.

Inglehart, R. & Baker, W.E. (2000) Modernization, cultural change and the persistence of traditional values. *American Sociological Review* **65**: 19–51.

Inkles, A. (1969) Making men modern: on the causes and consequences of individual change in sic developing countries. *American Journal of Comparative Sociology* **75**: 208–25.

Israel, B., Checkoway, B., Schulz, A. & Zimmerman, S. (1994) Helath Education and Community Empowerment: conceptualising and measuring perceptions of individual, organisational and community control. *Health Education Quarterly* 11: 1–47.

Jenkins, C.N.H., Le, T., McPhee, S.J., Stewart, S. & Ha, N.T. (1996) Health care access and prevention care among Vietnamese immigrants: Do traditional beliefs and practices pose barriers? *Social Science and Medicine* **43**: 1049–56.

Jilek, W.G. & Jilek-Aall, L.M. (1984) Intercultural psychotherapy: experiences from North American Indian patients. *Curare* 7: 161–6.

Kagitcibasi, C. (1996) *Family and Human Development Across Cultures: A view from the other side.* Hillsdale, NJ: Erlbaum.

Kalin, R. & Berry, J.W. (1995) Ethnic and civic self-identity in Canada. *Canadian Ethnic Studies* **27**: 1–15.

Kalp, C. (1999) Our quest to be perfect. *Newsweek*, 16 August.

Kanyangale, M. & MacLachlan, M. (1995) Critical incidents for refugee counsellors: An investigation of indigenous human resources. *Counselling Psychology Quarterly* 8(1): 89–101.

Kareem, J. (1992) The Nafsiyat Intercultural Therapy Centre: Ideas and experience in intercultural therapy. In: Kareem, J. & Littlewood, R. (eds) *Intercultural Therapy: Themes, interpretations and practice.* Oxford: Blackwell Scientific Publications.

Karlsen, S., Nazroo, J.Y. & Stephenson, R. (2002) Ethnicity, environment and health: putting ethnic inequalities in health in their place. *Social Science and Medicine* **55**: 1647–61.

Kazarian, S. & Evans, D. (2001) *Handbook of Cultural Health Psychology.* San Diego, CA: Academic Press.

Keel, P.K. & Klump, K.L. (2003) Are eating disorders culture-bound syndromes? *Psychological Bulletin* **125**: 747–69.

Kennedy, N. & McDonough, M. (2002) Koro: A case in an Eastern European asylum seeker in Ireland. *Irish Journal of Psychological Medicine* **19**: 130–1.

Kenny, M.G. (1985) Paradox lost: The Latah problem revisited. In: Simons, R.C. & Hughes, C.C. (eds) *Intercultural Therapy: Themes, interpretations and practice.* Dordrecht: D. Reidel, pp. 63–76.

Khandelwal, S.K., Sharan, P. & Saxena, S. (1995) Eating disorders: An Indian perspective. *International Journal of Social Psychiatry* **41**: 132–46.

Khanna, R., Kumar, A., Vaghela, J.F., Sreenivas, V. & Puliyel, J.M. (2003) Community based retrospective study of sex in infant mortality in India. *British Medical Journal* **327**: 126–9.

Kiernan, G., Gormley, M. & MacLachlan, M. (2004) Outcomes associated with participation in a therapeutic recreation camping programme for children from 15 European countries: Data from the 'Barretstown Studies'. *Social Science and Medicine* **59**: 903–13.

Kirmayer, L.J. & Santhanam, R. (2001) The anthropology of hysteria. In: Halligan, P.W., Bass, C. & Marshall, J.C. *Contemporary Approaches to Hysteria.* Oxford: Oxford University Press.

Kleinman, A. (1980) *Patients and Healers in the Context of Culture.* Berkeley, CA: University of California Press.

Klonoff, E.A. & Landrine, H. (2003) Is skin colour a marker for racial discrimination? In: LaVeist, A. *Race, Ethnicity, and Health: A public health reader.* New York: Jossey Bass.

Kluckhohn, C. & Kroeber, A. (1952) *Culture. Peabody Museum Papers* (Harvard University), 67(1).

Kobasa, S.C.O., Maddi, S.R., Puccetti, M.C. & Zola, M.A. (1985) Effectiveness of hardiness, exercise and social support as resources against illness. *Journal of Psychosomatic Research* **29**: 525–33.

Kohli, N. & Dalal, A.K. (1998) Culture as a factor in causal understanding of illness: A study of cancer patients. *Psychology and Developing Societies* **10**: 115–29.

Kopp, S. (1972) *If You Meet the Buddha on the Road, Kill Him!* CA: Sheldon Press.

Krause, J.S., Kemp, B. & Coker, J. (2000) Depression after spinal cord injury: relation to gender, ethnicity, aging and socioeconomic indicators. *Archives of Physical Medicine and Rehabilitation* **81**: 1099–109.

Krieger, N. & Sidney, S. (1996) Racial discrimination and blood pressure: The CARDIA study. *American Journal of Public Health* **86**: 1370–8.

Krieger, N., Sidney, S. & Coakley, E. (1998) Racial discrimination and skin color in the CARDIA study: Implications for public health research. *American Journal of Public Health* **88**: 1308–13.

La Roche, M.J. & Maxie, A. (2003) Ten considerations in addressing cultural differences in psychotherapy. *Professional Psychology: Research and Practice* **34**: 180–6.

Labonte, R. (2004) Challenges and Opportunities 2005: A Focus on the G8, Africa and Global Health. Workshop on Global Health Policy through 2005, Trinity College Dublin, Friday 9 July.

Lago, C. & Thompson, J. (1996) *Race, Culture and Counselling*. Buckingham: Open University Press.

Landrine, H. & Klonoff, E.A. (1992) Culture and health-related schemas: A review and proposal for interdisciplinary integration. *Health Psychology* **11**: 267–76.

Langford, R.A., Ritchie, J., & Ritchie, J. (1998) Suicidal behaviour in a bicultural society: A review of gender and cultural differences in adolescents and young personnel of Aotearoa/New Zealand. *Suicide and Life-Threatening Behaviour* **28**(1): 94–105.

LaVeist, T.A. (2002a) Introduction: Why we should study race, ethnicity, and health. In: LaVeist, T.A. (ed.) *Race, Ethnicity and Health: A public health reader*. New York: Jossey Bass.

LaVeist, T.A. (2002b) Beyond dummy variables and sample selection: What health service researchers ought to know about race as a variable. In: LaVeist, T.A. (ed.) *Race, Ethnicity and Health: A public health reader*. New York: Jossey Bass.

Lazarus, R.S. (1997) Acculturation isn't everything: Commentary on immigration, acculturation, and adaptation by J. Berry. *Applied Psychology: An International Review* **46**: 39–43.

Lazarus, R.S. & Folkman, S. (1984) *Stress, Appraisal and Coping*. New York: Springer.

Lee, A.M. & Lee, S. (1999) Disordered eating in three communities in China: A comparative study of high school students in Hong Kong.

Lee, K. (2004) Tobacco and Globalisation. Conference on Global Health: The Challenges. Centre Global Health Trinity College Dublin, July 10–12.

Lee, S. (2001) From diversity to unity: The classification of mental disorder in 21st century China. *Psychiatric Clinics of North America* **24**: 421–31.

Leit, A., Pope, H.G. & Gray, J.J. (2001) Cultural expectations of muscularity in men: The evolution of Playgirl centerfolds. *International Journal of Eating Disorders* **29**: 90–3.

Levine, R.V. & Bartlett, K. (1984) Pace of life, punctuality, and coronary heart disease in six countries. *Journal of Cross-Cultural Psychology* **15**: 233–55.

Leviton, L. (1996) Integrating psychology and public health: Challenges and opportunities. *American Psychologist* **51**: 42–51.

Lewin, K. (1952) Group decision and social change. In: Newcomb, T. & Hartley, E. (eds) *Readings in Social Psychology*. New York: Holt, Rhinehart & Winston, pp. 459–73.

Li, Y. (1998) *Subcultures of Homosexuality*. Beijing: China Today Press. (In Chinese and cited in Gao, 2005.)

Liang, R., Chiu, E., Chan, T.K. & Hawkins, B. (1994) An unrelated marrow donor registry in Hong Kong. *Bone Marrow Transplantation* **13**: 697–8.

Lieberman, M.D., Hariri, A., Jarcho, J.M., Eisenberger, N.I. & Bookheimer, S.Y. (2005) An fMRI investigation of race-related amygdala activity in African-American and Caucasian individuals. *Nature Neuroscience* **8**: 720–2.

Lipton, J.A. & Marbach, J.J. (1984) Ethnicity and the pain experience. *Social Science and Medicine* **19**: 1279–98.

Littlewood, R. (1992a) Towards an intercultural therapy. In: Kareem, J. & Littlewood, R. (eds) (*Intercultural Therapy: Themes, interpretations and practice*. Oxford: Blackwell Scientific Publications.

Littlewood, R. (1992b) How universal is something we can call therapy? In: Kareem, J. & Littlewood, R. (eds) (*Intercultural Therapy: Themes, interpretations and practice*. Oxford: Blackwell Scientific Publications.

Lobo, A., Garcia-Campayo, J., Campos, R. et al. (1996) Somatisation in primary care in Spain. I: Estimates of prevalence and clinical characteristics. *British Journal of Psychiatry* **168**: 344–53.

Lupton, D. (2003) *Medicine as Culture*, 2nd edn. London: Sage.

McAuliffe, E. (2004) Opening Remarks. Conference on Global Health: The Challenges. Centre for Global Health Trinity College Dublin, July 10–12.

McAuliffe, E. & MacLachlan, M. (1994) No great expectations (V): Back to the future. *Changes: International Journal of Psychology and Psychotherapy* **12**: 175–82.

McAuliffe, E. & McLachlan, M. (2005) Turning the ebbing tide: Knowledge flows and health in low-income countries. *Higher Education Policy*, **18**: 231–42.

McCrea, P.R. (2000) Trait psychology and the revival of personality-and-culture studies. *American Behavioral Science* **44**: 10–31.

McDonald-Scott, P., Machizawa, S. & Satoh, H. (1992) Diagnostic disclosure: a tale of two cultures. *Psychological Medicine* **22**: 147–57.

McGrath, M.H. & Mukerji, S. (2000) Plastic surgery and the teenage patient. *Journal of Pediatric and Adolescent Gynecology* **13**: 105–18.

McKinlay, J.B. & McKinlay, S.M. (1981) Medical measures and the decline of mortality. In: Conrad, P. & Kern, R. (eds) *The Sociology of Health and Illness*. New York: St Martin's Press, pp. 12–30.

MacLachlan, M. (1987) Self-esteem in affective disorder. In: Dent, H. (ed.) *Clinical Psychology: Research and developments*. London: Croom Helm.

MacLachlan, M. (1993) sustaining human resource development in Africa: The influence of expatriates. *Management Education and Development* **24**: 167–71.

MacLachlan, M. (1996a) From sustainable change to incremental improvement: the psychology of community rehabilitation. In: Carr, S.C. & Schumaker, J.F. (eds) *Psychology and the Developing World*. Westport, CT: Greenwood Publishing Group.

MacLachlan, M. (1996b) *Identifying Problems in Community Health Promotion: An illustration of the nominal group technique in AIDS*.

MacLachlan, M. (ed.) (2001) Cultivating health. In MacLachlan, M. *Cultivating Health: Cultural perspectives on promoting health*. Chichester: Wiley.

MacLachlan, M. (2002) Die Arbeit mit Psychotrauma: Personliche, kuterelle and kontextuelle Probleme [Working with psychotrauma: personal, cultural and contextual reflections]. In Ottomeyer, K. & Peltzer, K. (eds) *Uberleban am Abgrund: Psychotrauma und Menschenrechte*. Klagenfurt/Celovec: Drava Verlag, pp. 231–44.

MacLachlan, M. (2003a) Health, empowerment and culture. In: Murray, M. (ed.), *Critical Health Psychology*. London: Sage.

MacLachlan, M. (2003b) Cultural dynamics: transition and identity in modern Ireland. In: *Mosaic or Melting Pot? Living with diversity*. Dublin: European Cultural Foundation & Royal Irish Academy.

MacLachlan, M. (2004) *Embodiment: Clinical, critical and cultural perspective on health and illness*. Milton Keynes: Open University Press.

MacLachlan, M. (2005) *Social Health Sciences and the Integration of Culture*.

MacLachlan, M. & Carr, S.C. (1994a) From dissonance to tolerance: towards managing health in tropical cultures. *Psychology and Developing Societies* **6**: 119–29.

MacLachlan, M. & Carr, S.C. (1994b) Managing the AIDS crisis in Africa: In support of pluralism. *Journal of Management in Medicine* **8**(4): 45–53.

MacLachlan, M. & Carr, S.C. (2005) *The Human Dynamics of Aid*. Paris: OECD Development Centre Policy Insights No. 10.

MacLachlan, M. & McAuliffe, E. (1993) Critical incidents for psychology students in a refugee camp: Implications for counselling. *Counselling Psychology Quarterly* **6**: 3–11.

MacLachlan, M. & McAuliffe, E. (2003) Poverty and process skills. In: Carr, S.C. & Sloan T.S. (eds) *Poverty and Psychology*. Netherlands: Kluwer Academic/Plenum Publishers, pp. 267–84.

MacLachlan, M. & McAuliffe, E. (2005) New ways of delivering health care are needed in developing countries. *British Medical Journal* **331**: 48.

MacLachlan, M. & O'Connell, M. (eds) (2000) *Cultivating Pluralism: Psychological, social and cultural perspectives on a changing Ireland*. Dublin: Oak Tree Press.

MacLachlan, M., Ager, A. & Brown, J. (1997) Health locus of control in Malawi: A failure to support the cross-cultural validity of the HLOCQ. *Psychology and Health* **12**: 33–8.

MacLachlan, M., Chimombo, M. & Mpemba, N. (1997) AIDS education for youth through active learning: A school-based approach from Malawi. *International Journal of Educational Development*.

MacLachlan, M., Nyando, M.C. & Nyirenda, T. (1995) Attributions for admission to Zomba Mental Hospital: Implications for the development of mental health services in Malawi. *International Journal of Social Psychiatry* **41**(2): 79–87.

MacLachlan, M., Carr, S.C., Fardell, S., Maffesoni, G. & Cunningham, J. (1997) Transactional Analysis of Communication Styles in HIV/AIDS Advertisements. *Journal of Health Psychology* **2**(1): 67–74.

MacLachlan, M., Smyth, C.A., Breen, F. & Madden, T. (2004) Temporal acculturation and mental health in modern Ireland. *International Journal of Social Psychiatry* **50**: 345–50.

Magnusson, A. & Axelsson, J. (1993) The prevalence of seasonal affective disorder is low among descendants of Icelandic emigrants in Canada. *Archives of General Psychiatry* **50**: 947–51.

Mallaby, S. (2002) *Washington Post*, October 14, p. A29.

Marin, M.P.U. (1999) Where development will lead to mass suicide. *The Ecologist* **29**: 42–6.

Marks, D. (2004) Rights to health, freedon from illness: A life and death matter. In: Murray, M. (ed.) *Critical Health Psychology*. London: Palgrave.

Markus, H.R. & Kitayama, S. (1991) Culture and the Self: Implications for cognition, emotion and motivation. *Psychological Review* **98**: 244–53.

Masi, R. (1993) Multicultural health: Principles and policies. In: Masi, R. Mensah, L. & McLeod, K.A. (eds) *Health and Cultures I: Policies, professional practice and education*. London: Mosaic Press.

Matarrazzo, J.D. (1980) Behavioural health and behavioural medicine: Frontiers for a new health psychology. *American Psychologist* **35**: 807–17.

Matcha, D.A. (2000) *Medical Sociology*. Boston: Allyn & Bacon.

Mensah, L. (1993) Transcultural, cross-cultural and multicultural health perspectives in focus. In: R. Masi, L. Mensah and K.A. (eds) *Health and Culture, Exploring the Relationship: Policies, professional practice and education*. New York: Mosaic Press.

Meyerowitz, B.E., Richardson, J., Hudson, S. & Leedham, B. (1998) Ethnicity and cancer outcomes: behavioural and psychosocial considerations. *Psychological Bulletin* **123**: 74–80.

Miranda, A.O. & Fraser, L.D. (2002) Culture-bound syndromes: Initial perspectives from individual psychology. *Journal of Individual Psychology* **58**: 422–33.

Moghaddam, F.M., Taylor, D.M. & Wright, S.C. (1993) *Social Psychology in Cross-Cultural Perspective*. London: Freeman.

Moore, R.J. & Spiegel, D. (2000) Users of guided imagery for pain control by African-American and white women with metastatic breast cancer. *Integrative Medicine* **2**: 115–26.

Morselli, H. (1903) *Suicide: An Essay in Comparative Moral Statistics*. New York: Appleton.

Mumford, D.B. & Whitehouse, A.M. (1988) Increased prevalence of bulimia nervosa among Asian schoolgirls. *British Medical Journal* **297**: 718.

Mumford, D.B., Nazir, M., Jilani, F. & Baig, I.Y. (1996) Stress and psychiatric disorder in the Hindu Kush: A community survey of mountain villages in Chitral, Pakistan. *British Journal of Psychiatry* **168**: 299–307.

Murdock, G.P. (1980) *Theories of Illness: A world survey*. Pittsburgh: University of Pittsburgh Press.

Murray, C.J. & Lopez, A. (1996) *Global Burden of Diseases and Injuries*, Vol. 1. Geneva: WHO.

Murray, M. & Chamberlain, K. (1998) Qualitative research in health psychology. *Journal of Health Psychology* **3**: 291–5.

Nakanishi, N., Tatara, K. & Fujiwara, H. (1996) Do preventive health services reduce eventual demand for medical care? *Social Science and Medicine* **43**: 999–1005.

Nasser, M. (1999) The new veiling phenomenon – is it an anorexic equivalent? A Polemic. *Journal of Community and Applied Social Psychology* **9**: 407–12.

Nasser, M. (2001) Contributions to: Nasser, M. and Di Nicoola, V. Changing bodies, changing cultures: An intercultural dialogue on the body as the final frontier. In: Nasser, M., Katzman, M.A. & Gordon, R.A. (eds) *Eating Disorders and Cultures in Transition*. Hove: Brunner-Routledge.

National Institute for Clinical Excellence (NICE) (2004) *The Management of Post-traumatic Stress Disorder in Primary and Secondary Care*. London: NICE.

Neeleman, J. & Wessely, S. (1999) Ethnic minority suicide: a small area geographical study in south London. *Psychological Medicine* **29**: 429–36.

Nettleton, S. (1995) *The Sociology of Health and Illness*. Cambridge: Polity Press.

Neville, H.A. (2000) Psychological adaptation among racial and ethnic minority individuals following spinal cord injury: A proposed culturally inclusive ecological model. *Rehabilitation Psychology* **45**: 89–100.

Novins, D.K., Beals, J., Roberts, R.E. & Manson, S.M. (1999) Factors associated with suicide ideation among American Indian adolescents: Does culture matter? *Suicide and Life-Threatening Behaviour* **28**(1): 94–105.

Nsamenang, A.B. (1992) *Human Development in Cultural Context: A third world perspective*. Newbury park, CA: Sage.

Nsamenang, A.B. (1995) Factors influencing the development of psychology in Sub-Saharan Africa. *International Journal of Psychology* **30**: 729–39.

Nsamenang, A.B. & Dawes, A. (1998) Developmental psychology as political psychology in Sub-Saharan Africa: The challenge of Africanisation. *Applied Psychology: An International Review* **47**: 73–87.

Nussbam, M.C. (1997) *Cultivating Humanity: A classical defense of reform in liberal education*. Cambridge, MA: Harvard University Press.

Oakley, P. (1989) *Community Involvement in Health Development: An examination of the critical issues*. Geneva: WHO.

Oberg, K. (1960) Cultural shock: Adjustment to new cultural environments. *Practical Anthropology* **7**: 177–88.

O'Connell, M. (2001) *Changed Utterly: Ireland and the new Irish psyche*. Dublin: The Liffey Press.

O'Conners, W.A. & Lubin, B. (eds) (1984) *Ecological Approaches to Clinical and Community Psychology*. Malabar, FL: Robert E. Krieger Publishing Co.

Ogden, J. (2000) *Health Psychology: A textbook*, 2nd edn. Buckingham: Open University Press.

Olivardia, R. (2002) Body image and muscularity. In: Cash, T.F. & Pruzinsky, T. (eds) *Body Image: A handbook of theory, research, and practice*. New York: Guilford Press.

Ornstein, R. & Sobel, D. (1987) *The Healing Brain*. New York: Simon & Schuster.

Pargament, K.I. (2002) The bitter and the sweet: An evaluation of the costs and benefits of religiousness. *Psychological Inquiry* **13**: 168–81.

Parker, G., Gladstone, G. & Tsee Chee, K. (2001) Depression in the planet's largest ethnic group: The Chinese. *American Journal of Psychiatry* **158**: 857–64.

Paterson, C. & Dieppe, P. (2005) Characteristic and incidental (placebo) effects in complex interventions such as acupuncture. *British Medical Journal* **330**: 1202–4.

Pedersen, P.B. & Ivey, A. (1993) *Culture-Centered Counseling and Interviewing Skills: A practical guide*. Westport, CT: Praeger.

Peltzer, K. (1995) *Psychology and Health in African Cultures: Examples of ethnopsychotherapeutic practice*. Frankfurt: IKO Verlag.

Peltzer, K. (2002) Personality and social behaviour in Africa. *Social Behaviour and Personality* **30**(1): 83–94.

Philips, D.P., Ruth, T.E. & Wagner, L.M. (1993) Psychology and survival. *Lancet* **342**: 1142–5.

Poliakoff, M. (1993) Cancer and Cultural Attitudes. In Masi, R., Mensah, L. & McLeod, K.A. (eds) *Health and Cultures I: Policies, professional practice and education*. New York: Mosaic Press.

Prilleltensky, I. (2001) Cultural assumptions, social justice and mental health: Challenging the status quo. In: Schumaker, J. & Ward, T. (eds) *Cultural Cognition and Psychopathology*. Westport, CT: Praeger, pp. 251–65.

Prince, R. (1987) The brain-fag syndrome. In: Peltzer, K. & Ebigbo, P.O. (eds) *Clinical Psychology in Africa*. Enug, Nigeria: Working Group for African Psychology.

Proctor, R. (1988) *Racial Hygiene: Medicine under the Nazis*. London: Harvard University Press.

Pyszczynski, T., Greenberg, J., Solomon, S., Arndt, J. & Schimel, J. (2004) Why do people need self-esteem? A theoretical and empirical review. *Psychological Bulletin* **130**: 435–68.

Radley, A. (1994) *Making Sense of Illness: The social psychology of health and disease*. London: Sage.

Range, L.M., Leach, M.M., McIntyre, D. et al. (1999) Multicultural perspectives on suicide. *Aggression and Violent Behaviour* **4**: 413–30.

Rintala, M. & Mutajoki, P. (1992) Could mannequins menstruate? *British Medical Journal* **305**: 1575–6.

Ritchie, J. & Ritchie, J. (1979) *Growing up in Polynesia*. Sydney: Allen & Unwin.

Rix, J. (2005) *Rites and wrongs. Society Guardian*, p. 10, 1 June 2005.

Robinson, M. (2004) *One Human Family: Ethical globalisation in our times*. Michael Littleton Lecture, RTE Radio 1, 1 January.

Rogers, E. M. (1982) *Diffusion of Innovations*, 3rd edn. New York: The Free Press.

Rogers, W. (1991) *Explaining Health and Illness: An exploration of diversity*. Hertfordshire: Harvester Wheatsheaf.

Rogler, L.H., Malgady, R.G., Costantino, G. & Blumenthal, R. (1987) What do culturally sensitive mental health services mean? The case of Hispanics. *American Psychologist* **42**: 565–70.

Roup, J. (2004) Lost for words. *Financial Times – Weekend*, Saturday 8 May, pp. 1–2.

Ruderman, F.A. (1981) What is medical sociology? *Journal of the American Medical Association* **245**: 927–9.

Rudmin, F.W. (2003) Critical history of the acculturation psychology of assimilation, separation, integration and marginalization. *Review of General Psychology* **7**: 3–37.

Rushton, J.P. (1995) Construct validity, censorship, and the genetics of race. *American Psychologist* **50**: 40–41.

Russel, K., Wilson, M. & Hall, R. (1992) *The color complex: The politics of skin color among African Americans*. New York: Harcourt Brace Jovanovich.

Ryan, D. (2005) Psychological stress and the asylum process in Ireland. Unpublished doctoral thesis. Dublin: University College Dublin.

Ryan, R.M. & Deci, E.L. (2004) Avoiding death or engaging life as accounts of meaning and culture: Comment on Pyszczynski et al. *Psychological Bulletin* **130**: 473.

Sachs, L. (1989) *Evil Eye or Bacteria? Turkish migrant women and Swedish healthcare.* Stockholm: University of Stockholm.

Sarson, S.B. (1974) *The Psychological Sense of Community: Prospects for a community psychology.* San Francisco, CA: Jossey-Bass.

Sartorius, N. (1989) The World Health Organisation's view on the prevention of mental disorders in developed countries. In: Cooper, B. & Helgason, T. (eds) Epidemiology and the Prevention of Mental Disorders. London: Routledge.

Saussure, F. (1999) Course in general linguistic. In: *Literary Theory: An Anthology*, 76–91.

Schumaker, J. (1996) Understanding psychopathology: Lessons from the developing world. In: Carr, S.C. & Schumaker, J.F. (eds) *Psychology and the Developing World.* Westport, CT: Greenwood Publishing Group.

Schumaker, J.F. (2001) *The Age of Insanity: Modernity and mental health.* Westport, CT: Praeger.

Schwartz, T. (1992) Anthropology and psychology: An unrequited relationship. In: Schwartz, T., White, G.M. & Lutz, C.A. (eds) New *Directions in Psychological Anthropology.* Cambridge: Cambridge University Press.

Schwarzer, R., Jerusalem, M. & Hahn, A. (1994) Unemployment, social support and health complaints: a longitudinal study of stress in East German refugees. *Journal of Community and Applied Social Psychology* **4**: 31–45.

Searle, W. & Ward, C. (1990) The prediction of psychological and sociological adjustment during cross-cultural transitions. *International Journal of Intercultural Relations* **14**: 449–64.

Showalter, E. (1997) *Hystories: Hysterical epidemics and modern culture.* London: Picador.

Shreve-Neiger, A.K. & Edelstein, B.A. (2004) Religion and anxiety: a critical review of the literature. *Clinical Psychology Review* **24**: 379–97.

Shweder, R.A. (1991) *Thinking through Cultures: Expeditions in cultural psychology.* Cambridge, MA: Harvard University Press.

Simons, R.C. (1985) The resolution of the Latah paradox. In: Simons, R.C. & Hughes, C.C. (eds) *The Culture Bound Syndromes: Folk illnesses of psychiatric and anthropological interest.* Dordrecht: R. Reidel, pp. 43–62.

Simons, R.C. & Hughes, C.C. (eds) (1985) *The Culture Bound Syndromes: Folk illnesses of psychiatric and anthropological interest.* Dordrecht: R. Reidel.

Singer, M., Flores, C., Davison, L., Burke, G., Castillo, Z., Scanlon, K. & Rivera, M. (1990) SIDA: The economic, social, and cultural context of AIDS among Latinos. *Medical Anthropology Quarterly* **4**: 72–114.

Siperstein, G.N., Norins, J., Corbin, S. & Shriver, T. (2003) *Multinational Study of Attitudes towards Individuals with Intellectual Disabilities: General findings and calls to action.* Washington DC: Special Olympics.

Skultans, V. & Cox, C. (2000) *Anthropological Approaches to Medicine: Crossing bridges.* London: Knightly Press.

Smaje, C. (1995) Ethnic residential concentration and health – Evidence for a positive effect. *Policy and Politics* **23**: 251–69.

Smith, P. & Bond, M. (1993) *Social Psychology Across Cultures: Analysis and perspectives.* London: Harvester Wheatsheaf.

Smyth, C., MacLachlan, M. & Clare, A. (2003) *Cultivating Suicide? Destruction of self in a changing Ireland.* Dublin: The Liffey Press.

Solomon, S., Greenberg, J. & Pyszczynski, T. (1991) A terror management theory of social behaviour: the psychological functions of self-esteem and cultural worldviews. *Advances in Experimental Social Psychology* **24**: 93–159.

Solomon, S., Greenberg, J. & Pyszczynski, T. (1998) Tales from the crypt: on the role of death in life. *Zygon* 33: 9–43.

Sommers, J. (1996) Debt: The new colonialism. In: *75/25: Ireland in an increasingly unequal world.* Dublin: Dochas.

Souad (2004) *Burned Alive: The shocking, true story of one woman's escape from an 'honour' killing.* London: Bantam Press.

Steptoe, A. (1991) The links between stress and illness. *Journal of Psychosomatic Research* **35**: 633–44.

Steptoe, A. & Wardle, J. (eds) (1994) *Psychosocial Processes and Health*: A reader. Cambridge: Cambridge University Press.

Sue, S. (1994) Delivering mental health services. Paper presented at the Conference, Madrid, July 1994.

Suminski, R.R., Poston, W.S., Jackson, A.S. & Foreyt, J.P. (1999) Early identification of Mexican American children who are at risk of becoming obese. *International Journal of Obesity-Related Metabolic Disorders* **23**: 823–9.

Summerfield, D. (2005) The invention of post-traumatic stress disorder and the social usefulness of a psychiatric category. *British Medical Journal* **332**: 95–8.

Swanson, B., Keithley, J.K., Zeller, J.M. & Cronin-Stubbs, D. (2000) Complementary and alternative therapies to manage HIV-related symptoms. *Journal of the Association of Nurses in AIDS Care* **11**(5): 40–60.

Swartz, L. (1998) *Culture and Mental Health: A Southern African view*. Cape Town: Oxford University Press.

Tajfel, H. (ed.) (1978) *Differentiation between Social Groups: Studies in the social psychology of intergroup relations*. London: Academic Press.

Taylor, A.L., Ziesche, S., Yancy, C. et al. (2004) Combination of isosorbide dinitrate and hydralazine in blacks with heart failure. *New England Journal of Medicine* **351**: 2049–57.

Taylor, B. (2001) HIV, stigma and health: integration of theoretical concepts and the lived experiences of individuals. *Journal of Advanced Nursing* **35**: 792–8.

Taylor, S. (2003) *Health Psychology: Biopsychosocial interactions*. New York: McGraw Hill.

Thekaekera, M.M. (2005a) Combating Caste: The stink of untouchability and how those most affected are trying to remove it. *New Internationalist* 380 (July): 9–12.

Thekaekera, M.M. (2005b) View from the top. *New Internationalist* 380 (July): 16–17.

Thomas, R. (2003) *Society and Health: Sociology for health professionals*. New York: Kluwer/Plenum.

Timimi, S. (2005) Effect of globalisation on children's mental health. *British Medical Journal* **331**: 37–9.

Triandis, H.C. (1990) Theoretical concepts that are applicable to the analysis of ethnocentricism. In: Brislin, R.W. (ed.) *Applied Cross-Cultural Psychology*. Newbury Park, CA: Sage.

Triandis, H.C. & Gelfand, J. (1998) Converging evidence of horizontal and vertical individualism and collectivism. *Journal of Personality and Social Psychology* **74**: 118–28.

Triandis, H.C. & Suh, E.M. (2002) Cultural influences on personality. *Annual Review of Psychology* **53**: 133–60.

Triandis, H.C., Bontempo, R., Villareal, M.J., Asai, M. & Lucca, N. (1988) Individualism and collectivism: Cross-cultural perspectives on self in-group relationships. *Journal of Personality and Social Psychology* **54**: 323–38.

Tuft, T. (2002) Education and participation. Paper presented at the IAMCR Conference, Barcelona: 21–26 July (cited in Gao, 2005).

Uchino, B.N. & Garvey, T.S. (1997) The availability of social support reduces cardiovascular reactivity to acute psychological stress. *Journal of Behavioral Medicine* **20**: 15–27.

Uchino, B.N., Cacioppo, J.T. & Kiecolt-Glaser, J.K. (1996) The relationship between social support and physiological processes: a review with emphasis on underlying mechanisms and implications for health. *Psychological Bulletin* **119**: 488–531.

UNAIDS/WHO (2004) AIDS Epidemic Update – December 2004. Geneva: UNAIDS/WHO.

UNDP (1998) *Human Development Report*. Geneva: UNDP.

UNESCO (2001) *A Cultural Approach to HIV/AIDS Prevention and Care*. Paris: UNESCO.

UNESCO (2005) Downloaded from UNESCO 'Aids & Culture' web page: http://portal.unesco.org/ on 22/6/2005.

UNHCR (2005) *Asylum levels and Trends in Industrialized Countries – First Quarter 2005.* Geneva: UNHCR.

United Nations (2000) *The Millenium Declaration.* New York: United Nations.

Van der Gaag, N. (2005) Caste out. *New Internationalist* 380 (July): 14–16.

Van Ryn, M. & Burke, J. (2002) The effect of patient race and socioeconomic status on physicians' perceptions of patients. In: LaVeist, T.A. (ed.) *Race, Ethnicity and Health: A public health reader.* New York: Jossey Bass.

Varma, V.K. (1988) Culture, personality and psychotherapy. *International Journal of Social Psychiatry* **34**: 142–9.

Vega W.A. & Murphy, J. (1990) Projecto Bienestar: An example of a community based intervention. In: *Culture and the Restructuring of Community Mental Health: Contributions in psychology.* Series No. 16; Westport, CT: Greenwood Press, pp. 103–22.

Vincent, C. & Furnham, A. (1996) Why do patients turn to complementary medicine? An empirical study. *British Journal of Clinical Psychology* **35**: 37–48.

Vinck, J. (1994) The role of health psychology in the promotion of public health. International Congress of Applied Psychology, Madrid.

Wang, S. & Keats, D. (2001) Cultivating health and preventing HIV/AIDS in the dual employment system of China. In: MacLachlan, M. (ed.) Cultivating Health: Cultural Perspectives on Health Promotion. Chichester: Wiley.

Ward, C., Bochner, S. & Furnham, A. (2001) *The Psychology of Culture Shock,* 2nd edn. London: Routledge.

Watters, P., Carr, S.C. & MacLachlan, M. (2002) Non-linear regression modelling of traditional and biomedical approaches to HIV/AIDS prevention in Malawi. *Journal of Psychology in Africa* **12**: 55–64.

Weinman, J., Petrie, K.J., Moss, R. & Horne, R. (1996) The Illness Perception Questionnaire: A new method for assessing the cognitive representation of illness. *Psychology and Health* **11**: 431–45.

Weiss, M.G., Raguram, R. & Channabasavanna, S.M. (1995) Cultural dimensions of psychiatric diagnosis: A comparison of DSM-III-R and illness explanatory models in South India. *British Journal of Psychiatry* **166**: 353–9.

Weisz, J.R., Suwanlert, S., Chaiyasit, W. & Walter, B.R. (1987) Over and undercontrolled referral problems among children and adolescents from Thailand and the United States: The wat and wai of cultural differences. *Journal of Consulting and Clinical Psychology* **55**: 719–26.

Westbrook, M., Legge, V. & Pennay, M. (1993) Attitudes towards disabilities in a multicultural society. *Social Science and Medicine* **36**: 615–23.

Westbrook, M., Legge, V. & Pennay, M. (1994) Causal attributions for deafness in a multicultural society. *Psychology and Health* **10**: 17–31.

Westermeyer, J. (1989) *Mental Health for Refugees and other Migrants: Social and preventive approaches.* Springfield, IL: Charles Thomas Books.

White, K. (2002) *An Introduction to the sociology of health and illness.* London: Sage Publications.

Wilkinson, M. (1992) *A Mental Health Handbook for Malawi.* Blantyre: Assemblies of God.

Wilkinson, R. & Marmot, M. (2003) *Social Determinants of Health – The Solid Facts,* 2nd edn. Geneva: WHO.

Willcox, B.J., Willcox, D. & Suzuki, M. (2001) *The Okinawa Way: How to improve your health and longevity dramatically.* Ney York: Michael Joseph.

Williams, D.R., Lavisso-Mourey, R. & Warren, R.C. (1994) The concept of race and health status in America. *Public Health Reports* **109**: 28–41.

Willis, L.A., Coombs, D.W., Cockerham, W.C. & Frison, S.L. (2002) Ready to die: a postmodern interpretation of the increase of African–American adolescent male suicide. *Social Science and Medicine* **55**: 907–20.

Wilson, B.D. & Miller, R.L. (2003) Examining strategies for culturally grounded HIV prevention: A review. *AIDS Education and Prevention* **15**(2): 184–202.

Winett, R.A., King, A.C. & Altman, D.G. (1989) He*alth Psychology and Public Health: An integrative approach.* New York: Pergamon Press.

World Health Organization (1948) *Constitution of the World Health Organization.* Geneva: WHO.

World Health Organization (1988?) *International Classification of Disease*, 10th revision. Geneva: WHO.

Wray, I. (1986) Buddhism and psychotherapy: a Buddhist perspective. Cited in Wren (1962).

Wrenn, C.G. (1962) The culturally encapsulated counsellor. *Harvard Educational Review* **32**: 444–9.

Zola, I. (ed.) (1983) Oh where, oh where has ethnicity gone? *Sociomedical Inquiries.* Philadelphia: Temple University Press.

Index